Antiepileptic Drugs and Pregnancy

MJ Eadie • FJE Vajda

Antiepileptic Drugs and Pregnancy

A Guide for Prescribers

Adis

MJ Eadie
Emeritus Professor of Clinical Neurology and Neuropharmacology, University of Queensland, and Honorary Consultant Neurologist, Royal Brisbane and Women's Hospital
Brisbane, QLD
Australia

FJE Vajda
Department of Medicine and Neurology
Director of the Australian Epilepsy and Pregnancy Register, University of Melbourne and Royal Melbourne Hospital
Melbourne
Australia

ISBN 978-3-319-21433-7 ISBN 978-3-319-21434-4 (eBook)
DOI 10.1007/978-3-319-21434-4

Library of Congress Control Number: 2015949390

Springer Cham Heidelberg New York Dordrecht London

Printed on acid-free paper

Adis is a brand of Springer
Springer International Publishing AG Switzerland is part of Springer Science+Business Media (www.springer.com)

Preface

A prospective reader might well wonder why, at the present time, anyone would devote a monograph to such a seemingly limited topic as that of antiepileptic drugs and pregnancy. This is particularly so when it is generally accepted that, as far as possible, the use of therapeutic drugs should be avoided in pregnant women. This latter belief originated some half a century ago when thalidomide use in pregnant women was recognised to be responsible for the development of foetal malformations and when the prescription of stilbestrol for threatened miscarriage was found to result in gynaecological malignancies in the daughters of the women so treated. The short answer to the question posed above is that the use of antiepileptic drug therapy in pregnancy continues to be perhaps the most frequently encountered situation in which the use of therapeutic drugs in pregnant women appears clinically and ethically justified. As a result of the virtual embargo on the unnecessary use of therapeutic drugs in pregnant women, there is not a great deal of information available regarding the possible effects that pregnancy might have on the body's handling of these drugs or on the effect that these drugs may have on pregnant women and their foetuses. Therefore, the availability of information about these matters in relation to antiepileptic drugs, necessarily gathered in opportunistic studies rather than in deliberate controlled investigations, offers the possibility of obtaining knowledge from which principles can be derived that may prove more widely applicable in the future to new drugs as they become available and their possible use in human pregnancy is considered.

Over the course of almost half a century of such piecemeal accumulation of information concerning antiepileptic drugs in human pregnancy, sufficient relevant material appears to have been amassed for a reasonably systematic and probably fairly complete account of the current situation to be possible. It is hoped that such an account may prove of interest to those who manage patients with epilepsy, particularly neurologists and general physicians, and also obstetricians, and that it may also contain material that would also be useful to basic and clinical pharmacologists and to other medical professionals who appear to be increasingly using antiepileptic drugs to treat disorders other than epilepsy, in particular certain psychiatric illnesses.

All of the illustrations used in this book have been prepared by one or any of the authors and, except for the diagrams of metabolic pathways, are based on personal data. Where this material has been published previously, it has appeared in journals whose publishers do not require explicit permission for reproduction by the authors of illustrations that they have prepared. However, nearly all the graphs in this book have been redrawn to bring them into a common format. At first sight, some may appear similar to previously published illustrations, but the figures have been redrawn to include the additional data available in the Australian Pregnancy Register at the end of 2014.

A significant portion of the data presented in this volume has emanated from an ongoing collaboration between the authors over a period of more than 40 years. During the past 15 years, this collaboration has involved the collection and analysis of the prospective data related to the use of antiepileptic drugs in the management of women with epilepsy that are collected in the Australian Register of Antiepileptic Drugs in Pregnancy. In relation to the latter endeavour, we are greatly indebted to our colleagues in Australia, viz. TJ O'Brien, CM Lander, J Graham, A Hitchcock, A Roten Wood and C Nadebaum for their excellent and continuing participation in, and support of, the activities of the Register. Our thanks are due also to European colleagues, T Tomson, D Battino, D Lindhout, A Sabers, J Craig, D Bonnizzoni and E Perucca, S Thomas, for the tremendous collaborative facility they have created in the EURAP registry. We also wish to acknowledge support for the Australian Register from a variety of sources including the Australian National Health and Medical Research Council, the Epilepsy Society of Australia, the Royal Melbourne Hospital Neuroscience Foundation and the pharmaceutical industry, including the firms of Sanofi, Sci-Gen, UCB, Genzyme, Janssen, Eisai, Novartis and previously Pfizer, Glaxo, Roche, Schering, Marion Merrell Dow, Hoechst and CSL.

Thanks are also due to Simon Raoul Vajda for computer-related technical assistance and to Margaret Eadie for general support of the work.

The authors are most grateful for the initiative of Sue Pochon, of Springer, in suggesting that this book be written, and would wish to thank Ellen Blasig, Prasad Gurunadham and Meena Govindan for their roles in editing the typescript, converting it into forms suitable for hard copy and also electronic publication and then seeing it through the press.

Brisbane, QLD, Australia MJ Eadie
Melbourne, VIC, Australia FJE Vajda

Contents

Chapter 1
Introduction

Abstract It is now widely accepted that, as far as possible, the intake of therapeutic drugs is better avoided during pregnancy because of their possible harmful effects on the developing foetus. However, in some clinical situations, the benefit achieved by preserving maternal health may justify continuing therapeutic drug intake during pregnancy. One such commonly encountered situation is the treatment of epilepsy. A good deal of information has accumulated regarding pregnant human bodies' handling of antiepileptic drugs and their effects on the physical and intellectual development of the foetus. The present book attempts to provide an account of this information and to discuss its application in the management of pregnant women with seizure disorders, recognising that the principles that apply in this situation are likely to also be valid in guiding the management of other disorders, particularly psychiatric ones, in which this class of drugs may also need to be used during human pregnancy

For more than half a century, there has been an increasing awareness in the wider community that, as far as practicable, the intake of drugs, including therapeutic drugs, should be avoided during pregnancy to prevent possible drug-related injury to the foetus in utero. However, there are situations in which the hazards of maternal illness that would be treatable with available drugs will be judged to outweigh the possible disadvantages of exposing the foetus to these drugs. Leaving aside the short-term use of drugs to treat intercurrent illness, the prevention of epileptic seizures is one of the more frequently encountered situations in which it is usually considered that therapeutic drug use throughout pregnancy is justifiable.

This is not the only situation in which use of therapeutic drugs throughout pregnancy appears to offer greater overall advantages than disadvantages, but there probably is more scientific information available about the use of antiepileptic drugs than the amount that is available for most other classes of drug during pregnancy. However, over the years antiepileptic drugs have been used in managing disorders other than epilepsy, and this non-epilepsy use is increasing. Phenobarbitone was already being employed as a sedative in 1912 when its antiepileptic efficacy happened to be recognised (Hauptmann 1912). Phenytoin still finds occasional use apart from its role in treating epilepsy, while carbamazepine remains the usual agent of first choice in managing idiopathic trigeminal neuralgia and other neuropathic

M.J. Eadie, F.J.E. Vajda, *Antiepileptic Drugs and Pregnancy: A Guide for Prescribers*, DOI 10.1007/978-3-319-21434-4_1

pains, some of which may afflict pregnant women. Furthermore, though at first sight it may appear a little surprising, in a substantially sized population of pregnant women in the United States between 2001 and 2007, Bobo et al. (2012) found that the main use of what are classed as antiepileptic drugs proved to be for psychiatric illness rather than for epilepsy. There also was substantial use of these drugs in pain management. The psychiatric use seemed to be mainly for the purpose of mood stabilisation in bipolar disorders, a role in which carbamazepine, valproate and lamotrigine had been the preferred agents (Bobo et al. 2012). There is evidence that withdrawal of these agents to avoid drug intake in pregnancy is associated with an increased risk of relapse of the psychiatric disorder that was being treated (Viguera et al. 2007; Newport et al. 2008).

Despite this developing, if not already developed, preponderance in the use of antiepileptic drugs for indications apart from epilepsy, virtually all the scientific investigations of the clinical pharmacology of these agents have been carried out in relation to epilepsy, and writers such as Viguera et al. (2007) have acknowledged that the use of the drugs in psychiatry has depended on the experience of their use in epilepsy. Therefore, in this book, issues in relation to antiepileptic drugs and pregnancy have almost always been considered in relation to the use of the drugs for human epilepsy.

In the past, decisions regarding antiepileptic drug use in pregnancy were often based mainly on transmitted clinical wisdom and personal instinct. However, increasingly, statistical data have become available that, by and large, both justify existing therapeutic policies and also permit their refinement to yield better outcomes for both mother and foetus. Ex cathedra pronouncements as to optimal management employing these agents have been increasingly replaced by numerical estimates of efficacy and hazard; advice can be better tailored to the individual woman's situation, while the earlier idea that the antiepileptic drugs behaved in pregnant women as members of a single drug class with similar properties has given way to a realisation that the individual drugs are not all handled in identical ways by the pregnant female body. The increasing understanding of what happens to individual antiepileptic drugs in the woman's body during and after pregnancy has by and large confirmed what might have been predicted from existing knowledge of the physiology of pregnancy and lactation. This pharmacological knowledge permits the likely behaviour of other drugs, when used in pregnancy for other disorders, to be predicted with reasonable probability.

Drug treatment prescribed in relation to pregnancy involves the administered drug's simultaneous effects on one existing and on one (sometimes more) potential human being. During pregnancy, the existences of a woman and her foetus(es) are closely intertwined, and drugs intended for the benefit of the pregnant woman are likely to also affect the contents of her womb. At childbirth, the existences of a woman and her offspring immediately become physically separate though, if breast feeding occurs, they remain linked to decreasing extents for the duration of the breast feeding since part of any drug she is taking is likely to be excreted in her milk. Consequently, appropriate antiepileptic drug prescribing in relation to pregnancy may require judicious balancing of the interests of the woman concerned with those of her foetus(es) throughout pregnancy and during the period of lactation. There are also the woman's current and likely future life situations to be considered in any therapeutic decision, but in the present book, it has not seemed practicable to go into the varieties of the life situations that may apply in different women in any detail.

Pregnancy is a continuously progressive rather than a static physiological state. Therefore findings that apply at one stage of pregnancy, and also in the early weeks after pregnancy, may not necessarily apply at other stages. Pregnancy also is a situation in which clinically unnecessary investigations are better avoided, mainly in the interests of foetal safety and maternal comfort and convenience. As a result, not a great deal of systematic investigation into how the pregnant female body handles drugs has been carried out, in particular studies in the same woman at different stages of the course of her pregnancy. Formal pharmacokinetic investigations have rarely been practicable, though a few such studies in strategically fortuitous circumstances or employing stable (nonradioactive) isotope-labelled drug have been possible. Much of the available pharmacokinetic and drug metabolism information in relation to pregnancy seems to have been collected piecemeal and often opportunistically. While this has permitted trends to be identified with reasonable confidence, particular published pharmacokinetic parameter values in pregnancy have tended to show rather wide ranges of variation, partly due to their often having been determined at different stages of the nine months of pregnancy, even in the one study, with the time relationship to the stage of pregnancy not being made explicit.

The evidence regarding the behaviour of epileptic seizure disorders during pregnancy is also beset by limitations. Few women are prepared to keep seizure diaries not only during the whole duration of a pregnancy but for months beforehand and perhaps afterwards and, even if they are willing, succeed in sustaining the endeavour. The reliabilities of some published numerical data concerning the frequencies of minor seizures during pregnancy may be a little suspect, though information regarding generalised convulsive seizures, and particularly loss of control of previously inactive seizure disorders, is probably more likely to be correct.

Foetal malformations associated with antiepileptic drug exposure in utero appear to be comparatively rare events. Therefore, to obtain sufficient material to warrant drawing conclusions, publications concerning such maldevelopments have often been based on data collections drawn from various original sources. Those reporting such material have sometimes had to assume the reliability of the primary data in these collections because of sheer logistic practicalities involved in their actually collecting and verifying in person the original information.

Despite these various limitations, the accumulated information relating antiepileptic drugs and pregnancy has now achieved a sufficient mass to permit what are probably reliable conclusions regarding clinically important issues. There are still matters to be clarified and details to be completed, but the current state of knowledge allows assembling and assessing critically the available facts relating to antiepileptic drug use and pregnancy. This the present book attempts, working with data available in the literature to the end of February 2015 and with personal material, much of it already published. The approach chosen in presenting the material has been determined by the following consideration.

Unless her seizure disorder has begun during pregnancy, a woman with epilepsy will probably have been taking antiepileptic drug therapy prior to pregnancy, will take it throughout pregnancy and will continue to take it after her baby is born. To manage her situation optimally, it would be desirable to know: (a) whether her underlying seizure disorder and its drug treatment will affect the possibilities of her becoming pregnant and (b) what is likely to happen during and after pregnancy to (i) the antiepileptic drug or drugs involved and their effectiveness, (ii) the natural history of her seizure disorder in its own right, (iii) her obstetric management and (iv) the intrauterine and postnatal development of her foetus. On the basis of such knowledge, it should be possible to devise appropriate therapeutic policies for managing epileptic seizure disorders in women considering pregnancy, while pregnant and after pregnancy. These considerations have determined the sequence of the remaining chapters of this book, which deal in turn with:

- Antiepileptic drugs and the possibilities of becoming pregnant
- Antiepileptic drug disposition in pregnancy, in principle and in relation to individual antiepileptic drugs
- Antiepileptic drugs and epileptic seizure control in pregnancy
- Antiepileptic drugs and foetal malformations
- Antiepileptic drugs and foetal neurodevelopment
- The clinical use of antiepileptic drugs:

    (i) Before pregnancy
    (ii) During pregnancy
    (iii) After pregnancy

- Future possibilities in relation to antiepileptic drugs and pregnancy

References

Bobo WV, Davis RL, Toh S et al (2012) Trends in the use of antiepileptic drugs among pregnant women in the US, 2001–2007: a medication exposure in pregnancy risk evaluation program study. Paediatr Perinat Epidemiol 26:578–588

Hauptmann A (1912) Luminal bei Epilepsie. Munch Med Wochenschr 59:1907–1909

Newport DJ, Stowe ZN, Viguera AC et al (2008) Lamotrigine in bipolar disorder: efficacy during pregnancy. Bipolar Disord 10:432–436

Viguera AC, Whitfield T, Baldessarini RJ et al (2007) Risk of recurrence in women with bipolar disorder during pregnancy: prospective study of mood stabilizer discontinuation. Am J Psychiatry 164:1817–1824

Chapter 2
Antiepileptic Drugs and Becoming Pregnant

Abstract There is published evidence that intake of antiepileptic drugs may affect the possibility of a woman becoming pregnant. Use of the drugs in her male partner may tend to decrease his libido and sexual activity, thus diminishing the chances of pregnancy occurring. A similar effect on libido may occur in the woman being treated with antiepileptic drugs, and the treatment may be responsible for circulating sex hormone concentration alterations that result in menstrual disturbances, this combination of effects tending to lessen fertility. Taking antiepileptic drugs in the non-pregnant state, particularly the older agents that induce formation of enzymes that catalyse the metabolism of steroidal sex hormones, also tends to decrease the circulating concentrations of steroidal hormones used for contraceptive purposes. This effect may increase the chances of undesired pregnancies occurring.

This book attempts to deal with the interplay between pregnancy, antiepileptic drugs and the disorders, in particular epilepsy, for which these drugs are prescribed. To begin at the beginning, the first aspects of the interplay are the issues of whether the drugs may alter a woman's potential for becoming pregnant and for avoiding undesired pregnancy. Achieving pregnancy involves not only the drug's effects in the woman concerned but also its possible effects in her male partner, whereas avoiding pregnancy, at least in contemporary society, is more often a matter for the woman involved than for her male counterpart.

Achieving Pregnancy

The Situation in the Male

Even if the woman involved does nothing to alter the prospects of her becoming pregnant, could antiepileptic drug intake in her male partner increase or decrease the prospects of her achieving pregnancy if the drugs were to alter his sexual capacity or behaviour? There seems to be little in the medical literature to suggest that antiepileptic drug intake may be responsible for male sexual hyperactivity, though Grabowska-Grzyb et al. (2006) did describe two males who, after lamotrigine was added to their current antiepileptic drug (in one oxcarbazepine and the other

M.J. Eadie, F.J.E. Vajda, *Antiepileptic Drugs and Pregnancy: A Guide for Prescribers*, DOI 10.1007/978-3-319-21434-4_2

carbamazepine), developed dose-related but reversible hypersexuality. In appropriate circumstances, this could have increased the likelihoods of pregnancy in any female partners that they had.

Much more commonly, the literature has reported that males taking antiepileptic drugs exhibit diminished sexual function. For instance, Artama et al. (2006) found a statistically significantly lower birth rate to males with epilepsy who were treated with carbamazepine, oxcarbazepine or valproate, as compared with the birth rate in a reference population of males who did not have epilepsy. In many of the reports, the interpretation of the lower birth rate in relation to antiepileptic drug-treated males is confounded by the fact that the drugs were used to treat epilepsy, and epilepsy itself might have altered male fertility. Overt and also probably subclinical focal seizures, particularly ones arising in mesial temporal lobe structures, can spread into the hypothalamus. In that brain region, the epileptic discharges may alter neuroendocrine function and, through this mechanism, possibly influence male fertility. If the degree of reduced fertility correlated with changes in the dose or circulating concentration of the antiepileptic drug or drugs concerned, one could be moderately confident that the drugs played a causal role in decreasing male fertility. Even then, the possibility remains that intracerebral spread of epileptic seizure discharges to neuroendocrine nuclei may also have contributed.

Over 40 years ago, Livingstone (1972), in his monograph, described the occurrence of sexual impotence in a few men treated with primidone. Later Mattson et al. (1985), in their large-scale study of US male war veterans, reported that use of this drug was sometimes associated with a decreased libido and with complaints of impotence. Unfortunately, it is difficult to know whether at the time of the Mattson et al. study the primidone had been prescribed in awareness of the long elimination half-life of the phenobarbitone that is formed from it within the body. Too rapid primidone dosage escalation might have produced excessive sedation, thereby decreasing libido. The subsequent literature has not infrequently contained the statement that males with epilepsy tend to be less fertile than their fellows and have diminished libidos. However, there has been at least one report to the contrary, in relation to continued intake of carbamazepine and valproate (Røste et al. 2003). By way of contrast, Reis et al. (2013) compared reports of sexual function in 63 males taking carbamazepine and in 55 healthy male control subjects. There was an increased occurrence of erectile dysfunction and decreased coital frequency in the antiepileptic drug-exposed males. Luef et al. (2009) observed that previously persisting sexual dysfunction improved in 79.4 % of 228 antiepileptic drug-treated men when agents that did not induce drug-metabolising enzymes were substituted for antiepileptic drugs that did induce the enzymes.

The possible hormonal background to diminished male sexual function associated with antiepileptic drug intake was investigated by Isojärvi et al. (2004), who were aware of the reported decreased fertility of males with epilepsy. They studied 15 men taking carbamazepine, 18 taking oxcarbazepine and 27 taking valproate, comparing the concentrations of certain circulating sex hormones in these men with the concentrations that were present in 41 normal male control subjects. They found that carbamazepine use was associated with decreased circulating concentrations of dehydroepiandrosterone sulphate and valproate use with increased concentrations of androstenedione. There were increased tendencies for low sperm counts and the presence of more functionally abnormal sperm in the males taking carbamazepine. Valproate exposure was also associated with sperm abnormalities. As well, men taking this drug tended to have smaller testes. Verrotti et al. (2011) pointed out that antiepileptic drugs which induced the body's drug-metabolising enzyme systems also tended to cause increased formation of sex hormone-binding globulin, whose higher concentrations would result in decreased circulating levels of free (i.e. plasma protein unbound) relative to total testosterone. This reduction in free hormone levels might cause a lessened libido and potency. These authors also knew that valproate use was associated with increased circulating concentrations of dehydroepiandrosterone and decreased concentrations of gonadotropins. At much the same time, Sivaraaman and Mintzer (2011) described how the proposed hypothalamic disturbance that resulted from the spread of clinical and subclinical mesial temporal seizure discharges mentioned above might alter gonadotropin secretion. They also pointed out that use of the older enzyme-inducing antiepileptic drugs would produce increased blood levels of sex hormone-binding globulin, resulting in lower circulating concentrations of unbound relative to total testosterone. This pair of authors recognised that substituting the newer, generally non-inducing, antiepileptic drugs for the older inducing ones would avoid the alteration in circulating unbound testosterone concentrations and thereby might decrease hormone-related impairment of male sexual function. However, Najafi et al. (2012) noticed that decreased circulating testosterone concentrations also occurred when the non-inducing antiepileptic agent lamotrigine was being taken and mentioned that valproate use was associated with increased circulating concentrations of androstenedione.

Verrotti et al. (2011), in their review of the topic, pointed out the difficulties in distinguishing between the roles of having epilepsy, of taking antiepileptic drugs and of these two factors in combination, in explaining the increased likelihood that abnormal concentrations of reproductive steroid hormones may occur in men with epilepsy. A potential hormonal basis thus appears to exist that could contribute to the diminished sexual activity, libido and fertility reported in males with antiepileptic drug-treated epilepsy. Also, because there is a little published evidence that the altered sexual behaviour tends to vary with the antiepileptic drug dose and with the enzyme-inducing capacity of drug used, it seems likely that antiepileptic drug intake can interfere with male sexual function. Nonetheless, it seems likely that various psychosocial factors, such as limitations on lifestyle and possible earning capacity consequent on suffering from epilepsy, also play significant roles in the situation. The available medical literature contains relatively little detailed information dealing with the contributions made by such psychosocial factors.

The Situation in the Female

As in the male, theoretical possibilities exist that antiepileptic drug therapy in the female may enhance or diminish sexual activity and that these alterations may influence her possibility of becoming pregnant. In the literature, almost all the available data pertain to decreased female sexual activity or lowered female fertility.

The statement has often been made that women with epilepsy, which in practice will nearly always be antiepileptic drug-treated epilepsy, exhibit decreases in fertility, libido, sexual arousal and orgasm and increases in the incidences of menstrual irregularity, tendencies to early menopause or premature ovarian failure and also face a heightened risk of suffering from the polycystic ovary syndrome. All these changes would militate against the chances of becoming pregnant (Klein et al. 2001; Harden 2006; Pennell 2009). However, in their material, Klein et al. could not correlate premature ovarian failure manifestations with antiepileptic drug intake. Some quantitative data are available in relation to the lowered fertility aspect. In females with epilepsy aged 15–44 years, Wallace et al. (1998) found a live birth rate of 47.1 per 1000 per year as compared with the national 1993 England and Wales live birth rate of 62.6 per 1000 per year. Artama et al. (2006), in two cohorts from the Finnish population, also found a lower birth rate in women with epilepsy treated with carbamazepine, oxcarbazepine and valproate as compared with a reference cohort, though the reduction in rate was not statistically significant. Kariuki et al. (2008) found a 3-year fertility rate of 46 live births per 1000 women with established epilepsy, a reduction by two-thirds as compared with the expected rate for the local African population. Jalava and Sillanpää (1997) followed up a cohort of childhood epilepsy sufferers and showed that, in the longer term, they had a lower marriage rate than would have been expected and also a lower rate of fertility.

The above alterations in fertility and in other aspects of female sexual function appear to have a hormonal basis. In three women, Isojarvi and Tapanainen (2000) drew attention to an apparent association between intake of valproate and the presence of polycystic ovaries and hyperandrogenism. Replacing the valproate with lamotrigine caused the polycystic ovaries to disappear in two of the women, and plasma testosterone concentrations fell in all three. Bilo et al. (2001) noted the presence of various reproductive disorders in 32 % of 50 women with (treated) epilepsy, the disorder encountered being polycystic ovaries in 26 %. These authors failed to detect a correlation between the abnormalities and the intake of any particular antiepileptic drug. They therefore suggested that having epilepsy per se might be responsible. Despite the latter suggestion, it seems to have become fairly widely accepted that there is a real association between the use of valproate and the occurrence of polycystic ovaries (Crawford 2009).

The use of antiepileptic drugs that induce drug-metabolising enzymes increases the concentration of sex hormone-binding globulin in women as well as in men. This increase may decrease the concentrations of circulating unbound (and therefore biologically active) oestrogen relative to total oestrogen concentrations, an effect which could contribute to the presence of menstrual disorders in some women with epilepsy (Isojärvi 2008). As well, the use of valproate in women causes increased circulating testosterone concentrations, which also might disturb the menstrual cycle and as well contribute to the development of polycystic ovaries. These various altered circulating steroid hormone concentrations may contribute to the decreased fertility of women with epilepsy. Hamed (2008) suggested that antiepileptic drugs may also modulate hormone release from the hypothalamic–pituitary axis and, through this additional means, diminish fertility in women.

Jankovic et al. (2006) investigated a further matter that might be relevant to impaired fertility in antiepileptic drug-treated women. In a laboratory study, they found that carbamazepine and lamotrigine, at concentrations within the ranges encountered in the treatment of epilepsy, inhibited motility in surgically removed human fallopian tubes. This effect could contribute to the diminished fertility of women with epilepsy, by reducing the opportunity for contact between the sperm and the ovum at an appropriate time and anatomical site.

It is highly probable that various psychological and social factors that vary between individual women with epilepsy will also have major influences on fertility and also on some of the other aspects of altered sexual function that have been mentioned above. For instance, it is not difficult to appreciate that a woman with uncontrolled seizures may have problems in sustaining enduring personal relationships and may also be reluctant to undertake pregnancy because of uncertainties about her ability to care for a young infant.

Avoiding Pregnancy

Although in present-day society other methods of preventing the occurrence of pregnancy are sometimes employed by women or their partners, the oral use of synthetic steroidal hormones is probably the most frequent approach to contraception, though parenterally or intravaginally administered progestogen-type preparations that slowly release their hormonal contents enjoy some popularity. Ethinyl oestradiol is the oestrogen employed in the great majority of oral contraceptive combinations, together with various progestogens.

Not long after combined (oestrogen plus progestogen) oral contraceptives came into general use, when the contraceptives were used in conjunction with the then available antiepileptic drugs (mainly ones which induced microsomal drug-metabolising enzymes), the so-called pill failure began to be reported (e.g. Coulam and Annegers 1979). Such reports have continued to appear and a good deal of information has accumulated regarding the effects of various antiepileptic drugs on the concentrations of the orally administered steroidal sex hormones. Because this is a matter of considerable importance both to the pharmaceutical industry and to prescribers, to say nothing of women with drug-treated epilepsy, in recent years investigations have been carried out at relatively early stages in the development and use of new antiepileptic agents to determine whether or not they alter circulating concentrations of synthetic hormones derived from contraceptive preparations.

As a generalisation, it appears that antiepileptic drugs which induce microsomal drug-metabolising enzymes tend to cause reduced circulating concentrations and increased clearances of synthetic oestrogens and progestogens, as well as natural progesterone (sometimes employed as a contraceptive). There is a certain amount of apparently conflicting information in the literature, but Crawford (2009) summarised the situation as follows: phenobarbitone and drugs metabolised to it, phenytoin, carbamazepine, oxcarbazepine, lamotrigine and topiramate interact with oral contraceptives to decrease circulating steroidal sex hormone levels, whereas the other antiepileptic drugs in common contemporary use do not. The extent of the interaction may not be sufficient to consistently reduce the overall sex hormonal effects to the extent that ovulation and implantation of a fertilised embryo can occur, but the likelihood of this happening is increased. For instance, Davis et al. (2011) reported that a carbamazepine dose of 600 mg a day interacted with an oral contraceptive combination comprising ethinyl oestradiol 20 μg and levonorgestrel 100 μg to allow ovulation to occur in five of the ten menstrual cycles that were followed. Breakthrough bleeding occurred in eight of the ten cycles, as compared with two of ten cycles when a placebo instead of antiepileptic drug was taken together with the hormonal contraceptive combination. There seems to be a general impression in the literature that a 'pill' content of 50 μg ethinyl oestradiol offers a sufficient margin of contraceptive safety if an inducing antiepileptic drug is in use (Wang et al. 2012). However, that is not to say that such a margin is always necessary to avoid conception.

Studies that have investigated possible interactions in which antiepileptic drugs may have been responsible for altered plasma concentrations and/or clearances of exogenous steroid hormone are summarised in Table 2.1. The inducing antiepileptic drugs also interact with the hormone released from etonorgestrel and levonorgestrel implants (Schindlbeck et al. 2006; Gaffield et al. 2011).

Table 2.1 Effects of antiepileptic drugs on plasma concentrations of combined oral contraceptive hormonal components

Antiepileptic drug	Ethinyl oestradiol	Levonorgestrel	Norethindrone	Norgestrel	Author
Carbamazepine	Decreased	Decreased			Davis et al. (2011)
Eslicarbazepine	Decreased	Decreased			Falcão et al. (2013)
Felbamate	No change			Decreased	Saano et al. (1995)
Gabapentin	No change		No change		Eldon et al. (1998)
Lacosamide	No change	No change			Cawello et al. (2013)
Lamotrigine	No change	Mild decrease			Sidhu et al. (2006)
Levetiracetam	No change	No change			Ragueneau-Majlessi et al. (2002)

(continued)

Table 2.1 (continued)

Antiepileptic drug	Ethinyl oestradiol	Levonorgestrel	Norethindrone	Norgestrel	Author
Oxcarbazepine	Decreased	Decreased			Fattore et al. (1999)
Phenobarbitone	Decreased	Decreased			Crawford et al. (1990)
Phenytoin	Decreased	Decreased			Crawford et al. (1990)
Primidone	Decreased				Crawford et al. (1990)
Topiramate[a]	No change		No change		Doose et al. (2003)
	Decreased		No change		Rosenfeld et al. (1997)
Valproate	No change	No change			Crawford et al. (1986)
Vigabatrin	No change	No change			Bartoli et al. (1997)
Zonisamide	No change	No change			Griffith and Dai (2004)

Names of antiepileptic drugs that induce hepatic drug-metabolising enzymes appear in bold typeface
[a]Topiramate's induction of the enzyme CYP 2C19 at high dosage

The material discussed in this chapter will probably result in an impression that considerably more information is available regarding the physical and chemical mechanisms that are involved in facilitating or avoiding pregnancy in women taking antiepileptic drugs than in the psychological and social factors that are inevitably involved in the situation. However, these latter factors probably play the major part in determining whether or not most such women become pregnant.

References

Artama M, Isojärvi JI, Auvinen A (2006) Antiepileptic drug use and birth rate in patients with epilepsy – a population-based cohort study in Finland. Hum Reprod 21:2290–2295

Bartoli A, Gatti G, Cipolla G et al (1997) A double-blind, placebo-controlled study on the effect of vigabatrin on in vivo parameters of hepatic microsomal enzyme induction and on the kinetics of steroid oral contraceptives in healthy female volunteers. Epilepsia 38:702–707

Bilo L, Meo R, Valentino R, Di Carlo C, Striano S, Nappi C (2001) Characterization of reproductive endocrine disorders in women with epilepsy. J Clin Endocrinol Metab 86:2950–2956

Cawello W, Rosenkranz B, Schmid B, Wierich W (2013) Pharmacodynamic and pharmacokinetic evaluation of coadministration of lacosamide and an oral contraceptive (levonorgestrel plus ethinylestradiol) in healthy female volunteers. Epilepsia 54:530–536

Coulam CB, Annegers JF (1979) Do anticonvulsants reduce the efficacy of oral contraceptives? Epilepsia 20:519–525

Crawford PM (2009) Managing epilepsy in women of childbearing age. Drug Saf 32:293–307

Crawford P, Chadwick D, Cleland P, Tjia J, Cowie A, Back DJ, Orme ML (1986) The lack of effect of sodium valproate on the pharmacokinetics of oral contraceptive steroids. Contraception 33:23–29

Crawford P, Chadwick DJ, Martin C, Tjia J, Back DJ, Orme M (1990) The interaction of phenytoin and carbamazepine with combined oral contraceptive steroids. Br J Clin Pharmacol 30:892–896

Davis AR, Westhoff CL, Stanczyk FZ (2011) Carbamazepine coadministration with an oral contraceptive: effects on steroid pharmacokinetics, ovulation, and bleeding. Epilepsia 52:243–247

Doose DR, Wang SS, Padmanabhan M, Schwabe S, Jacobs D, Bialer M (2003) Effect of topiramate or carbamazepine on the pharmacokinetics of an oral contraceptive containing norethindrone and ethinyl estradiol in healthy obese and nonobese female subjects. Epilepsia 44:540–549

Eldon MA, Underwood BA, Randinitis EJ, Sedman AJ (1998) Gabapentin does not interact with a contraceptive regimen of norethindrone acetate and ethinyl estradiol. Neurology 50:1146–1148

Falcão A, Vaz-da-Silva M, Gama H, Nunes T, Almeida L, Soares-da-Silva P (2013) Effect of eslicarbazepine acetate on the pharmacokinetics of a combined ethinylestradiol/ oral contraceptive in healthy women. Epilepsy Res 105:368–376

Fattore C, Cipolla G, Gatti G, Limido GL, Sturm Y, Bernasconi C, Perucca E (1999) Induction of ethinylestradiol and levonorgestrel metabolism by oxcarbazepine in healthy women. Epilepsia 40:783–787

Gaffield ME, Culwell KR, Lee CR (2011) The use of hormonal contraception among women taking anticonvulsant therapy. Contraception 83:16–29

Grabowska-Grzyb A, Nagańska E, Wolańczyk T (2006) Hypersexuality in two patients with epilepsy treated with lamotrigine. Epilepsy Behav 8:663–665

Griffith SG, Dai Y (2004) Effect of zonisamide on the pharmacokinetics and pharmacodynamics of a combination ethinyl estradiol-norethindrone oral contraceptive in healthy women. Clin Ther 26:2056–2065

Hamed SA (2008) Neuroendocrine hormonal conditions in epilepsy: relationship to reproductive and sexual functions. Neurologist 14:157–169

Harden CL (2006) Sexuality in men and women with epilepsy. CNS Spectr 11(8 Suppl 9):13–18

Isojärvi J (2008) Disorders of reproduction in patients with epilepsy: antiepileptic drug related mechanisms. Seizure 17:111–119

Isojarvi JI, Tapanainen JS (2000) Valproate, hyperandrogenism, and polycystic ovaries: a report of 3 cases. Arch Neurol 57:1064–1068

Isojärvi JI, Löfgren E, Juntunen KS, Pakarinen AJ, Päivänsalo M, Rautakorpi I, Tuomivaara L (2004) Effect of epilepsy and antiepileptic drugs on male reproductive health. Neurology 62:247–253

Jalava M, Sillanpää M (1997) Reproductive activity and offspring health of young adults with childhood-onset epilepsy: a controlled study. Epilepsia 38:532–540

Jankovic SM, Jankovic SV, Kostic J, Kostic I, Jakovljevic M (2006) Inhibitory effects of selected antiepileptics on spontaneous motility of isolated human oviducts. Eur J Clin Pharmacol 62:707–712

Kariuki JG, Joshi MD, Adam AM, Kwasa TO, Machoki M (2008) Fertility rate of epileptic women at Kenyatta National Hospital. East Afr Med J 85:341–346

Klein P, Serje A, Pezzullo JC (2001) Premature ovarian failure in women with epilepsy. Epilepsia 42:1584–1589

Livingstone S (1972) Comprehensive management of epilepsy in infancy, childhood and adolescence. Charles C Thomas, Springfield

Luef G, Krämer G, Stefan H (2009) Oxcarbazepine treatment in male epilepsy patients improves pre-existing sexual dysfunction. Acta Neurol Scand 119:94–99

Mattson RH, Cramer JA, Collins JF et al (1985) Comparison of carbamazepine, phenobarbital, phenytoin and primidone in partial and secondarily generalized tonic-clonic seizures. N Engl J Med 313:145–151

Najafi MR, Ansari B, Zare M, Fatehi F, Sonbolestan A (2012) Effects of antiepileptic drugs on sexual function and reproductive hormones of male epileptic patients. Iran J Neurol 11:37–41

Pennell PB (2009) Hormonal aspects of epilepsy. Neurol Clin 27:941–965

Ragueneau-Majlessi I, Levy RH, Janik F (2002) Levetiracetam does not alter the pharmacokinetics of an oral contraceptive in healthy women. Epilepsia 43:697–702

Reis RM, de Angelo AG, Sakamoto AC, Ferriani RA, Lara LA (2013) Altered sexual and reproductive functions in epileptic men taking carbamazepine. J Sex Med 10:493–499

Rosenfeld WE, Doose DR, Walker SA, Nayak RK (1997) Effect of topiramate on the pharmacokinetics of an oral contraceptive containing norethindrone and ethinyl estradiol in patients with epilepsy. Epilepsia 38:317–323

Røste LS, Taubøll E, Haugen TB, Bjørnenak T, Saetre ER, Gjerstad L (2003) Alterations in semen parameters in men with epilepsy treated with valproate or carbamazepine monotherapy. Eur J Neurol 10:501–506

Saano V, Glue P, Banfield CR et al (1995) Effects of felbamate on the pharmacokinetics of a low-dose combination oral contraceptive. Clin Pharmacol Ther 58:523–531

Schindlbeck C, Janni W, Friese K (2006) Failure of Implanon contraception in a patient taking carbamazepin for epilepsia. Arch Gynecol Obstet 273:255–256

Sidhu J, Job S, Singh S, Philipson R (2006) The pharmacokinetic and pharmacodynamic consequences of the co-administration of lamotrigine and a combined oral contraceptive in healthy female subjects. Br J Clin Pharmacol 61:191–199

Sivaraaman K, Mintzer S (2011) Hormonal consequences of epilepsy and its treatment in men. Curr Opin Endocrinol Diabetes Obes 18:204–209

Verrotti A, Loiacono G, Laus M, Coppola G, Chiarelli F, Tiboni GM (2011) Hormonal and reproductive disturbances in epileptic male patients: emerging issues. Reprod Toxicol 31:519–527

Wallace H, Shorvon S, Tallis R (1998) Age-specific incidence and prevalence rates of treated epilepsy in an unselected population of 2,052,922 and age-specific fertility rates of women with epilepsy. Lancet 352:1970–1973

Wang H, Bos JH, de Jong-van den Berg LT (2012) Co-prescription of antiepileptic drugs and contraceptives. Contraception 85:28–31

Part I
Antiepileptic Drug Pharmacokinetics in Pregnancy

Chapter 3
Antiepileptic Drug Disposition in Pregnancy

Abstract The progressive physiological changes that occur in the female body during pregnancy, and their reversal in the weeks after the delivery of the foetus and placenta at the time of childbirth, have consequences for the body's handling of drugs. The physiological changes have little effect on the absorption of the orally administered drugs, but the expanded extracellular fluid volume of pregnancy and the increasing bulk of the uterus and its contents have a diluting effect on circulating drug concentrations. Also, in later pregnancy, plasma protein concentrations decrease, resulting in a relative increase in plasma-unbound drug concentrations relative to total drug concentrations. Overall, the magnitude of these effects is small relative to the effects of pregnancy on drug elimination. Increased glomerular filtration during pregnancy increases the excretion of antiepileptic drugs that are cleared from the body predominantly as unchanged molecules, while the increasing circulating steroidal sex hormone concentrations of pregnancy induce formation of the liver enzymes that metabolise antiepileptic drugs that are cleared from the body by biotransformation. The overall result of these two processes is for circulating concentrations of antiepileptic drugs to fall relative to drug dose during pregnancy, potentially compromising the control of the seizure disorders for which the drugs have been prescribed.

After childbirth, antiepileptic drugs seem to enter maternal milk by a process of passive transfer along concentration gradients, with factors such as the fat and protein content of the milk affecting the drugs' concentrations in that fluid. These concentrations are generally lower than those simultaneously present in maternal plasma.

The understanding of the way the human body handles antiepileptic drugs has depended to a considerable extent on the ability to measure the concentrations of these drugs that are present in the body during therapeutic use. Despite at least one earlier attempt, reasonably satisfactory assays that permitted these measurements did not become available until 1956. Then Dill et al. (1956) devised an assay for measuring phenytoin and Plaa and Hine (1956) one for measuring both phenytoin and phenobarbitone simultaneously. These particular methods have since been superseded by numerous more convenient, more specific and more sensitive techniques. Once the ability to undertake the measurements existed, interested

M.J. Eadie, F.J.E. Vajda, *Antiepileptic Drugs and Pregnancy: A Guide for Prescribers*, DOI 10.1007/978-3-319-21434-4_3

clinicians began to employ them to help guide the treatment of epilepsy, while the more pharmacologically minded began to utilise the drug concentration data that became available to enhance the understanding of the dispositions of antiepileptic drugs in the human body.

By the 1970s, enough knowledge was available to permit the publication of two collections of papers describing the measurement techniques and some of their applications in clinical practice (Meijer et al. 1973; Pippenger et al. 1978). Around this time, the first reports appeared of measurements of the behaviour of the concentrations of antiepileptic drugs in the serum or plasma of women during the course of pregnancy (Dam et al. 1976; Lander et al. 1977). The drugs that were then measured were phenytoin and phenobarbitone, at that time the most commonly used antiepileptic agents. Both sets of investigators obtained similar findings, ones that were perhaps a little unanticipated in view of the comparatively stable concentration values relative to drug dose that were present over considerable periods of time in individual women while they were not pregnant. The Danish workers showed that, in all 23 women taking phenytoin (with 14 also taking phenobarbitone), plasma phenytoin concentrations relative to drug dose fell appreciably as pregnancy progressed. The plasma ratio of phenobarbitone concentration to dose also fell, though not so much. The changes could begin as early as the 6th week of pregnancy. Postnatally, the concentration to dose ratios for the drugs tended to return progressively to their pre-pregnancy values (the plasma concentration to dose ratio is the reciprocal of the pharmacokinetic parameter, the steady-state clearance, expressed as volume per unit of time). The Australian workers also showed that plasma phenytoin concentrations fell progressively relative to drug dose as pregnancy progressed (in 9 of 10 women taking the drug), with the concentration to dose ratios returning to their pre-pregnancy values in the 7 of the 9 women whose drug concentrations had been followed into the puerperium (Fig. 3.1). In 5 women taking phenobarbitone, or a structurally related barbiturate molecule that is metabolised to it (methylphenobarbitone or primidone), the plasma phenobarbitone concentration to dose ratios also fell during pregnancy.

The Danish investigators suggested that women developed an increased capacity to metabolise phenytoin during pregnancy. The Australian workers proposed a similar interpretation but in addition raised the possibility that the increased maternal body volume resulting from the presence of the placental–foetal unit together with the possible additional drug-metabolising capacity of that unit, and the known effect of prescribed folic acid intake in reducing plasma phenytoin concentrations, might also contribute to the phenomenon. Because the concentration to dose ratios did not return to pre-pregnancy values immediately after the foetus and placenta became abstracted from the maternal body at the time of childbirth, they favoured the view that changes in the mother rather than the contributions of the foetus and placenta were the main factor involved in the increased clearances of the two drugs during pregnancy.

By the 1970s, the centuries-old notion that drugs acted by means of some mysterious inherent property had almost completely given way to the realisation that the body handled exogenous chemicals, including drugs, through the same physico-

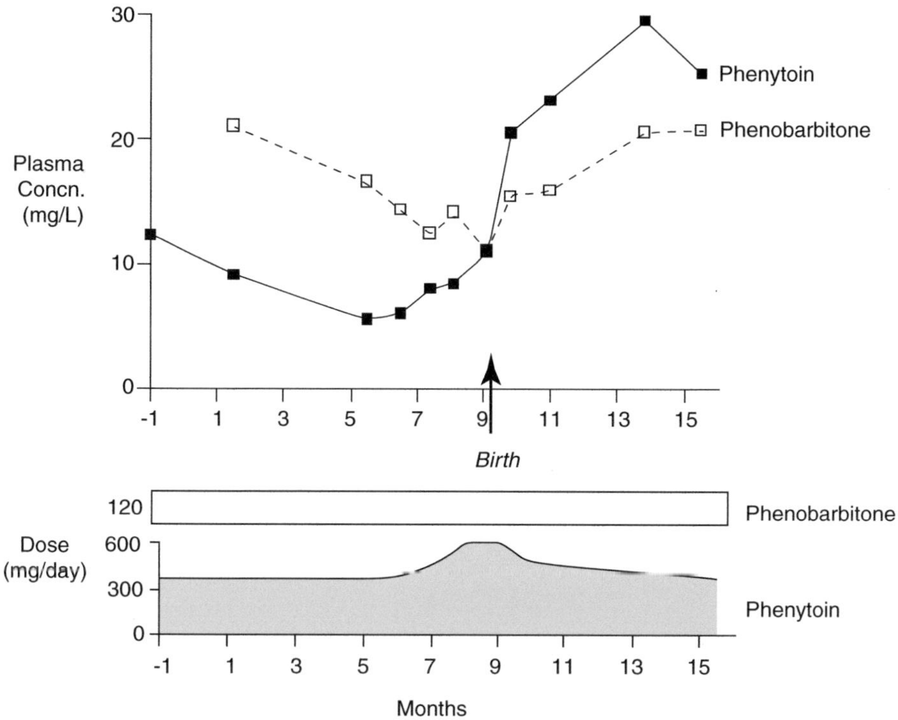

Fig. 3.1 The courses of plasma phenytoin and phenobarbitone concentrations during pregnancy and the puerperium in one woman who took a constant dose of phenobarbitone throughout but whose phenytoin doses were adjusted to try to maintain its plasma concentration in the range 10–20 mg/L (Redrawn from the data of Lander et al. (1977))

chemical mechanisms that it employed in dealing with endogenous molecules. The similarities of the findings of the two papers referred to above and the subsequently publications of these two groups with additional case material (Mygind et al. 1976; Eadie et al. 1977) made it likely that both groups had described a genuine phenomenon related to human pregnancy and that the explanation of its mechanism would lie in knowledge of the changes that occur in a woman's body during and after pregnancy. From this knowledge, principles might be derived that would be applicable more generally to drugs taken during pregnancy.

Body Changes During Pregnancy

Without going into the physiology of pregnancy in more than superficial detail, fertilisation of the ovum followed by implantation of the embryo in the endometrium initiates a series of changes in a woman's body. The forming trophoblast begins to secrete chorionic gonadotropin, while the corpus luteum does not regress as it does in the latter stage of the normal menstrual cycle. Instead, the corpus continues to secrete progesterone in increasing amounts, while ovarian secretion of oestrogens continues. The resulting raised circulating steroidal sex hormonal levels begin to produce various tissue changes in the maternal body. After about 10 weeks of pregnancy, the corpus luteum secretion of progesterone diminishes. By this time the placenta has largely taken over the secretion of this hormone and also that of oestrogens. The circulating levels of these steroidal hormones continue to rise till near term. The process of childbirth relatively abruptly removes the foetus and placenta, with their associated oestrogen- and progesterone-secreting capacities, from the overall maternal–foetal complex. After childbirth, the maternal pituitary secretion of prolactin increases, initiating lactation. This series of progressive steroidal sex hormonal events during pregnancy produces various changes in the anatomy, physiology and biochemistry of the female body. Those changes likely to be relevant to the body's handling of antiepileptic drugs are mentioned below.

Changes in Physiology

By late pregnancy (Heidemann and McClure 2003), the maternal plasma volume will have increased by about 45 % over its pre-pregnancy value, because rising circulating concentrations of progesterone and oestrogen cause the increased secretion of renin and aldosterone. These latter increases produce sodium retention and consequent expansion of the plasma volume. The circulating red cell mass increases by about 20 % during pregnancy so that plasma haemoglobin concentrations fall because of the disproportionately greater expansion in plasma water volume. By two weeks after childbirth, the maternal plasma volume will normally have returned to its pre-pregnancy value. The increased circulating concentrations of oestrogen and progesterone during pregnancy lead to vasodilatation. A hyperkinetic circulatory state develops, with a 50 % increase in cardiac output being present by later pregnancy. The increased cardiac output results in increased regional plasma flow and a raised renal glomerular filtration rate. Maternal tissue growth occurs, particularly involving the breasts and uterus. During pregnancy, no consistent change appears to occur in gastric emptying time or in other measures of alimentary tract motility.

Changes in Biochemistry

During pregnancy there is an overall increase in energy production that is required to sustain the growth of maternal and foetal tissues. Pancreatic insulin secretion increases, but a degree of tissue insulin resistance develops. The renal tubules become less able to resorb glucose from tubular urine. There are changes that involve mainly, but are not necessarily restricted to, the maternal liver. These changes influence the extent of the body's capacity to synthesise various proteins. Circulating levels of enzymes such as γ-glutamyl transpeptidase, alanine transaminase, aspartate transaminase and lactate dehydrogenase tend to rise in pregnancy, though not to concentrations that would be regarded as pathological in other circumstances. By late pregnancy, overall liver protein synthesis has decreased by up to 25 %, resulting in lowered plasma albumin and α_1-acid glycoprotein levels. What is particularly pertinent to the foetal–maternal unit's handling of many drugs is that changes occur in the synthesis of various enzymes that are normally responsible for the inactivation and elimination of certain endogenous molecules and also that of various xenobiotics (including most of the antiepileptic drugs).

Laboratory studies carried out in human liver cells have shown that oestriol induces the synthesis of CYP450 isoenzymes such as CYP2A6, CYP2B6 and CYP 3A4, the latter being responsible for the metabolism of oestrogens and progestogens (Reddy 2010). Progesterone also induces the synthesis of these isoenzymes and also that of CYP2C8 and CYP3A5 (Choi et al. 2013). There is induction of the synthesis of hepatic CYP2C9 and CYP2C19 (Fahmi et al. 2010). In contrast to the increased synthesis of the above isoenzymes, there is decreased synthesis of CYP1A2 (Papageorgiou et al. 2013). This decrease becomes recognisable by 14–18 weeks of pregnancy, a time when the increased synthesis of the other CYP isoenzymes is becoming detectable (Tracy et al. 2005).

Cytochrome P450 enzymes are also synthesised in the human placenta (Myllynen et al. 2007). In that organ CYP19 becomes detectable from the 17th week of pregnancy (Fokina et al. 2011). CYP3A4 , CYP3A5 and CYP3A7 mRNAs are present in the human placenta, amnion and chorion/decidua at term, with the level of CYP3A4 mRNA being highest in the placenta and the levels of the mRNAs for the other CYP450 isoenzymes in the chorion/decidua (Maezawa et al. 2010). Placental tissue also contains the conjugating enzymes glucuronosyl transferase and sulphatase (Wang et al. 2008; Wloch et al. 2009; Reimers et al. 2011). These latter enzymes are detectable in the placenta during the first trimester of human pregnancy (Collier et al. 2002). The molecular transport molecule P-glycoprotein is also present in the placenta (Syme et al. 2004).

In addition, Wloch et al. (2009) have shown that certain of these isoenzymes are present in the foetal liver (CYP2A6, CYP2E1, CYP3A7).

Thus, as pregnancy progresses, there is evidence that the human foetus and placenta develop the metabolic capacities to inactivate various xenobiotic molecules, supplementing that already present in the maternal liver and other tissues.

Lactation

Once initiated by rising circulating prolactin concentrations after childbirth, the process of lactation usually continues until terminated by maternal decision. The secretion of milk is an active process which results in added loss of fluid from the maternal body. Various endogenous and also xenobiotic molecules enter milk by a process of passive transfer along concentration gradients. Some of the transferred molecules may bind to the proteins secreted into the milk, while others may dissolve in the fat content of the milk, which may differ at various stages of lactation. The review of Davanzo et al. (2013) provides further details concerning the presence of antiepileptic drugs in human milk.

Drug Disposition in Pregnancy and Lactation

A drug's presence within the human body at any particular time results from the algebraic sum of three processes, viz. (1) its entry into the body, i.e. absorption, (2) its distribution within the body (including its delivery to the sites where the drug's action occurs) and (3) its elimination from the body by (a) excretion in unchanged form and (b) metabolism, i.e. transformation into other molecules, generally but not invariably pharmacologically inactive ones. The expected effects on antiepileptic drug disposition resulting from the alterations in the physiology and biochemistry of the female body during and after pregnancy, and from the presence of the foeto–placental complex, are summarised below.

Drug Absorption

Pregnant women nearly always take their antiepileptic drugs by mouth. If for some reason antiepileptic drugs cannot be swallowed, they will almost always be administered by intravenous injection. The intramuscular and subcutaneous injection routes are usually both inefficient and undesirable for repeated use. With intravenous administration, the whole drug dose should enter the circulation directly so that the drug's bioavailability is complete. Alimentary tract function usually remains unaltered in pregnancy, apart from the possible effects of morning sickness. Therefore the absorption of orally administered antiepileptic drugs is likely to be as complete as is permitted by the properties of the pharmaceutical preparations in which they are marketed. An exception to this generalisation may occur if an orally administered drug is absorbed from the alimentary tract by means of a substance-specific active transport mechanism, whose transfer capacity becomes saturated at higher oral drug dosages. Despite full absorption, drugs that are extensively metabolised in the gut wall or during their initial passage through the liver in portal venous blood may still have calculated incomplete oral bioavailabilities. This is so because it is only the drug that reaches the general circulation in unmetabolised form that is measured in determining bioavailability. If pregnancy alters the body's capacity for pre-systemic metabolism of such a drug, the value of its oral bioavailability during pregnancy may differ from that in the same woman when not pregnant.

Drug Distribution

Simply through a dilutional effect, the expansion in maternal plasma and body fluid volume and in the volume of foetal body fluids that develops during pregnancy will tend to reduce the concentration of an antiepileptic drug in maternal plasma relative to the drug dose when compared with the concentration that would have applied outside pregnancy in the same woman. The degree of reduction in concentration will be greater for drugs with very small volumes of distribution, i.e. ones that are largely restricted to blood plasma or extracellular water. The expected reduction will tend to be less marked if the drug is more widely distributed through total body water in both mother and foetus. If the drug is also concentrated in a particular body region or tissue, the calculated value of the apparent volume of distribution may exceed that of the actual total physical volume of the body. In such instances, the dilution effect on maternal plasma drug concentrations associated with pregnancy may be small.

As already mentioned, a decrease in plasma albumin concentrations develops in the later stages of pregnancy. For drugs bound to plasma proteins, this decrease results in there being proportionately more unbound (and potentially biologically active) drug in plasma relative to the total drug concentration in that fluid. Failure to realise this may confound the interpretation of total (i.e. protein bound plus unbound) drug concentration in plasma in the last trimester of pregnancy. In that situation, measurements of the concentration of the drug in plasma water rather than in whole plasma may be more informative.

Many drugs seem to cross the placenta and enter foetal tissues by a process of bidirectional passive transfer along concentration gradients until an equilibrium is reached. However, the presence of P-glycoprotein in the placenta suggests that this organ may be able to exclude some molecules from access to the foetus by means of a process of active extrusion. There have been suggestions that this latter possibility could apply to some antiepileptic drugs, though its actual occurrence does not seem to have been demonstrated in humans.

As mentioned earlier in this chapter, for the most part, the entry of drugs into maternal breast milk appears to be a passive transfer process along concentration gradients. Therefore there should be an ongoing equilibrium between drug concentrations in maternal plasma water and in the aqueous phase of milk. However, there could be higher overall drug concentrations in whole breast milk, depending on the solubility of the drug in the lipids of milk and on the protein concentration in milk if the drug binds to milk proteins. Anderson (2006) and Davanzo et al. (2013) have published data for the ratios found between the milk and maternal plasma concentrations of various antiepileptic drugs.

Drug Elimination

Drugs may be eliminated from the body by excretion as the intact molecule or by being metabolised (biotransformed).

Excretion of Unmetabolised Drug

The increased maternal glomerular filtration rate that develops in early pregnancy should enhance the renal excretion of any unmetabolised antiepileptic drug or biologically active drug metabolite that is present in plasma water. Special renal tubular transport mechanisms may exist and increase the excretion from the body of certain drugs or enhance their retention within the body. After childbirth, the relatively rapid restoration of normal plasma volumes and circulatory function during the first few postnatal days might be expected to allow renal excretion of unmetabolised antiepileptic drugs to return to its pre-pregnancy value relatively quickly.

Drug Metabolism

During pregnancy, in the maternal liver and probably in other maternal tissues and also in the placenta and the foetal liver (see above), there is induction of many of the CYP450 isoenzymes that are responsible for catalysing drug oxidations. Although Myllynen et al. (2007) have listed the drug-metabolising enzymes that have been reported as present in the human placenta, the quantitative contribution to drug metabolism made by the placenta and foetus is uncertain. In pregnancy there also is increased formation of the glucuronosyl transferase enzymes that catalyse the formation of water-soluble and nearly always pharmacologically inactive glucuronide metabolites of drugs and of their phase 1 oxidative biotransformation derivatives. Relative to drug dose, these various substrate-specific inductions of metabolic capacity during pregnancy would be expected to reduce the amount of active antiepileptic substance within the maternal body, in particular lowering circulating concentrations of antiepileptic drugs that are eliminated mainly by metabolism. The enhanced maternal metabolic capacity appears to develop relatively early in the course of pregnancy, with that of the placenta and the foetus appearing later. The collective effects of these processes in reducing the amount of drug in the maternal and foetal body would be expected to increase as pregnancy progresses.

At the time of childbirth, there is an abrupt deletion of a probably quantitatively significant component of the overall drug-metabolising capacity of the previous maternal–foetal unit. This might be expected to produce a fairly quick, though partial, reversion towards the pre-pregnancy state of the maternal body's drug-metabolising capacity. Probably the decreasing circulating oestrogens and progesterone concentrations postnatally are then responsible for progressive de-induction of the residual enhanced drug-metabolising capacity that was present during pregnancy. The de-induction process probably runs its course over some days to a few weeks, though more exact information as to the timing in relation to individual drugs does not seem to be available.

The data mentioned earlier in this chapter, where the courses of the plasma concentrations of two antiepileptic drugs were followed through a number of human pregnancies, and afterwards, appear to fit with what could have been predicted on the basis of the above information. It now remains to be seen (Chaps. 4, 5 and 6) whether these principles continue to hold for the knowledge that is available concerning the pharmacokinetics of the other currently available antiepileptic drugs during pregnancy.

References

Anderson GD (2006) Using pharmacokinetics to predict the effects of pregnancy and maternal-infant transfer of drugs during lactation. Clin Pharmacokinet 2:947–960

Choi SY, Koh KH, Jeong H (2013) Isoform-specific regulation of cytochrome P450 expression by estradiol and progesterone. Drug Metab Dispos 41:263–269

Collier AC, Tingle MD, Paxton JW, Mitchell MD, Keelan JA (2002) Metabolizing enzyme localization and activities in the first trimester human placenta: the effects of maternal gestational age, smoking and alcohol consumption. Hum Reprod 17:2564–2572

Dam M, Mygind KI, Christiansen J (1976) Antiepileptic drugs: plasma clearance during pregnancy. In: Janz D (ed) Epileptology. Thieme, Stuttgart, pp 179–183

Davanzo R, Bo SD, Bua J, Copertine M, Zanelli E, Matarazzo L (2013) Antiepileptic drugs and breast feeding. Ital J Pediatr 39:50

Dill WA, Kazenko A, Wolf LM, Glazko AJJ (1956) Studies on 5-5′-diphenylhydantoin (Dilantin) in animals and man. J Pharmacol Exp Ther 118:270–279

Eadie MJ, Lander CM, Tyrer JH (1977) Plasma drug level monitoring in pregnancy. Clin Pharmacokinet 2:427–436

Fahmi OA, Kish M, Boldt S, Obach RS (2010) Cytochrome P450 3A4 mRNA is a more reliable marker than CYP 3A4 activity for detecting pregnane X receptor-activated induction of drug-metabolizing enzymes. Drug Metab Dispos 38:1605–1611

Fokina VM, Patrikeeva SL, Zharikova OL, Nanovskaya TN, Hankins GV, Ahmed MS (2011) Transplacental transfer and metabolism of buprenorphine in preterm human placenta. Am J Perinatol 28:25–32

Heidemann BH, McClure JH (2003) Changes in maternal physiology during pregnancy. Br J Anaesth CEPD Rev 3:65–68

Lander CM, Edwards VE, Eadie MJ, Tyrer JH (1977) Plasma anticonvulsant concentrations during pregnancy. Neurology 27:128–131

Maezawa K, Matsunaga T, Takezawa T, Kanai M, Ohira S, Ohmori S (2010) Cytochrome P450 3As gene expression and testosterone 6 beta-hydroxylase activity in human fetal membranes and placenta at full term. Biol Pharm Bull 33:249–254

Meijer JWA, Meinardi H, Gardner-Thorpe C, van der Kleijn E (1973) Methods of analysis of anti-epileptic drugs. Excerpta Medica, Amsterdam

Mygind KI, Dam M, Christiansen J (1976) Phenytoin and phenobarbitone plasma clearance during pregnancy. Acta Neurol Scand 54:160–166

Myllynen P, Pasanen M, Vakakangas K (2007) The fate and effects of xenobiotics in the human placenta. Expert Opin Drug Metab Toxicol 3:331–346

Papageorgiou I, Grepper S, Unadkat JD (2013) Induction of hepatic CYP3A enzymes by pregnancy-related hormones: studies in human hepatocytes and hepatic cell lines. Drug Metab Dispos 41:281–290

Pippenger CE, Penry JK, Kutt H (1978) Antiepileptic drugs: quantitative analysis and interpretation. Raven, New York

Plaa GL, Hine CC (1956) Hydantoin and barbiturate blood levels observed in epileptics. Arch Int Pharmacodyn Ther 128:375–382

Reddy DS (2010) Clinical pharmacokinetic interactions between antiepileptic drugs and hormonal contraceptives. Expert Rev Clin Pharmacol 3:183–192

Reimers A, Osttby L, Struen I, Sundby E (2011) Expression of UDP glucuronosyltransferase 1A4 in human placenta at term. Eur J Drug Metab Pharmacokinet 35:79–82

Syme MR, Paxton JW, Keelan JA (2004) Drug transfer and metabolism by the human placenta. Clin Pharmacokinet 43:387–514

Tracy TS, Venkataramanan R, Glover DD, Cariris SN (2005) Temporal changes in drug metabolism (CYP1A2, CYP2D6 and CYP3A activity) during pregnancy. Am J Obstet Gynecol 192:633–639

Wang H, Ping J, Peng RX et al (2008) Changes of multiple phase I and phase II enzyme activities in human fetal adrenals during fetal development. Acta Pharmacol Sin 29:231–238

Wloch S, Palasz A, Kaminski M (2009) Active and passive transport of drugs in the human placenta. Ginekol Pol 80:772–777

Chapter 4
The Older Antiepileptic Drugs

Abstract This chapter outlines the pharmacokinetics and clinical pharmacology of the longer established antiepileptic drugs that continue to be reasonably often used in pregnancy, to provide a background to considering the alterations pregnancy and its aftermath produce in these parameters. The four drugs considered, viz. phenobarbitone, phenytoin, carbamazepine and valproate, are cleared from the body mainly by virtue of metabolism, and the clearance values of all increase progressively during pregnancy, though the change for carbamazepine is relatively small unless it is co-administered with another antiepileptic drug that induces the activity of drug-metabolising enzymes. The literature contains information regarding the individual metabolic pathways for phenytoin and carbamazepine biotransformation during pregnancy, indicating that the increased clearances of these drugs are due mainly to the development of increased capacities of already existing metabolic pathways rather than the appearance of new metabolic pathways. Relatively little information has been published concerning the dispositions of these drugs in the neonate, though there are data on their concentration ratios between maternal plasma and breast milk.

This chapter and the following two attempt to deal with the clinical pharmacology of the antiepileptic drugs for which useful pregnancy-related data are available in the current literature. In the accounts that follow, the main emphasis is given to the pharmacokinetics of the drugs, because pregnancy alters antiepileptic drug pharmacokinetics rather than other aspects of their pharmacology. At the end of the section, considering each individual drug in what it is hoped will be sufficient detail for background purposes, there is a separate portion concerning the effects of pregnancy on the drug's pharmacokinetics. These portions considering the situation in pregnancy are referenced in some detail, whereas the referencing of the remainder of the material for each drug is less exhaustive, both to conserve space and because detailed contemporary accounts of the topic outside pregnancy are available (e.g. Levy et al. 2002; Engel and Pedley 2008; Shorvon et al. 2009). A few overall reviews of the pharmacokinetics of the antiepileptic drugs in pregnancy have been published (e.g. Pennell 2003; Tomson et al. 2013).

M.J. Eadie, F.J.E. Vajda, *Antiepileptic Drugs and Pregnancy: A Guide for Prescribers*, DOI 10.1007/978-3-319-21434-4_4

In Chaps. 4 (older drugs), 5 (newer drugs) and 6 (less commonly used drugs), the individual antiepileptic drugs are dealt with largely in the order of their first appearance in clinical use, though drugs that have had comparatively small usages in women of childbearing age, and those for which relatively little information relevant to pregnancy is available, are considered after the more widely used agents have been discussed.

It should be appreciated that the values of the pharmacokinetic parameters of a given drug in the non-pregnant state may remain relatively constant over long periods in adult life, whereas the values change throughout the course of pregnancy. Hence, because the published values may have been determined at different stages of pregnancy (with the stage sometimes not being specified), the parameter values for pregnant women tend to show wider ranges of variation than those that apply in the relatively unchanging non-pregnant state.

Certain pharmacokinetic parameters, in particular drug clearance, have sometimes been expressed in the literature relative to body weight, and sometimes not, and also over periods of either an hour or a day. In the following chapters, clearances have been expressed on a per hour basis in the interests of uniformity, but it has not been possible to express them consistently on, or not on, a body weight basis because of lack of the requisite weight data in some published studies.

Phenobarbitone

Phenobarbitone (phenobarbital) is the oldest antiepileptic drug that remains in reasonably frequent present-day use. Its ability to prevent seizures was recognised as long ago as 1912. The drug's use in Western countries is diminishing even though it is a reasonably effective agent. Because of its low cost, it remains one that is still widely employed in many other parts of the world. Over the years, a number of its molecular derivatives have been synthesised and used to treat epilepsies. The only derivative still employed, though now only on a modest scale, is primidone (desoxy-phenobarbitone) which probably acts mainly through the phenobarbitone to which it is biotransformed. However, the primidone molecule possesses sedative actions in its own right and is believed to be useful in treating essential tremor. The other phenobarbitone congener that had some recent use was *N*-methylphenobarbitone, which has an interesting stereospecific pattern of metabolism. Only phenobarbitone itself is considered further in this chapter, with a few comments added concerning available primidone data.

Chemistry

Phenobarbitone (5-ethyl-5-phenyl barbituric acid) is usually provided for oral use as 30, 50 and 100 mg tablets. The corresponding more water-soluble sodium salt is usually employed in parental preparations of the drug. Phenobarbitone has a pKa value of 7.2 and a molecular weight of 232.23.

Pharmacodynamics

At a molecular level, the antiepileptic effects of phenobarbitone are thought to depend on its binding to specific receptors on the $GABA_A$–chloride ion channel mechanism in neuronal cell membranes. The binding prolongs the opening of the ion channel and so hyperpolarises the cell membrane. Phenobarbitone's effects tend to be somewhat similar to those of GABA-ergic agents. At supratherapeutic doses the drug may also bind to voltage-dependent cell membrane Na^+ ion channels.

Clinically, phenobarbitone is reasonably effective against all of the commonly encountered types of focal and primary generalised epileptic seizure types apart from absences.

Pharmacokinetics

Absorption

The available information suggests that orally administered phenobarbitone has a fairly rapid absorption rate. However peak plasma phenobarbitone levels may not occur for several hours after oral drug intake. This happens because the drug's slow elimination results in the amount absorbed per unit time after each dose exceeding the amount being cleared from the body for a relatively long period. Unlike several other injectable antiepileptic drugs, phenobarbitone seems to be absorbed relatively quickly after intramuscular injection. No values for the oral bioavailability of the drug seem to be readily available, but clinical experience suggests that it is reasonably fully absorbed from the available preparations of the drug that are marketed for oral administration.

Distribution

Phenobarbitone's apparent volume of distribution is around 0.5 L per kilogram, consistent with its being distributed throughout body water without there being any major accumulation in a particular body component. In infants and neonates, the value of the apparent volume of distribution seems to be higher. The plasma protein binding of the drug is lower in the neonate than in the adult, in whom about 50 % of the drug in plasma is protein bound. The binding percentage in plasma remains constant over the drug concentration range of 20–100 mg/L. The drug's concentrations in cerebrospinal fluid, saliva and milk are largely similar to the simultaneous concentrations of the protein-unbound drug in plasma.

Elimination

At therapeutic concentrations, phenobarbitone appears to be eliminated by processes which follow linear kinetics. The elimination half-life in adults is 3–4 days, though it is shorter in children (mean 37 h as compared with 73 h in adults; Garrettson and Dayton 1970).

Guelen et al. (1975) cited a phenobarbitone oral clearance value of around 0.012 l per kilogram per hour in young children, falling to around 0.004 L per kilogram per hour by the age of 12–15 years and thereafter remaining reasonably constant throughout adult life.

Excretion Unchanged

The range of published values for the proportion of a phenobarbitone dose excreted unchanged in urine has been rather wide, the most reliable average figure being around 25 %, consistent with the drug being cleared mainly by metabolism.

Metabolism

Part of a phenobarbitone dose (perhaps some 30 %) follows a rather unusual metabolic pathway, being excreted in urine after conversion to an *N*-glucoside conjugate. This, together with unmetabolised drug, probably accounts for a little over half of a phenobarbitone dose under steady-state conditions. Much of the remainder of the dose is converted to various hydroxy derivatives (Fig. 4.1). None of phenobarbitone's metabolites appear to possess pharmacological activity.

Clinical Pharmacokinetics

Phenobarbitone at plasma levels around 10 mg/L has some effectiveness in controlling seizures in the types of epilepsy that respond to the drug. Above that threshold value, the proportion of patients whose seizures respond increases with increasing plasma drug concentrations. The upper level of the beneficial concentration of the drug varies from person to person. A representative, though perhaps conservative figure for the upper limit, might be 30 mg/L. Patsalos et al. (2008) cited a therapeutic range of 10–40 mg/L. Schmidt et al. (1986) found that a mean plasma phenobarbitone concentration of 18 mg/L was associated with full control of the tonic–clonic seizures of primary generalised epilepsies, but a mean plasma level of 37 mg/L was required before control of simple or complex partial seizures was achieved, whether or not these seizures became secondarily generalised.

Travers et al. (1972) reported that, relative to the phenobarbitone dose, females tended to have lower plasma levels of the drug than males, though the difference was not statistically significant. Eadie et al. (1976, 1977) noted no difference in the steady-state relationship between plasma phenobarbitone concentration and drug dose between 4-year-old and older males and females. However, compared with their male counterparts, younger females required substantially lower phenobarbitone doses to attain the same steady-state plasma phenobarbitone concentrations.

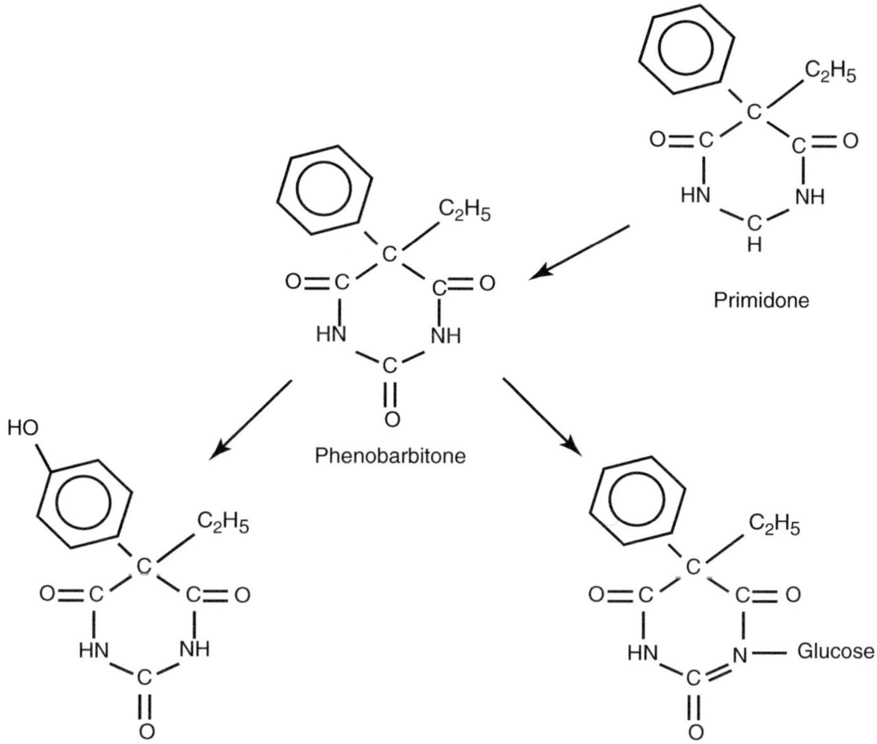

Fig. 4.1 The relationship between the molecular structures of phenobarbitone and primidone, and the two main phase I metabolites of phenobarbitone

Interactions

Phenobarbitone is one of the classic inducers of the microsomal mono-oxygenase enzyme system that catalyses the oxidative metabolisms both of numerous endogenous substances and also exogenous molecules, including various therapeutic drugs (Gillette 1963; Conney 1967). Lecamwasam et al. (1975) showed that continuous administration of phenobarbitone to humans for more than 7 days caused increased formation of liver microsomal protein and heightened activities of various cytochrome P450 enzymes, including CYP3A4 which catalyses numerous drug biotransformations. As a result of this enzyme induction, continuing phenobarbitone intake is associated with decreased plasma concentrations of endogenous molecules such as bilirubin, cortisol, folate and unconjugated oestriol. Carbamazepine, ethinyl oestradiol, phenytoin, valproate and warfarin are among the more relevant drugs whose clearances are affected by the induction, but there are numerous others. As mentioned in Chap. 2, the decreased circulating levels of oestrogenic hormones resulting from concurrent administration of phenobarbitone may compromise the effectiveness of certain oral contraceptives that have relatively low oestrogen contents. The kinetics of vitamin K are not affected by phenobarbitone-mediated enzyme induction. More extensive accounts of the drug's interactions are available in the reviews of Patsalos and Perucca (2003a, b).

Several authors have noticed that phenytoin intake tends to cause a rise in plasma phenobarbitone concentrations (Morselli et al. 1971; Lambie et al. 1976; Windorfer and Sauer 1977). In contrast, co-administered carbamazepine and clonazepam have little effect on circulating phenobarbitone levels. Simultaneous administration of valproate causes a notable increase in plasma phenobarbitone concentrations (Vakil et al. 1976; Wilder et al. 1978; Bruni et al. 1980). Kapetanovic et al. (1981) showed that the co-administration of valproate lengthened the half-life of phenobarbitone and decreased its clearance. This change is associated with falls in the urinary excretions of its oxidative metabolite *p*-hydroxy phenobarbitone and the drug's *N*-glucoside conjugate (Bernus et al. 1994). Folic acid administration has been reported not to alter plasma phenobarbitone levels (Baylis et al. 1971) but there have been contrary findings (Mattson et al. 1973; Eadie et al. 1977).

Adverse Effects

Phenobarbitone has dose-related sedative effects which trouble some patients even at quite low plasma drug concentrations. Some tolerance to the sedation may develop if low phenobarbitone dosages are used at the outset and increased very gradually, recognising that the rather long half-life of the drug means that new steady-state conditions may not apply until more than 2 weeks after a dosage change. Different patients respond to the sedation from the drug in different ways. Some simply become rather depressed, miserable and relatively inert; others become irritable and aggressive as they struggle against the slowing of their mental processes produced by the drug. In those with epilepsy, Reynolds and Travers (1974) found a statistical correlation between increasing plasma phenobarbitone concentrations in the range that is usually considered to be associated with therapeutic benefit and psychomotor slowing and personality change. In frank overdosage with the drug, increasing drowsiness, nystagmus, double vision and ataxia of gait occur.

Long-continued phenobarbitone administration can be accompanied by reduced plasma folate concentrations and rarely by macrocytic anaemia (Chanarin et al. 1958; Davis and Woodliff 1971). Hypocalcaemia and decreased bone mineral density have been reported. Critchley et al. (1976) found a 56 % incidence of Dupuytren's contracture in the hands of chronic epileptic patients treated with phenobarbitone in a residential centre, but there do not seem to have been subsequent reports of this effect. Intake of the drug may precipitate attacks of porphyria in those predisposed to that disorder. Other complications such as skin rashes, agranulocytosis, aplastic anaemia and hepatitis are considerable rarities.

Teratogenicity

This matter is considered in Chap. 9.

Pregnancy

The Mother

As mentioned in Chap. 3, in pregnant women Lander et al. (1977) noted that there was a changing relationship between phenobarbitone oral dosage and steady-state plasma phenobarbitone concentrations that was consistent with the apparent clearance of the drug increasing as pregnancy progressed. Employing the term 'apparent clearance' is necessary in this connexion, because in this study no proof was provided that the full oral dosage of the drug had been absorbed. In the previous year, Mygind et al. (1976) and Dam et al. (1976) had found no increase in the drug's clearance in pregnancy, but during the following decade, Bardy et al. (1982), Hosokawa et al. (1984), Kan et al. (1984) and Yerby et al. (1990) all found that the behaviour of the phenobarbitone dose to plasma concentration relationship in pregnancy was consistent with the drug's clearance being increased, particularly in the later stages of pregnancy. There seems to have been little subsequent exploration of the matter, but it now seems fairly generally accepted that phenobarbitone's clearance usually increases in pregnancy and returns to its baseline value after childbirth. Increased biotransformation probably accounts for the increased clearance, but studies demonstrating this do not seem to have been reported. It would be interesting to know what happens to the capacity of the drug's unusual *N*-glucosidation pathway during pregnancy.

Battino et al. (1984) noted a tendency for plasma primidone levels to rise, relative to drug dose, in the second trimester of pregnancy, coinciding with a decrease in plasma phenobarbitone concentrations derived from the drug. There appears to be no further information available regarding the mechanisms involved in the change. With the declining use of primidone, it seems unlikely that an explanation will become available.

The Foetus

In ex vivo studies in perfused human placenta cotyledons obtained shortly after delivery, Kluck et al. (1988) found that phenobarbitone was comparatively rapidly transferred across the placenta to the foetal compartment. They obtained no evidence that the placenta could metabolise the drug. De Carolis et al. (1992) reported that, in five mother–infant pairs at the time of birth, plasma phenobarbitone concentrations in maternal and umbilical cord plasma were very similar. Earlier, Melchior et al. (1967) and Ishizaki et al. (1981) had both shown that phenobarbitone concentrations in the neonate's umbilical cord plasma were some 95 % of the simultaneous concentrations in maternal plasma.

Breast Milk

Coradello (1973) could not detect measurable phenobarbitone concentrations in the milk of lactating women who were taking the drug. However, in a series of studies, Kaneko et al. (1979, 1982, 1984) found that the mean milk to maternal plasma phenobarbitone concentration ratios were, respectively, 45.9, 36.1 and 34.6 %. Davanzo et al. (2013) cited a figure of 40–60 % for the parameter.

The Neonate

Phenobarbitone has been used to control seizures in the neonate and some information is available regarding its pharmacokinetic properties in that age group. The drug's apparent volume of distribution appears to be proportionately greater than in the adult. Painter et al. (1977) quoted a value of 0.97 ± 0.20 L per kg for the parameter, Pitlick et al. (1978) a very similar value and Fischer et al. (1981) a mean value of 0.81 L per kg. In neonates, some 57–64 % of the drug in plasma is not protein bound (Bossi 1982). Boreus et al. (1975) observed that the elimination half-life of phenobarbitone in neonates was inversely related to the plasma phenobarbitone concentration. Pitlick et al. (1978) found that the elimination half-life shortened from a mean of 115 h at the end of the first neonatal week to a mean of 67 h by the end of the fourth week. Fischer et al. (1981) cited a half-life value of 103.4 h and Ishizaki et al. (1981) a mean half-life value of 74.0 h. The parameter values cited earlier in this paragraph apply to the initial dose of phenobarbitone received by neonates not previously exposed to the drug. No information is available concerning the metabolic pathways involved in eliminating the drug in this age group. It is unclear whether the elimination rates would be similar in neonates whose mothers had taken the drug throughout pregnancy, in which case the neonate's drug-metabolising capacity may have already been induced before birth.

Phenytoin

Phenytoin was developed as an antiepileptic agent in the late 1930s as the outcome of an attempt to discover new chemicals with molecular structural resemblances to phenobarbitone and with similar or greater antiepileptic efficacies. The drug remains in widespread use after more than two-thirds of a century, though in more affluent societies it is less often employed than formerly.

Chemistry

Phenytoin (5,5′-diphenylhydantoin), a white crystalline material (pK_a ~ 8.4), is marketed for oral use as the free acid (molecular weight 252.3) or as the sodium salt (molecular weight 274.3). The latter is more water soluble, though still poorly so. Oral suspensions of the drug, and a few solid dosage forms, contain the drug as the free acid. Most oral dosage forms contain the sodium salt. Sodium phenytoin preparations contain about 8 % less active substance than preparations containing the same weight of drug but in the form of the corresponding free acid. The solution of the sodium salt for intravenous or intramuscular injection has a pH of around 12.

Pharmacodynamics

In the past, numerous possible biochemical mechanisms were proposed to explain the antiseizure action of phenytoin, but it now appears clear that, at therapeutically relevant concentrations, the drug's antiepileptic action is mediated through its effects on cell membrane voltage-dependent Na^+ ion channels (Mantegazza et al. 2010). Phenytoin binds to, and then prolongs the inactivation state of, Na^+ channels (mainly α-subtypes 1.1, 1.2, 1.3 and 1.6 – Qiao et al. 2014). This is particularly the case when the channels are in their fast-inactivated state (Karoly et al. 2010). The drug's effect is greater when the cell membrane is already depolarised and in an inactive state than when the membrane is hyperpolarised (Thomas and Petrou 2013). The Na^+ channel block becomes use dependent if the cell membrane is depolarised repeatedly. Phenytoin's inactivation of voltage- and frequency-dependent Na^+ channels renders partly depolarised axons less able to transmit rapid trains of action potentials (as occurs in epileptic discharges) but has less effect on relatively infrequent and more physiological action potential traffic along axons. The drug binds to the same site in the inner pore of sodium channel as carbamazepine and lamotrigine do (Lipkin and Fozzard 2010).

At high concentrations, phenytoin may inhibit axonal and axon terminal calcium channels, thereby potentially stabilising the cell membranes and decreasing the release of excitatory neurotransmitters, in particular glutamate, from axon terminals which have been activated by the arrival of action potentials. It also increases chloride conductance at $GABA_A$ receptors. This, at least in theory, might have an antiseizure effect. Phenytoin has no action at the T-type calcium channels in the thalamus that are involved in the genesis of absence seizures (Kuo 1998).

Phenytoin's rather selective inhibition of fast action potential traffic along axons seems to account for its ability to impede the spread of epileptic activity while having relatively little effect on more physiological rates of transit of neuronal axon traffic. It also helps explain the observation that the drug tends not to prevent seizure discharge initiation but deters discharges spreading.

Clinically, phenytoin is useful in controlling most forms of epileptic seizure disorder, though not the absence seizures of idiopathic, i.e. genetic, generalised epilepsy. The drug's action on cell membrane Na^+ channels has also been utilised to treat cardiac arrhythmias, myotonia and certain other disorders.

Pharmacokinetics

The clinical pharmacokinetics of phenytoin was reasonably fully worked out a generation ago. Little additional knowledge has subsequently become available.

Absorption

The available information concerning the oral bioavailability of phenytoin was reviewed by Neuvonen (1979). The occurrence of a formulation-related bioavailability issue in Australasia nearly 50 years ago should have alerted the medical community to the drug's potential bioavailability issues, but reports of generic phenytoin tablets whose oral bioavailabilities appear incomplete and also possibly inconsistent continue to appear in the literature (e.g. Berg et al. 2008). Storage of the drug under conditions of high temperature and humidity may impair its bioavailability.

Intramuscular administration of phenytoin is too inefficient to be useful clinically, because the drug is absorbed very slowly and inconsistently from its administration site. Fosphenytoin, a water-soluble phenytoin prodrug, is better absorbed after intramuscular administration (Fischer et al. 2003). Intravenously injected phenytoin is fully bioavailable, but the solution is highly alkaline and contains polyethylene glycol. Consequently, it must be administered very slowly to minimise unwanted effects. Furthermore, the drug may crystallise from solution if injected into an intravenous fluid reservoir containing a solution at a more physiological pH, e.g. glucose saline.

Distribution

In humans, phenytoin is distributed throughout total body water. Published values for the drug's apparent volume of distribution have been in the range 0.5–0.8 L/kg. There seems to be little or no selective regional concentration of the drug. Its concentrations in plasma are a little higher than those in red blood cells. Brain phenytoin levels are slightly higher than simultaneous drug concentration in plasma. Under steady-state conditions, the drug's concentration is higher in cerebral white than grey matter. Phenytoin is transported out of the brain by a P-glycoprotein mechanism situated in cells in the blood–brain barrier. Animal studies have shown that, if this extrusion mechanism is well developed or is induced following repeated seizures, brain phenytoin concentrations become disproportionately low relative to simultaneous plasma water drug concentrations. This effect may be associated with apparent treatment resistance in experimental animals with seizures (Loscher 2007). It is not yet clear whether a similar situation applies in human epilepsy (French 2013).

About 90 % of the phenytoin in adult plasma is bound to plasma proteins, mainly albumin. The protein-unbound fraction of the drug in plasma is higher in neonates than adults and also increases a little with advanced age, in late pregnancy, in the presence of hypoalbuminaemia from various causes and in that of high glycated albumin levels, as occur in diabetics. Phenytoin concentrations in cerebrospinal fluid and routinely collected saliva, tears and sweat are very similar to the unbound concentrations of the drug in plasma. However saliva phenytoin concentrations vary with saliva flow rate and are affected by the presence of gum disease (Kamali and Thomas 1994).

Elimination

Phenytoin is unusual among drugs in present-day therapeutic use in that, at clinically relevant dosages, it exhibits Michaelis–Menten rather than linear elimination kinetics. Nevertheless, the linear kinetic parameters of elimination half-life and clearance are often cited for the drug. The numerical values of the latter parameters are not constant in a given individual but vary with the phenytoin concentration range over which the values have been determined. The calculated half-life is longer and the clearance lower, at higher plasma drug concentrations than at lower ones in the same person. A commonly quoted value for the drug's half-life over the concentration range likely to be encountered in human therapeutics is 22 ± S.D. 9 h, with a clearance value for adults of 0.02 L/kg/h, and for children below 5 years of age, one of 0.06 L/kg/h.

Most published values for the Michaelis constant (K_m) of phenytoin have ranged between 3 and 30 mg/L, with the mean around 6 mg/L (24 μmol). This is a lower concentration than the conventional lower limit of the therapeutic range of plasma concentrations of the drug (10 mg/L). The saturable elimination of the drug produces a non-linear relationship between phenytoin dosage and steady-state plasma phenytoin concentration. Relatively small dose increases are associated with disproportionately large increases in plasma phenytoin concentrations. Published values for the maximum velocity of phenytoin elimination (V_{max}) have been in the range 6–16 mg/kg/day [17.5–46.7 mg/h]. The values are higher on a body weight basis in young children than in adults (Bauer and Blouin 1983).

Excretion Unchanged

Less than 5 % of a phenytoin dose is excreted in urine unchanged, the drug being eliminated mainly through metabolism.

Metabolism

The main known metabolite of the drug, accounting for 60–80 % of the dose, is the pharmacologically inactive oxidation product *p*-hydroxy phenytoin (5-phenyl, 5′-*p*-hydroxyphenylhydantoin, HPPH). The conversion of the parent molecule to *p*-hydroxy phenytoin, via a postulated short-lived arene oxide intermediate, is catalysed by the CYP450 isoforms CYP2C9 and CYP 2C19 and, in the skin, possibly by CYP2C18. Much of the *p*-hydroxy phenytoin formed in the phase I biotransformation stage appears in urine as a glucuronide conjugate formed in a reaction catalysed by UDP glucuronosyl transferase 1A isoforms (Nakajima et al. 2002). Other quantitatively minor oxidation products are known, e.g. phenolic, dihydrodiol, catechol and O-methyl catechol derivatives (Fig. 4.2). The liver is responsible for nearly all of the biotransformation of the drug, but some may occur in the gums, skin and other peripheral tissues.

At conventional dosages in humans, CYP2C9 activity is responsible for some 90 % of the hydroxylation of phenytoin, the [S]-isomer of *p*-hydroxy phenytoin being formed preferentially. The [R]-isomer of *p*-hydroxy phenytoin is formed via activity of CYP2C19. Poor metabolisers of the now superseded hydantoin derivative mephenytoin (methoin) form relatively little [R]-*p*-hydroxy phenytoin (Ieiri et al. 1995). CYP2C9 polymorphisms may account for the occasional individuals in Western populations and the more frequent ones of Asian extraction, who cannot tolerate conventional phenytoin dosages (Kesavan et al. 2010).

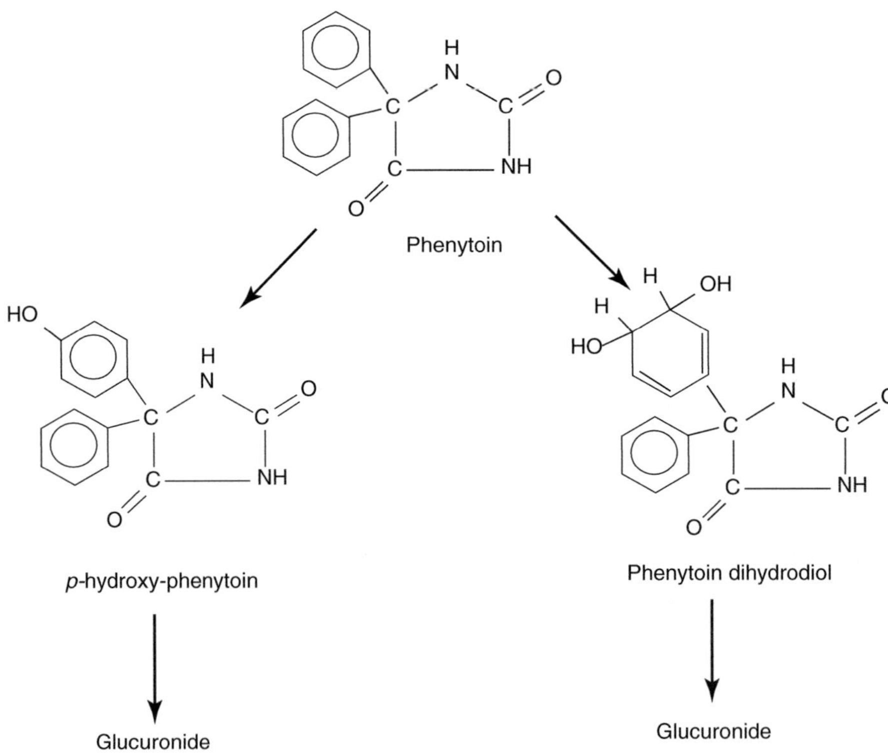

Fig. 4.2 Main pathways of phenytoin metabolism. The *heavier arrows* indicate the pathways whose capacity is increased in pregnancy

Clinical Pharmacokinetics

Kutt et al. (1964) nominated a range of plasma phenytoin concentration between 10 and 20 mg/L (40–80 μmol) as being usually associated with the best chance of achieving seizure control without producing drug overdosage manifestations. This concentration range has come to be regarded as the 'therapeutic' or 'target' range for the drug. However, other authors have proposed different lower and upper limits of the range, e.g. from 7 mg/L (28 μmol) to 25 mg/L (100 μmol) (Loiseau et al. 1977). In some patients, seizures are controlled at plasma concentrations above or below the 10–20 mg/L range, without unwanted effects of the drug occurring (Patsalos et al. 2008). Schmidt et al. (1986) found that a mean plasma phenytoin concentration of 14 mg/L (56 μmol) sufficed to control generalised tonic–clonic seizures, but a mean concentration of 23 mg/L (92 μmol) was required to control partial seizures. The therapeutic range values for the drug in plasma water (i.e. the unbound plasma concentration) and in saliva are approximately one-tenth of those that apply for whole plasma.

For plasma phenytoin concentrations in the 'therapeutic' or 'target' range, new steady-state conditions should apply 4–8 days after a phenytoin dosage change. At higher circulating drug concentrations steady-state conditions may be more delayed after a dosage change (up to about 2 weeks). Under steady-state condition, the peak-to-trough fluctuation in therapeutic range plasma phenytoin concentration in adults is likely to be of the order of ± 10 % over a 12 h dosage interval. There are greater inter-dosage fluctuations over the same time interval in children.

In a population taking commonly used adult dosages of phenytoin (300 or 400 mg/day), there is a wide range of steady-state plasma phenytoin concentrations. An appreciable proportion of the values falls outside the therapeutic range. Expressing drug dosage relative to body weight improves the correlation. In the average adult, a phenytoin dose of 5 mg/kg/day will be associated with a mean mid-therapeutic range steady-state plasma phenytoin concentration of 15 mg/L (60 μmol). Prepubertal children, with their higher velocities of elimination of the drug, are likely to require double that dosage to achieve a similar mean steady-state plasma drug concentration. Neonates and children in the first few months of life and the elderly require slightly lower doses on a body weight basis than the average adult.

As mentioned above, if a patient's phenytoin dosage has to be increased, it is important to realise that the Michaelis–Menten elimination kinetics of the drug will cause plasma levels of the drug to increase more than if linear elimination kinetics had been applied.

If the presence of a reduced plasma protein-binding capacity for phenytoin is suspected, measurement of unbound plasma phenytoin or salivary phenytoin concentrations is likely to provide a more reliable basis for interpreting the clinical situation than the whole plasma drug concentration value.

Some workers have reported that, for a give phenytoin dose, adult females have statistically significantly lower plasma phenytoin levels than adult males (Sherwin et al. 1974; Richens 1975). Others have not detected such differences (Eadie et al. 1973; DeLeacy et al. 1979). The latter workers noted that when oral contraceptives were being taken, plasma phenytoin concentrations tended to be higher relative to drug dose than in women not taking these agents.

In some women, plasma phenytoin levels tend to fall, relative to the drug dose, around the time of menstruation (Rościszewska et al. 1986). Shavit et al. (1984) showed that the clearance of phenytoin tended to be higher and the elimination half-life shorter, at the time of menstruation as compared with the values of these parameters at the mid-interval of the menstrual cycle.

Interactions

Over the years, numerous interactions between phenytoin and endogenous substances and co-administered drugs have been described (Nation et al. 1990; Patsalos and Perucca 2003a, b; Patsalos 2013). Nearly all the interactions are pharmacokinetic in nature and mainly involve altered rates of metabolism of one or both of the substances involved. The interactions that have been described are too numerous for detailed individual consideration here.

Interactions Altering Phenytoin Concentrations

A few interactions involve altered phenytoin absorption, but these are unlikely to prove an issue during pregnancy. Certain endogenous substances and various acidic drugs (e.g. salicylates, valproic acid, heparin) may displace phenytoin from its plasma protein-binding sites. These interactions are also unlikely to cause subsequent difficulties during pregnancy unless free (i.e. protein-unbound) drug concentrations are used as a guide to the adequacy of antiepileptic therapy, as may be done particularly in late pregnancy.

Interactions that alter phenytoin metabolism are a different matter. Taking drugs which inhibit phenytoin metabolism may cause raised phenytoin concentrations and possibly overdosage manifestations. For example, co-administration of antiepileptic drugs such as ethosuximide, felbamate, oxcarbazepine and sulthiame may result in increased plasma phenytoin levels relative to the drug dose. Interactions which involve induction of phenytoin metabolism, thus lowering its plasma concentrations, are more common. Such interactions may go unnoticed, unless plasma phenytoin concentrations are monitored or seizure control deteriorates. Primidone, vigabatrin, carbamazepine and phenobarbitone may be responsible for such interactions. However, the opposite effect sometimes occurs when carbamazepine or phenobarbitone is added to phenytoin therapy. The effects of valproic acid on plasma phenytoin levels appear to be inconsistent.

Phenytoin Affecting Other Substances

Phenytoin may alter the elimination of other substances by inducing: (1) the synthesis of the CYP isoenzymes responsible for their metabolism, including not only CYP2C isoforms but also CYP3A4 (which catalyses many drug oxidations) and CYP1A12, and (2) the synthesis of certain glucuronyl transferases involved in drug conjugation. As well, co-administered phenytoin may inhibit the metabolism of other CYP2C9 or CYP2C19 eliminated drugs. Drugs that may be encountered in pregnant women, and whose plasma concentrations are likely to be reduced in the presence of phenytoin include, among antiepileptic agents, carbamazepine, clobazam, clonazepam, felbamate, lamotrigine, primidone, tiagabine, topiramate, valproic acid, ethosuximide and zonisamide. Phenytoin's effect on circulating phenobarbitone concentrations is variable. Plasma levels and clinical effectiveness of many cardiovascular agents, chemotherapeutic agents, hormonal agents, psychotropic agents and other substances may be reduced by concurrent phenytoin administration.

The references cited at the beginning of the present chapter provide additional information regarding the drug's numerous described interactions.

Adverse Effects

Numerous adverse effects of phenytoin have been described over its long period of extensive use in humans. Some adverse effects are clearly dose related; others probably involve hypersensitivity reactions, possibly related to immune-mediated processes.

Nervous System

Phenytoin overdosage tends to produce manifestations of vestibulocerebellar disturbance before sedation becomes troublesome. There may be horizontal nystagmus, typically at plasma phenytoin concentrations above 20 mg/L (80 μmol). At concentrations above 30 mg/L (120 μmol), ataxia of gait and double vision occur. At concentrations above 40 mg/L (160 μmol), drowsiness, sometimes with nausea and vomiting, and, at still higher concentrations, coma develop (Kutt et al. 1964). There are considerable interindividual differences in the correlation between phenytoin concentration and adverse effects. Some patients experience unwanted effects even at plasma levels below the conventional therapeutic range. Other patients appear untroubled at plasma phenytoin levels above 30 mg/L (120 μmol). Occasional patients may experience mood disorders, mainly depression, as the dose of the drug is increased. Paradoxically, seizure control may deteriorate in some patients as plasma phenytoin levels become 'supratherapeutic' or if the drug has been prescribed for epilepsy syndromes that involve absence or myoclonic seizures. Rarely, phenytoin overdosage results in various dyskinetic and dystonic involuntary movements, asterixis or ophthalmoplegia. Shorvon and Reynolds (1982) reported that the drug may cause subclinical, and occasionally clinically recognisable, peripheral neuropathy.

Skin and Gums

Within the first few days of phenytoin intake, 5–10 % of patients given the drug develop a measles-like rash, usually appearing first on the trunk. If phenytoin intake is not ceased promptly, more extensive and serious skin and internal organ involvement can develop. Other cutaneous reactions, e.g. Stevens–Johnson syndrome, systemic lupus erythematosus, exfoliative dermatitis and toxic epidermal necrolysis, are less frequent. Continued phenytoin intake may cause an overgrowth of body hair, particularly in dark-haired women. Acne and coarsening of facial features can develop.

Intravenous administration of phenytoin may lead to a 'purple glove' syndrome with progressive skin discoloration, oedema and pain which involve the hand and forearm distal to the administration site (O'Brien et al. 1998). Too rapid intravenous infusion of the drug is better avoided. As well, thrombophlebitis may develop in the vein into which the drug has been administered. The incidence of this adverse effect appears to be lower when intravenous fosphenytoin is used (Fischer et al. 2003).

Gum hyperplasia may develop in between 13 and 40 % of those taking phenytoin. The topic has been reviewed on several occasions (Meraw and Sheridan 1998; Ayra and Gulati 2012). The severity of the gum hyperplasia seems related to the plasma phenytoin level, though poor dental hygiene makes the hypertrophy more obvious.

Bone

Long-term phenytoin intake, alone or together with another older antiepileptic drug, can be responsible for the development of reduced bone mineral density and sometimes overt osteomalacia resulting from increased bone turnover. Plasma calcium levels may fall and alkaline phosphatase levels increase, with reduced plasma 25-hydroxycholecalciferol concentrations. The problem is likely to be worse if the diet is poor in vitamin D content and if there is little exposure to sunlight. Induction of vitamin D metabolism by the drug, and possibly impaired intestinal absorption of dietary calcium, appears to be responsible.

Lymphoid Tissue

Rarely, a widespread but reversible lymphadenopathy, a pseudolymphoma syndrome, can develop after long-term phenytoin use. Histologically the appearance of the affected lymph glands resembles that of Hodgkin's disease. Even more rarely, true lymphoma has been reported in association with the drug.

Folates

Continued phenytoin intake may cause reduced plasma and red blood cell folate levels, the extent of the reduction being related to the plasma phenytoin concentration. The mechanisms involved are not fully elucidated. In patients taking long-term phenytoin therapy, the folate deficiency may occasionally result in megaloblastic anaemia.

Cardiovascular Effects

Oral phenytoin therapy in usual dosages is very unlikely to cause cardiovascular disturbances. Intravenous administration of the drug is potentially hazardous, there being dangers of hypotension, cardiovascular collapse and central nervous system depression.

Other Effects

Phenytoin intake can precipitate attacks of porphyria in sufferers from the disorder. If paroxysmal hypoglycaemic symptoms from an insulinoma are misdiagnosed as manifestations of epilepsy and treated with phenytoin, the real diagnosis may be further delayed because phenytoin can diminish pancreatic insulin secretion. As a result, the drug for a time may appear to provide successful therapy. Rare adverse effects of the drug include hepatitis, vasculitis, interstitial lung infiltration, interstitial nephritis, myopathy, thyroiditis, arthritis and the suppression of the formation of particular lines of blood cell.

Phenytoin intake can produce various asymptomatic biochemical effects. These include raised plasma levels of γ-glutamyl transpeptidase, alkaline phosphatase, high-density lipoprotein (HDL) cholesterol, caeruloplasmin, copper, prolactin and sex hormone-binding globulin. It may also cause reduced plasma concentrations of folate (discussed above), IgA, IgG, IgE, IgM, fibrinogen, thyroxine, triiodothyronine (but not free T_4 and T_3), protein-bound iodine, vitamin K, vitamin E, vitamin D metabolites (mentioned above), cortisol, oestrogens, progesterone, free testosterone, pyridoxal phosphate, tryptophan and thiamine. As mentioned in Chap. 2, the reduced circulating steroidal sex hormone levels may be associated with a diminished libido and with other disturbances of sexual functioning.

Teratogenicity

This topic is considered in Chap. 9.

Pregnancy

The Mother

Once the altered relationship between phenytoin dose and plasma phenytoin concentrations during pregnancy was recognised in the 1976–1977 period (see Chap. 3), the explanation for the changes was sought. One possibility was that the oral bioavailability of the drug was decreased during pregnancy. Ramsay et al. (1978) described a single instance in which this may have occurred. In the 22nd week of her pregnancy, the woman involved appeared to excrete 56 % of her daily phenytoin dose (of 900 mg) unchanged in faeces. At 3 months and subsequently at 30 months postpartum, by which time the oral dose of the drug had fallen to 400 mg a day, the proportion of the dose lost in faeces had decreased, initially to 40 % and finally to 23 % of the oral dose. No further instances of such altered phenytoin absorption from the alimentary tract during pregnancy have been reported. Lander et al. (1984) carried out an opportunistic formal bioavailability investigation in five women who suffered their first epileptic seizures during pregnancy. Before commencing regular phenytoin intake, each woman received an initial intravenous dose of phenytoin followed a week later by an oral dose of the same magnitude. Except for folate, which all the women were taking, none of the women took any other agent known to affect plasma phenytoin concentrations. The calculated oral bioavailability fraction for the drug ranged from 0.79 to 1.01, with a mean value of 0.91 ± 0.10 (Fig. 4.3). It therefore appears unlikely that an incomplete oral bioavailability is the usual explanation for the drug's altered dose to steady-state concentration relationship during pregnancy.

An increased apparent volume of distribution, related both to the water retention of pregnancy and to the increased volume of the overall maternal–foetal unit, always seemed likely to make some contribution to the reduced plasma phenytoin levels relative to phenytoin dose in pregnancy. However, it seemed more likely that the main factor involved would be increased elimination of the drug. Several published measurements have demonstrated increased numerical clearance values for phenytoin during pregnancy. However, as mentioned when discussing the interpretation of clearance values for a drug whose elimination is better described by Michaelis–Menten kinetics than linear ones, the quantitative significance of phenytoin clearance value changes can be somewhat uncertain. Being aware of this, Dickinson et al. (1989) carried out studies at stages between the 20th and 36th week of pregnancy and again between eight and 16 weeks postpartum, in five women taking regular phenytoin therapy. These women received single intravenous 50 mg doses of stable isotope-labelled phenytoin on their study days, while continuing to take their usual oral phenytoin dosage, less the equivalent of the 50 mg intravenous dose,

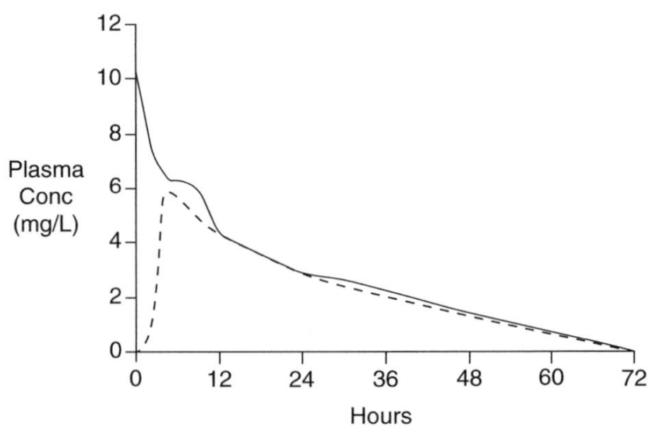

Fig. 4.3 The time courses of plasma phenytoin concentrations following intravenous (*solid line*) and oral administration (*broken line*) of a 250 mg phenytoin dose in a pregnant woman (Redrawn from the data of Lander et al. (1984))

on that day. Plasma stable isotope and total phenytoin concentrations were measured at intervals over the next 72 h. Simultaneous fitting of equations to the paired concentration–time data sets on each occasion permitted calculation of the Michaelis–Menten parameters of the drug during and after pregnancy in the same woman (Figs. 4.4 and 4.5). The mean maximum velocity of phenytoin elimination during pregnancy (1170 ± 600 mg per day) was statistically significantly higher than that after pregnancy (780 ± 470 mg per day). The Michaelis constant was also higher during pregnancy (18.2 ± 8.4 mg/L in whole plasma, 2.5 ± 0.85 mg/L in plasma water) than after pregnancy (10.2 ± 7.4 and 1.16 ± 0.65 mg/L respectively). The difference in the plasma water values for the Michaelis constant was also statistically significant. For what it is worth, the calculated clearance of the isotopic drug in pregnancy was also statistically significantly higher (0.025 ± 0.012 L per kg per hour) [1.75 L/h] than after pregnancy (0.021 ± 0.013 L per kg per hour) [1.47 L/h].

The increased elimination parameter values for the drug during pregnancy must represent consequences of increased biotransformation of the drug, since the intravenously administered isotopic drug was fully bioavailable.

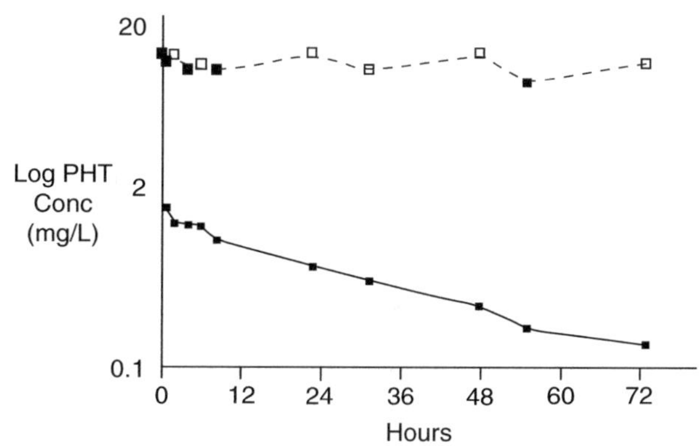

Fig. 4.4 Semilogarithmic plots of the time courses of non-isotopic plasma phenytoin (PHT) concentrations (*broken line*) and isotopic phenytoin concentrations (*continuous line*) after a 50 mg intravenous dose of isotopic phenytoin given to a pregnant woman (Redrawn from the data of Dickinson et al. (1989))

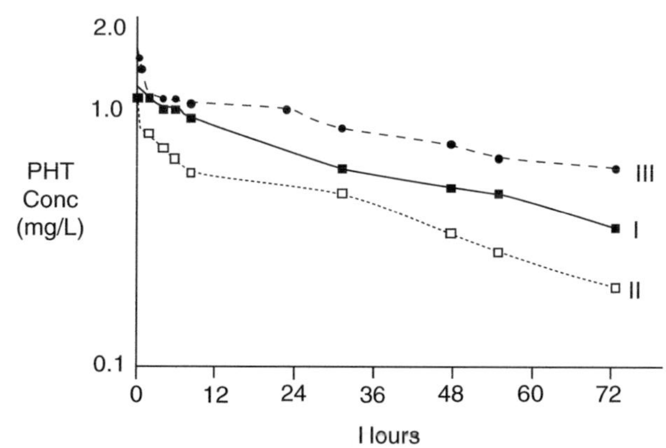

Fig. 4.5 Semilogarithmic plots of the time courses of isotopic plasma phenytoin concentrations after 50 mg intravenous doses of isotopic phenytoin given to a woman in the 20th (I) and 31st (II) week of pregnancy and in the 15th postnatal week (III) (Redrawn from the data of Dickinson et al. (1989))

Are the capacities of all the metabolic pathways for the drug's biotransformation enhanced during pregnancy or only those of particular pathways? On two occasions during pregnancy, and once postpartum, Eadie et al. (1992) studied five pregnant women who were not taking any other drug metabolism-inducing agent. They found that the urinary excretion of the main phenytoin metabolite, *p*-hydroxy phenytoin, accounted for a mean of 56.6 % of the dose in earlier pregnancy, one of 64.3 % of the dose in later pregnancy but only one of 52.9 % of the dose postpartum. Subsequently Bernus et al. (1997), with the ability to measure additional urinary excretion products of the drug, found in a larger group of women with epilepsy that during pregnancy there was increased urinary excretion of both the main para-hydroxylated metabolite of the drug and that of this metabolite's conjugates, mainly glucuronides, in urine. However, there was no increase in the excretion of the diol derivative of the drug and also no significant increase in the excretion of unmetabolised phenytoin (see Fig 4.2).

Near term, the plasma protein binding of phenytoin tends to be decreased (Dean et al. 1980; Ruprah et al. 1982).

The Foetus

Phenytoin concentrations are similar in neonatal umbilical cord plasma and in simultaneously collected maternal plasma (Mirkin 1971; Ishizaki et al. 1981).

Breast Milk

Phenytoin concentrations in human breast milk are lower than simultaneous concentrations of the drug in whole plasma. Kaneko et al. (1979, 1982, 1984) in a series of measurements found that the mean values for phenytoin concentration in breast milk ranged between 18.1 and 18.8 % of those in maternal plasma. Bar-Oz et al. (2000) found that breast milk phenytoin concentrations were between 3 and 55 % of maternal plasma ones. Davanzo et al. (2013) in a recent review stated that the drug's milk to plasma ratio was 0.18–0.45 (the figure varying to an extent with the fat and protein content of the milk). A breast-fed infant would be unlikely to receive enough phenytoin from breast milk to produce overdosage effects, unless the mother was herself considerably overdosed with the drug.

The Neonate

The unbound fraction of the drug in plasma is higher in the neonate than in the adult.

In the neonate exposed to phenytoin during pregnancy, blood coagulation defects, probably due to a relative deficiency of vitamin K-catalysed clotting factors, have been claimed to cause bleeding on the first neonatal day unless the mother receives vitamin K before delivery and/or the baby receives prophylactic vitamin K immediately after birth. Presumably phenytoin induces the conversion of the vitamin to inactive products. The more recent literature suggests that the risk of this adverse effect may not be as great as was earlier thought. Kaaja et al. (2002) failed to find evidence of any increased bleeding tendency in neonates exposed to enzyme-inducing antiepileptic drugs during pregnancy.

Carbamazepine

Carbamazepine came into use as an antiepileptic agent in the 1960s and at much the same time found a place as an effective treatment for trigeminal neuralgia (tic douloureux). It remains in widespread use half a century later and is sometimes considered to be the gold standard against which to assess the efficacies of more recently developed agents for treating focal (partial) epilepsies.

Chemistry

Carbamazepine (5-carbamyl-5H-dibenz[*b,f*]azepine) is a white crystalline material (MW 236.26). It is very poorly soluble in water, and no satisfactory parenteral formulation for human use has become available. The molecule is essentially neutral in pH and does not ionise in biological fluids.

Carbamazepine is marketed in solid dosage forms, mainly in 100 mg, 200 mg and 400 mg dosage units, some with modified release properties, and in oral suspensions.

Pharmacodynamics

The molecular mechanism of action of carbamazepine at the concentrations at which it is effective in human therapeutics appears to be rather similar to that of phenytoin, viz. blocking cell membrane voltage-dependent Na^+ ion channels. Carbamazepine has other known mechanisms of action, though the extents to which these contribute to its antiseizure and pain-suppressing effects are unclear. In experimental preparations, the drug binds to brain adenosine receptors and can cause their upregulation (Marangos et al. 1987).

The action of carbamazepine on the cell membrane voltage-dependent Na^+ channels in active tissues enables the drug to limit fast trains of axon impulses spreading from their neural sites of origin, rather than inhibiting the initiation of the impulse trains (Julien and Hollister 1975). This action appears capable of accounting for the usefulness of the drug in all forms of focal epilepsy and in the convulsive seizures of idiopathic, i.e. genetic, generalised epilepsy. The drug does not appear particularly effective in controlling myoclonic seizures and is not useful in treating absence seizures. The same mechanism of action appears to account for carbamazepine's efficacy in relieving the pain of trigeminal and glossopharyngeal neuralgias and for its ability to blunt the severity of other neuralgic-type pains, e.g. painful peripheral neuropathies. Carbamazepine may also be used to treat non-nephrogenic diabetes insipidus and myotonia. In recent years it has been increasingly employed in managing psychiatric illness.

Pharmacokinetics

Absorption

Both the speed and the extent of the absorption of orally administered carbamazepine in solid dosage forms are influenced by the particle size of the drug in the preparation studied (Dam et al. 1981; Neuvonen 1985). The drug is absorbed considerably faster when administered in solution than in solid dosage forms (absorption half-time 0.29 h versus 1.72 h – Levy et al. 1975). If the particle size is too coarse, the orally administered drug may not be fully bioavailable, and if the particle size is too small, the drug may be absorbed quickly enough to cause temporary symptoms after intake, e.g. unsteadiness of gait and double vision associated with nystagmus. Carbamazepine appears to be one of those drugs for which patients are well advised to continue to use the same manufacturer's preparation on all occasions. In good-quality preparations, the drug's oral bioavailability seems reasonably complete but may still be vulnerable to the vagaries of gastrointestinal tract motility.

A range of values has been reported for the time of achieving peak plasma levels of the drug after a single oral dose. The values have been between 2 and 9 h (Rey et al. 1979), 6 to 24 h (Morselli 1975) and 5 to 35 h (Cotter et al. 1977). Gerardin et al. (1976) found that the higher the carbamazepine dose used, the more delayed the time to achieve maximum plasma concentration became.

Distribution

Close to 75 % of the carbamazepine in plasma is bound to proteins (albumin and α_1-acid glycoprotein). Some 48–53 % (Morselli 1975) or 63±9 % (Elyas et al. 1986) of the drug's biologically active metabolite carbamazepine-10,11-epoxide is bound to plasma proteins.

Values for the volume of distribution of carbamazepine, assuming complete oral bioavailability of the drug, have ranged between 1.43±0.37 L per kilogram (Westenberg et al. 1978) and 0.74 L per kilogram (Bertilsson and Tomson 1986), the average probably being a little over 1.0 L per kilogram. Such values would be consistent with the drug being distributed fairly uniformly throughout body water, though perhaps achieving some selective storage in some body site or sites. The apparent volume of distribution of the epoxide metabolite is 0.74 L per kilogram (Bertilsson and Tomson 1986).

The drug's concentration in red blood cells is only 38.3 ± 17.9 % of its simultaneous concentration in plasma (Hooper et al. 1975). The epoxide metabolite does not enter red blood cells.

Carbamazepine concentrations in cerebrospinal fluid average some 20–25 % of those in plasma. Therefore the CSF concentration of the drug should provide a valid measure of its simultaneous plasma water one. Similarly, the salivary concentrations of the drug reflect its plasma water ones. Salivary concentrations of carbamazepine-10,11-epoxide average 14–70 % of those in plasma (MacKichan et al. 1981).

Elimination

The elimination of carbamazepine seems to follow simple linear kinetics. After a first dose of the drug, mean values of the elimination half-life are around 36 h. There is no evidence of dose dependence in the half-life over the dosage range of 3–9 mg per kilogram (Levy et al. 1975).

Because of uncertainty regarding the completeness of absorption of some orally administered carbamazepine preparations, only apparent clearance values for the drug are available. These have been in the range 0.7–1.8 L per hour, with Westenberg et al. (1978) citing a several times higher figure of 0.076 ± 0.032 L per kilogram per hour, though this figure was obtained in patients chronically treated with the drug and was expressed on a body weight basis. The explanation for this latter apparently aberrant value probably lies in the fact that, with continued intake, carbamazepine over some days or weeks induces its own metabolism and thereby increases its own clearance value. This auto-induction process causes steady-state plasma carbamazepine levels to increase less with consecutive dosage increases than would have been expected from the drug's plasma concentration at earlier lower doses.

Excretion Unchanged

Only some 2 % of a carbamazepine dose is excreted in urine without being metabolised. To some extent depending on the properties of the solid dosage form studied, up to 10–15 % of the orally administered drug may be present in faeces. It therefore appears that majority of the bioavailable drug must be eliminated through metabolism.

Metabolism

Carbamazepine is biotransformed via several known pathways (Fig. 4.6). The most important one, at least from the clinical point of view, is an oxidation that yields the reasonably stable epoxide intermediate, carbamazepine-10,11-epoxide. This substance

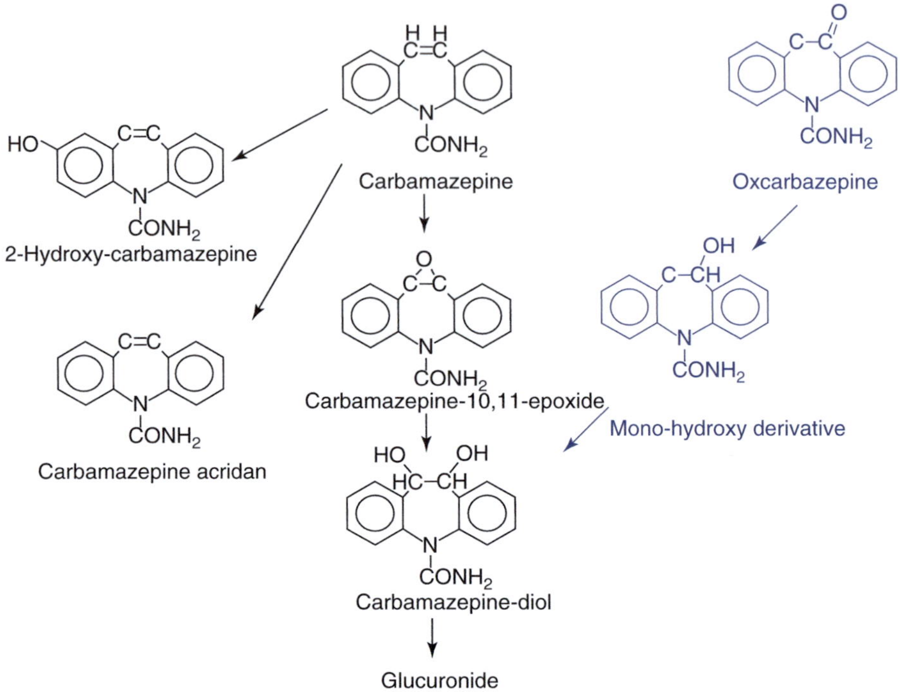

Fig. 4.6 Major known metabolic pathways for carbamazepine and for the structurally related antiepileptic drug oxcarbazepine

possesses activity against both epilepsy and trigeminal neuralgia (Morselli 1975). Its formation is catalysed by CYP3A4. Epoxide hydrolase activity then converts the epoxide to a dihydrodiol derivative which lacks pharmacological activity and is excreted in urine mainly as a glucuronide conjugate. Tomson et al. (1983) calculated that about 25 % of a carbamazepine dose is normally eliminated along this epoxide–diol pathway. Other carbamazepine metabolites include phenolic, catechol and O-methyl catechol derivatives that are produced by oxidations on one of the benzene rings of the molecule. These metabolites again appear in urine mainly as glucuronide conjugates.

Clinical Pharmacokinetics

As mentioned above, the epoxide metabolite of carbamazepine is biologically active. Therefore attempted correlations between plasma levels of the parent drug and measures of biological activity, in particular seizure control, should take into consideration the simultaneous concentrations of both drug and metabolite.

With regular oral carbamazepine intake, steady-state conditions would be expected to apply after some 7 or 8 days, if the elimination half-time for the parent molecule remained constant at its initial value of around 36 h. However, the drug's progressive auto-induction of its metabolism after any dosage change may shorten the time for steady-state conditions to apply. In practice, during continuous intake in monotherapy, the half-life of carbamazepine is likely to be around 15–20 h. Therefore there may be some inter-dosage fluctuation in plasma levels when the drug is taken twice daily. Using stable isotope-labelled drug during chronic therapy, Eichelbaum et al. (1982) calculated that the elimination half-life of the drug was 12.3 ± 0.8 h. Plasma carbamazepine–epoxide levels tend to parallel simultaneous plasma carbamazepine levels after an initial dose of the drug. This implies that the rate of decline in the concentrations of the metabolite is determined not by its elimination rate but by its formation rate. Plasma carbamazepine–epoxide levels relative to drug dose tend to be slightly higher in females than in males (McKauge et al. 1981).

There seems fairly general agreement that plasma carbamazepine levels of around 5 or 6–12 mg/L (Patsalos et al. 2008) are associated with the best chance of achieving control of epileptic seizures of the types likely to respond to the drug and also relief of trigeminal and other neuralgic pain syndromes, without unacceptable adverse effects being present. McKauge et al. (1981) attempted to measure simultaneous plasma concentrations of carbamazepine and its epoxide to see if the combined values yielded a better correlation with antiseizure effects than plasma concentrations of the parent drug did. No advantage accrued from the attempt.

An important issue clinically can arise if another drug, particularly the antiepileptic agent phenytoin, which induces CYP3A4 activity, is administered simultaneously with carbamazepine. The rate of elimination of carbamazepine is thus enhanced, and more carbamazepine is converted to its epoxide metabolite. As a result, steady-state plasma carbamazepine levels fall, but higher concentrations of the epoxide are present in plasma. In this situation some patients will not tolerate plasma carbamazepine levels of 8 mg/L or higher, and the clinician may need to work to a lower carbamazepine therapeutic range than the conventional 5 or 6–12 mg/L one. Also, after each dose, peak plasma carbamazepine levels will occur sooner than if the drug was used in the absence of a CYP3A4-inducing agent. Adding phenytoin to twice-daily carbamazepine therapy may lead to patients experiencing temporary carbamazepine toxicity 1–2 h after oral intake. Subdividing the carbamazepine dose so that the drug is taken three or four times a day will nearly always resolve this problem without needing to alter the total daily drug dose.

The correlation between steady-state plasma carbamazepine concentrations and drug dose in the treated population is relatively poor, partly because of the possible variables that may be involved in the situation, viz. the auto-induction and possible hetero-induction of drug-metabolising capacity, as well as the borderline oral bioavailability of some marketed carbamazepine preparations.

Interactions

Carbamazepine has been reported on several occasions to reduce circulating levels of both total and free thyroxine (e.g. Bensten et al. 1983). Serum immunoglobulin levels apart from that of IgG may be altered (Gilhus et al. 1982). The effects of carbamazepine administration on plasma phenytoin levels are inconsistent, in some individuals increasing, in some lowering and in others being associated with little or no changes in the levels. Carbamazepine appears to enhance the conversion of primidone to phenobarbitone (Battino et al. 1983) and increases the clearance of valproate, resulting in lowered circulating concentrations of the latter (Panesar et al. 1986). The drug increases the clearance of warfarin and may thus compromise the latter's anticoagulant effects.

Valproate, but not other antiepileptic drugs in common use, may displace carbamazepine from its plasma protein-binding sites (Mattson et al. 1982). The frequently encountered interaction between phenytoin and carbamazepine has been discussed above in the Clinical Pharmacokinetics section because of its importance in relation to interpreting plasma carbamazepine concentrations. Phenobarbitone administration also causes lowered plasma carbamazepine concentrations relative to drug dose, with a rise in plasma carbamazepine–epoxide levels. Valproate, too, may alter the relationship between circulating concentrations of carbamazepine and its epoxide.

Drugs apart from antiepileptic agents, e.g. propoxyphene, verapamil, diltiazem, isoniazid, nicotinamide, danazol and erythromycin, may interact with carbamazepine to raise its plasma levels. Many of these substances are inhibitors of CYP3A4.

Adverse Effects

Given in high enough dosages, or introduced so rapidly into treatment that there is not time for the effects of auto-induction to develop, carbamazepine can produce appreciable sedation with drowsiness and intellectual dulling, and sometimes irritability, aggressiveness and confusion, and also impaired psychomotor performance. In overdosage, nystagmus and ataxia of gait develop, with a sense of disequilibrium. At more substantial overdosage, double vision and drowsiness are present. Various forms of dyskinesia and dystonia have rarely been reported.

In the first week or two of exposure to carbamazepine, a skin rash may appear, most often an erythematosus macular one. If this happens, it is advisable to abandon the drug to avoid the development of more major hypersensitivity reactions such as hepatitis. There is a known association of pharmacogenomics importance between serious carbamazepine cutaneous hypersensitivity reactions and carriage of the HLA-B*15:02 and HLA-A*31:01 genes, both of which are common in Southeast Asian populations (Amstutz et al. 2014). In long-term carbamazepine use, delayed chronic skin lesions very occasionally develop.

Carbamazepine produces increased plasma antidiuretic activity, apparently by an effect at hypothalamic osmoreceptors. This action can be of therapeutic use in managing diabetes insipidus. It may also occasionally be responsible for symptomatic hyponatraemia, and this may activate epileptogenic foci to cause a recurrence of seizure activity. If this happens, additional carbamazepine may be prescribed if the culprit mechanism is not recognised.

When carbamazepine first came into use, there was concern that it might cause significant agranulocytosis and perhaps aplastic anaemia. The basis of these concerns was never clear; the fears were never realised and are now largely forgotten. The drug may cause bradycardia and a reversible hepatitis and can precipitate episodes of acute intermittent porphyria.

Teratogenesis

Carbamazepine-related teratogenesis is considered in Chap. 9.

Pregnancy

The Mother

It seems to be fairly widely accepted in the literature that plasma carbamazepine concentrations fall relative to drug dose as pregnancy progresses, e.g. Dam et al. (1979), and that the drug's apparent clearance is increased (Lander and Eadie 1991). However, the situation may not be quite that simple. Battino et al. (1985) commented that plasma carbamazepine levels were fairly stable throughout pregnancy and that the clearance of the drug between weeks 4 and 24 of pregnancy was higher than that between weeks 25 and 32. Yerby et al. (1985) noted that the intrinsic clearance of carbamazepine, i.e. the clearance of the protein-unbound fraction of the drug in plasma, remained fairly stable throughout pregnancy. The plasma protein binding of both carbamazepine and its 10,11-epoxide metabolite is slightly decreased in pregnancy, particularly in late pregnancy, compared with postnatally (Yerby et al. 1985).

Bernus et al. (1995) compared carbamazepine apparent clearances in ten women, when pregnant and when not pregnant. Four of the women were taking another potentially enzyme-inducing antiepileptic drug; the remaining six took carbamazepine in antiepileptic drug monotherapy. In the women receiving carbamazepine only, the mean clearance during pregnancy was 127.1 ± 35.9 L per day [5.30 L/h] and after pregnancy 116.9 ± 39.7 L per day [4.87 L/h], a slightly higher value in pregnancy that was not statistically significant. However, for the four women taking a potentially enzyme-inducing second antiepileptic drug, the corresponding values were 216.9 ± 58.1 L per day [9.04 L/h] and 154.3 ± 46.2 L per day [6.43 L/h], a difference of greater magnitude that was statistically significant. Possibly the various hormonally driven changes that accompany pregnancy add relatively little further induction to any already existing auto-induction of carbamazepine metabolism, but if a second drug with enzyme-inducing capabilities is present, there is a greater capacity for pregnancy to induce cytochrome P450 activity.

In the same group of women, Bernus et al. (1995) compared the actual clearances of carbamazepine to urinary excretion products along a number of metabolic pathways during pregnancy and in the non-pregnant state. In those receiving carbamazepine monotherapy, there was a considerable increase during pregnancy in carbamazepine-10,11-epoxide excretion and a decrease, though a relatively small one, in metabolism along the 2-hydroxy carbamazepine pathway. Otherwise there were no statistically significant changes. In the women also taking potentially inducing agents, there again was the increase along the urinary carbamazepine-10,11-epoxide excretion pathway but also a substantial increase in excretion along the carbamazepine–diol and the 2-hydroxy carbamazepine pathways, with a borderline increase in excretion of urinary carbamazepine–acridan. It therefore appears that, depending on the actions of various drug-metabolising enzyme-inducing agents which may or may not be co-administered during pregnancy, different carbamazepine metabolic pathways may be activated in pregnancy.

The Foetus

Little information is available regarding carbamazepine disposition in the foetus.

Breast Milk

Pynnonen and Sillanpaa (1975) reported that carbamazepine concentrations in human breast milk were some 60 % of maternal plasma ones and that carbamazepine–epoxide concentrations were 93 % of those in maternal plasma. However, Kaneko et al. (1979) found that the carbamazepine concentrations in breast milk averaged about 40 % of those present in maternal plasma. Davanzo et al. (2013) stated that milk carbamazepine concentrations were 69 % of those in maternal plasma.

The Neonate

The plasma protein binding of both carbamazepine and carbamazepine-10,11-epoxide is lower in the neonate than in the adult, having values of, respectively, 29.8–30.6 % and 47.5–52 % in the very young (Groce et al. 1985). Yerby et al. (1985) found that, at birth, maternal concentrations of carbamazepine and its epoxide were, respectively, 40 % and 48 % higher than those in the neonate.

Valproate

Valproate's antiepileptic properties were discovered accidentally in 1961 while it was being used as a solvent in the testing of other substances for their antiepileptic effects. The drug has been very extensively used in the treatment of epilepsy and in more recent times increasingly employed in psychiatry and for purposes such as migraine prophylaxis.

Chemistry

Valproic acid (pKa 4.95) is the trivial name for *n*-propyl pentanoic acid, sometimes called di-*n*-propyl acetic acid. It is often marketed as the sodium salt (MW 166.198), a hygroscopic white powder that is often provided in coated preparations to avoid uptake of atmospheric moisture if it is not stored in a sealed container. In some countries the drug is also available as the coordination complex sodium hydrogen valproate or in the form of the prodrug valproamide. After absorption from the alimentary tract, regardless of the chemical nature of the preparation used, the active ingredient is absorbed and exists in the body as the valproate ion.

As well as oral administration in solid or liquid dosage forms, the drug may be given rectally or by intravenous infusion. The solid dosage form is usually available in 100, 200 and 500 mg units.

Pharmacodynamics

Valproate has several known biochemical mechanisms of action that would be expected to contribute to its antiepileptic effects. Firstly, it blocks voltage-dependent cell membrane Na^+ ion channels, a mechanism of action which it shares with phenytoin, carbamazepine and lamotrigine. Secondly, at clinically relevant concentrations, the drug raises brain concentrations of the inhibitory neurotransmitter γ-aminobutyrate, mainly by inhibiting the enzyme succinate-semialdehyde dehydrogenase. The drug also reduces brain levels of the excitatory amino acid neurotransmitter aspartate.

This broader range of potential antiepileptic mechanism of action than those of the drugs previously discussed in this chapter probably correlates with the fact that valproate is effective against a wider range of epileptic seizure types than the antiepileptic drugs hitherto considered. Its spectrum of antiepileptic activity covers virtually all of the common types of human epileptic seizure disorder, including absences.

Pharmacokinetics

Absorption

Orally administered valproate appears to be both completely and rapidly absorbed from the alimentary tract. For practical purposes the drug's oral bioavailability is 100 %. Peak plasma valproate levels are likely to occur within 1–3 h of oral intake unless the drug is given in enteric-coated preparations which are designed to delay its release and thus prolong the presence of effective drug concentration in the body. If the drug is taken by mouth as the amide or the semi-sodium salt, the active ingredient seems to be released prior to absorption from the intestinal tract.

Absorption of the drug after rectal administration is reasonably efficient.

Distribution

Calculated values for the apparent volume of distribution of valproate have generally been in the range 0.15–0.20 L per kilogram, suggesting that the drug's distribution is largely restricted to extracellular water. Estimates of the parameter in young children yield somewhat higher values, raising the possibility that in this age group the drug enters intracellular water.

Like other fatty acids, valproate binds to plasma proteins and may compete with fatty acids for plasma protein-binding sites. The extent of the drug's protein binding varies with the valproate concentration. At concentrations in the range 50–100 mg/L, levels commonly encountered in human therapeutics, about 90 % of the drug is normally protein bound. The binding fraction begins to diminish once the valproate concentration exceeds 80 mg/L and can be as low as 70 % at valproate concentrations of 150 mg/L (Cramer et al. 1986). Less valproate appears to be bound to plasma protein in the elderly. The binding also decreases in the latter half of pregnancy.

Valproate concentrations in cerebrospinal fluid are generally similar to those in plasma water. Monaco et al. (1982) quoted a mean value of 11 % for the parameter. However concentrations of valproate in saliva appear to bear little relationship to simultaneous concentrations of the drug in either plasma water or whole plasma.

Elimination

Valproate has linear elimination kinetics, with an elimination half-life in the range of 8–15 h. The half-life tends to be shorter when enzyme-inducing antiepileptic drugs are present simultaneously.

The drug's clearance values are higher in children than in adults and also tend to be higher if other enzyme-inducing antiepileptic drugs are being taken. During chronic therapy, the mean valproate clearance value is 0.018 L per kilogram per hour.

Excretion Unchanged

Very little valproate is excreted unchanged in urine. Some investigators have not detected measurable amounts. Knowing the complete oral bioavailability of the drug, the almost negligible appearance in urine of the intact molecule indicates that the drug undergoes extensive biotransformation.

Metabolism

A considerable amount of investigation has been carried out into valproate biotransformation. The two main pathways involved are: (1) fatty acid β-oxidation and (2) direct conjugation of valproate with glucuronic acid, forming an ester glucuronide. However there are a number of quantitatively less significant pathways, as illustrated in Fig. 4.7. The valproate molecule itself may bind to carnitine, and it may be dehydrogenated at its δ, ω, ω-1 and γ-carbon atoms to yield a considerable array of derivatives which then undergo further metabolism. The niceties of this chemistry are unlikely to be important to the contemporary clinician.

At lower valproate doses, the main metabolic pathway of the drug is fatty acid β-oxidation which forms, consecutively, [E]-2-en-valproate (which seems to possess some biological activity), 3-hydroxy-valproate and finally 3-oxo-valproate, which enters the Krebs tricarboxylic acid cycle. At higher valproate doses, the drug load seems to outstrip the capacity of the β-oxidation pathway. The predominant biotransformation mechanism then increasingly becomes direct conjugation of valproate with glucuronic acid.

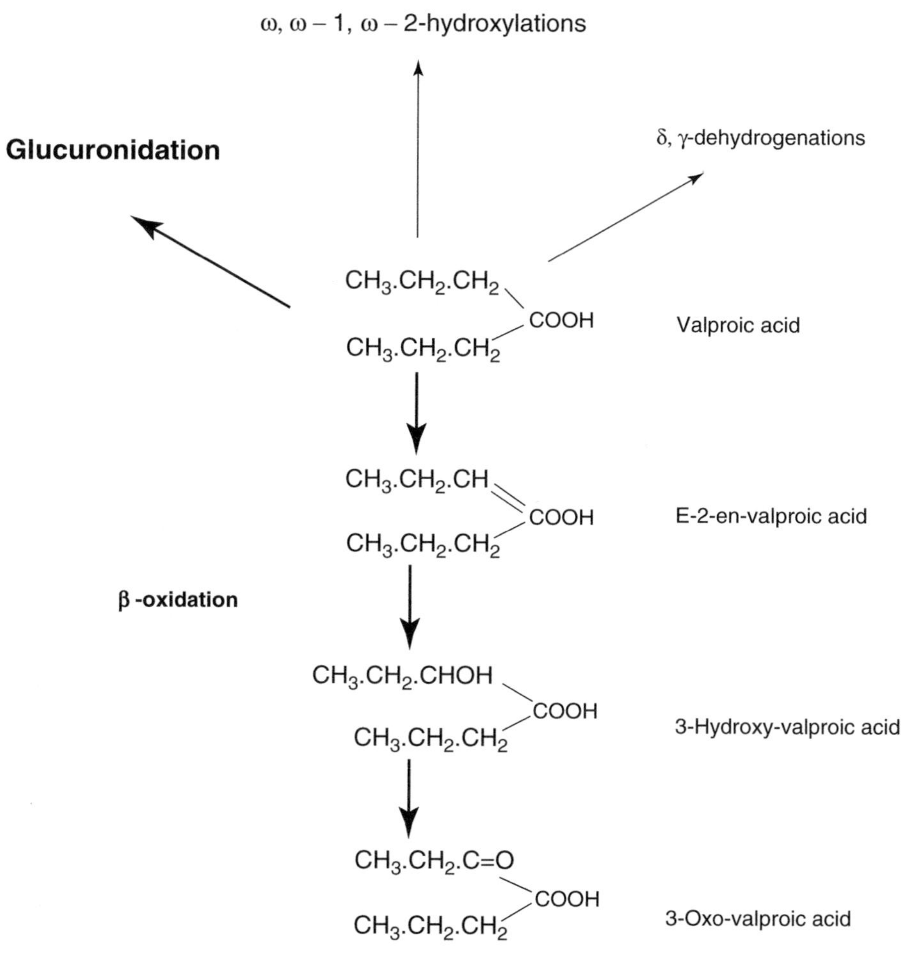

Fig. 4.7 Pathways of valproate biotransformation, showing molecular structures of its β-oxidation products. *Thick arrows* and *bold* type indicate the quantitatively major pathways of metabolism

Clinical Pharmacokinetics

Depending on whether or not modified release formulations of valproate are used, peak plasma levels of the drug may be expected anywhere from 2 to 5 h after drug intake. Steady-state conditions apply some 3 days after a dosage change. The therapeutic range of plasma concentration of the drug is often said to be 50–100 mg/L (Patsalos et al. 2008), but it is difficult to trace adequate quality studies on which this recommendation has been based. Because the drug is effective for different forms of epilepsy, it is possible that there may be different lower limits to the therapeutic ranges for different types of seizure disorder. A similar consideration may apply to the threshold concentration that provides benefit in treating other indications, e.g. the prevention of migraine. The upper limit of the therapeutic range for the drug tends to be determined by the development of adverse effects, commonly a noticeable ataxic tremor involving the upper limbs.

Interactions

Valproate may displace drugs such as phenytoin, carbamazepine, phenobarbitone and diazepam from their plasma protein-binding sites. The displacement of phenytoin might be expected to increase its clearance and therefore decreases its plasma concentrations. In practice, raised plasma phenytoin levels have sometimes been reported due to the interaction. If valproate is co-administered with phenobarbitone or a drug that is converted to phenobarbitone in the body, there can be a substantial rise in plasma phenobarbitone concentrations. This occurs because valproate inhibits the *N*-glucosidation pathway that accounts for the clearance of some 25 % of a phenobarbitone dose (Bernus et al. 1994). Valproate enhances the metabolism of carbamazepine along its epoxidation pathway (Pisani et al. 1986) and decreases the clearances of ethosuximide and diazepam. Crawford et al. (1986) found that valproate did not alter the plasma levels of ethinyl oestradiol and levonorgestrol, components of several oral contraceptive preparations.

Plasma valproate concentrations are reduced by concurrent phenytoin or phenobarbitone intake or by the presence of carbamazepine, which increases the valproate clearance. Plasma valproate levels are also decreased by oral contraceptive intake (Herzog et al. 2009).

Adverse Effects

Relative to the extent of its use, valproate has been responsible for rather few serious adverse effects. The drug tends to be less sedating than many other antiepileptic drugs, though it is not without sedative effects, particularly at high dosages. Occasionally it can cause disturbed behaviour in young people and also confusion, aggressiveness and sometimes stupor. It tends to make essential tremor more severe and can bring a previously latent essential tremor to clinical notice.

Occasional patients taking valproate complain of some thinning of scalp hair. Weight gain occurs with some frequency in those taking the drug. There may sometimes be a fall in circulating platelet numbers though this rarely has clinical consequences. As mentioned in Chap. 2, valproate has acquired a reputation for being associated with the presence of the polycystic ovary syndrome (e.g. Crawford 2009). However, Bauer et al. (2000) found that, at least in women with focal epilepsies, the incidence of the syndrome in women taking valproate was similar to that in association with carbamazepine exposure and also that present in untreated women.

Liver function tests may be altered by valproate intake. Usually this is of no clinical consequence if the alterations are of small magnitude. However, mainly in children, there have been instances of an unusual form of liver failure associated with valproate intake. This may not occur immediately after use of the drug commences and can be delayed for months, even years, during which the patient appears quite well. Pathologically, the affected liver may show either diffuse microvesicular steatosis like that of Reye's syndrome, or actual liver cell destruction with inflammatory cell infiltration of the liver stroma and portal tracts, and bilirubin retention. In recent times, reports of this condition seem to have become substantially less frequent. Its exact pathogenesis remains uncertain. There have been suggestions that the liver injury is a toxic reaction to high concentrations of the unsaturated valproate metabolite 4-en-valproate or that it is a consequence of a limited capacity of the drug's β-oxidation processes leading to diversion of the drug's metabolism towards γ-dehydrogenation. Even less commonly, acute pancreatitis may occur in association with valproate intake.

There have been reports of low fibrinogen levels in women taking valproate, and there has been a description of a newborn infant who died of uncontrollable bleeding (Majer and Green 1987).

Teratogenicity

This topic is discussed in Chaps. 8 and 9.

Pregnancy

The Mother

Philbert et al. (1985) noted a fall in plasma valproate concentrations relative to drug dose in late pregnancy, but there is a general impression that the whole plasma levels of the drug, when it is used in monotherapy, do not vary greatly over the course of pregnancy.

The Foetus

Valproate crosses the placenta (Dickinson et al. 1979), probably by a process of passive diffusion along concentration gradients (Bailey and Briggs 2005). Fowler et al. (1989) found no evidence that the drug was metabolised in ex vivo perfused human placental lobules. Omtzigt et al. (1992) measured the concentration of valproate and some of its metabolites in amniotic fluid and noted that their concentrations in that fluid were proportionate to their concentrations in maternal plasma.

Breast Milk

Philbert et al. (1985) stated that the valproate concentration in human milk was some 5–10 % of the concentration in maternal plasma. Kaneko et al. (1984) cited a similar value, but Davanzo et al. (2013) quoted a figure of 42 % for the parameter.

The Neonate

Nau et al. (1984) found that the ratio of umbilical cord venous to maternal plasma valproate concentrations was 1.7 ± 0.5 for whole plasma and 0.47 ± 0.24 for the protein-unbound drug. Philbert et al. (1985) stated that, at term, umbilical cord vein valproate levels were 145–219 % of simultaneous maternal venous plasma levels of the drug.

References

Amstutz U, Shear NH, Rieder MJ et al (2014) Recommendations for HLA-B*15:02 and HLA-A*31:01 genetic testing to reduce the risk of carbamazepine-induced hypersensitivity reactions. Epilepsia 55:496–506

Ayra R, Gulati S (2012) Phenytoin-induced gingival overgrowth. Acta Neurol Scand 125:149–155

Bailey DN, Briggs R (2005) Valproic acid binding to human serum and human placenta. Ther Drug Monit 27:375–377

Bardy AH, Teramo K, Hiilesmaa VK (1982) Apparent clearances of phenytoin phenobarbitone, primidone and carbamazepine during pregnancy: results of the prospective Helsinski study. In: Janz D, Bossi L, Helge H, Richens A, Schmidt D (eds) Epilepsy, pregnancy, and the child. Raven, New York, pp 141–145

Bar-Oz B, Nulman I, Koren G, Ito S (2000) Anticonvulsants and breast feeding. Paediatr Drugs 2:113–126

Battino D, Avanzini G, Bossi L, Croci D, Cusi C, Gomeni C, Moise A (1983) Plasma levels of primidone and its metabolite phenobarbital: effects of age and associated therapy. Ther Drug Monit 5:73–79

Battino D, Binelli S, Bossi L, Como ML, Croci D, Cusi C, Avanzini G (1984) Changes in primidone/phenobarbitone ratio during pregnancy and the puerperium. Clin Pharmacokinet 9:252–260

Battino D, Binelli S, Bossi L et al (1985) Plasma concentrations of carbamazepine and carbamazepine-10,11-epoxide during pregnancy and after delivery. Clin Pharmacokinet 10:279–284

Bauer LA, Blouin RA (1983) Phenytoin Michaelis-Menten pharmacokinetics in Caucasian pediatric patients. Clin Pharmacokinet 8:545–549

Bauer J, Jarre A, Klingmuller D, Eiger CE (2000) Polycystic ovary syndrome in patients with focal epilepsy: a study of 93 women. Epilepsy Res 41:163–167

Baylis EM, Crowley JM, Preece JM, Sylvester PE, Marks V (1971) Influence of folic acid on blood phenytoin levels. Br Med J 1:62–64

Bensten KD, Gram L, Veje A (1983) Serum thyroid hormones and blood folic acid during monotherapy with carbamazepine or valproate. Acta Neurol Scand 67:235–241

Berg MJ, Gross RA, Tomaszewski KJ, Zingaro WM, Haskins LS (2008) Generic substitution in the treatment of epilepsy: case evidence of breakthrough seizures. Neurology 71:525–530

Bernus I, Dickinson RG, Hooper WD, Eadie MJ (1994) Inhibition of phenobarbitone-N-glucosidation by valproate. Br J Clin Pharmacol 38:411–416

Bernus I, Hooper WD, Dickinson RG, Eadie MJ (1995) Metabolism of carbamazepine and co-administered anticonvulsants during pregnancy. Epilepsy Res 21:65–75

Bernus I, Hooper WD, Dickinson RG, Eadie MJ (1997) Effects of pregnancy on various pathways of human antiepileptic drug metabolism. Clin Neuropharmacol 20:13–21

Bertilsson L, Tomson T (1986) Clinical pharmacokinetics and pharmacological effects of carbamazepine and carbamazepine-10,11-epoxide: an update. Clin Pharmacokinet 11:177–198

Boreus LO, Jalling B, Kallberg N (1975) Clinical pharmacology of phenobarbital in the neonatal period. In: Garrattini S, Sereni F, Morselli PL (eds) Basic and therapeutic aspects of perinatal pharmacology. Raven Press, New York, pp 331–340

Bossi L (1982) Neonatal period including drug disposition in newborns: review of the literature. In: Janz D, Bossi L, Dam M, Helge H, Richens A, Schmidt D (eds) Epilepsy, pregnancy, and the child. Raven, New York, pp 327–341

Bruni J, Wilder BJ, Perschalski RJ, Hammond EJ, Villareal HJ (1980) Valproic acid and plasma levels of phenobarbital. Neurology 30:94–97

Chanarin I, Mollin DL, Anderson BB (1958) Folic acid and megaloblastic anaemia. Proc R Soc Med 51:757

Conney AH (1967) Pharmacological implications of microsomal enzyme induction. Pharmacol Rev 19:317–366

Coradello H (1973) Ueber die Ausscheidung von Antiepileptika in die Muttermilch. Wein Klin Wochenschr 85:695–697

Cotter LM, Eadie MJ, Hooper WD, Lander CM, Smith MT, Tyrer JH (1977) The pharmacokinetics of carbamazepine. Eur J Clin Pharmacol 12:451–456

Cramer JA, Mattson RH, Bennett DM, Swick CT (1986) Variable free and total valproic acid concentration in sole- and multi-drug therapy. Ther Drug Monit 8:411–415

Crawford P (2009) Managing epilepsy in women of childbearing age. Drug Saf 32:293–307

Crawford P, Chadwick D, Cleland P, Tjia J, Cowrie A, Back DJ, Orme M (1986) The lack of effect of sodium valproate on the pharmacokinetics of oral contraceptive steroids. Contraception 33:23–29

Critchley EMR, Vakil SD, Hayward HW, Owen VMH (1976) Dupuytren's contracture in epilepsy: result of prolonged administration of anticonvulsants. J Neurol Neurosurg Psychiatry 39:498–503

Dam M, Mygind KI, Christiansen J (1976) Antiepileptic drugs: plasma clearance during pregnancy. In: Janz D (ed) Epileptology. Thieme, Stuttgart, pp 179–183

Dam M, Christiansen J, Munck O, Mygind KI (1979) Antiepileptic drugs: metabolism in pregnancy. Clin Pharmacokinet 4:53–62

Dam M, Christiansen J, Kristensen CB, Helles A, Jaegerskou A, Schmiegelow M (1981) Carbamazepine: a clinical biopharmaceutical study. Eur J Clin Pharmacol 20:59–64

Davanzo R, Bo SD, Bua J, Copertino M, Zanelli E (2013) Antiepileptic drugs and breastfeeding. Ital J Pediatr 39:50

Davis RE, Woodliff HJ (1971) Folic acid deficiency in patients receiving anticonvulsant drugs. Med J Aust 2:1070–1072

De Carolis MP, Romagnoli C, Fressa S et al (1992) Placental transfer of phenobarbital: what is new? Dev Pharmacol Ther 19:19–26

Dean M, Stock B, Patterson RJ, Levy R (1980) Serum protein binding and after pregnancy in humans. Clin Pharmacol Ther 28:253–261

DeLeacy EA, McLeay CD, Eadie MJ, Tyrer JH (1979) Effect of subjects' sex and intake of tobacco, alcohol and oral contraceptives on plasma phenytoin levels. Br J Clin Pharmacol 8:33–36

Dickinson RG, Harland RC, Lynn RK, Smith WB, Gerber N (1979) Transmission of valproic acid (Depakene) across the placenta: half-life of the drug in mother and baby. J Pediatr 94:832–835

Dickinson RG, Hooper WD, Wood B, Lander CM, Eadie MJ (1989) The effect of pregnancy in humans on the pharmacokinetics of stable isotope labelled phenytoin. Br J Clin Pharmacol 28:17–27

Eadie MJ, Tyrer JH, Hooper WD (1973) Diphenylhydantoin dosage. Proc Aust Assoc Neurol 10:53–59

Eadie MJ, Lander CM, Hooper WD, Tyrer JH (1976) The effect of phenobarbitone dose on plasma phenobarbitone levels in epileptic patients. Proc Aust Assoc Neurol 13:89–96

Eadie MJ, Lander CM, Hooper WD, Tyrer JH (1977) Factors influencing plasma phenobarbitone levels in epileptic patients. Br J Clin Pharmacol 4:541–547

Eadie MJ, McKinnon GE, Dickinson RG, Hooper WD (1992) Phenytoin metabolism during pregnancy. Eur J Clin Pharmacol 43:389–392

Eichelbaum M, Kothe KW, Hoffman F, Von Uruth GE (1982) Use of stable labelled carbamazepine to study its kinetics during chronic carbamazepine treatment. Eur J Clin Pharmacol 23:241–244

Elyas AA, Patsalos PN, Agbato OA, Brett EM, Lascelles PT (1986) Factors influencing simultaneous concentrations of total and free carbamazepine and carbamazepine-10,11-epoxide in serum of children with epilepsy. Ther Drug Monit 8:288–292

Engel JJ, Pedley T (2008) Epilepsy. A comprehensive textbook, vol 2. Wolters Kluwer, Lippincott Williams and Wilkins, Philadelphia

Fischer JH, Lockman LA, Zaske D, Kriel R (1981) Phenobarbital maintenance dose requirements in treating neonatal seizures. Neurology 31:1042–1044

Fischer JH, Patel TV, Fischer PA (2003) Fosphenytoin: clinical pharmacokinetics and comparative advantage in the acute treatment of seizures. Clin Pharmacokinet 42:33–58

Fowler DW, Eadie MJ, Dickinson R (1989) Transplacental transfer and biotransformation studies of valproic acid and its glucuronide(s) in the perfused human placenta. J Pharmacol Exp Ther 249:318–323

French JA (2013) P-glycoprotein expression and antiepileptic drug resistance. Lancet Neurol 12:732–733

Garrettson LK, Dayton PG (1970) Disappearance of phenobarbital and diphenylhydantoin from serum of children. Clin Pharmacol Ther 11:674–679

Gerardin AP, Abadie FV, Campestrini JA (1976) Pharmacokinetics of carbamazepine in normal humans after single and repeated oral doses. J Pharmacokinet Biopharm 4:521–535

Gilhus NE, Strandjord RE, Aarli JA (1982) The effect of carbamazepine on serum immunoglobulin concentrations. Acta Neurol Scand 66:172–179

Gillette JR (1963) Metabolism of drugs and other foreign compounds by enzymatic mechanisms. Prog Drug Res 6:11–73

Groce JB III, Casto DT, Gal P (1985) Carbamazepine and carbamazepine-epoxide serum protein binding in newborn infants. Ther Drug Monit 7:274–276

Guelen PJM, van der Kleijn E, Woudstra U (1975) Statistical analysis of pharmacokinetic parameters in epileptic patients chronically treated with antiepileptic drugs. In: Janz D, Gardner-Thorpe C, Meinardi H, Sherwin AL, Schneider H (eds) Clinical pharmacology of antiepileptic drugs. Springer, Berlin, pp 2–10

Herzog AG, Blum AS, Farina EL et al (2009) Valproate and lamotrigine level variation with menstrual cycle phase and oral contraceptive use. Neurology 72:911–914

Hooper WD, Du Betz DK, Bochner F, Cotter LM, Smith GA, Eadie MJ, Tyrer JH (1975) Plasma protein binding of carbamazepine. Clin Pharmacol Ther 17:433–440

Hosokawa K, Takahashi S, Yamamoto M (1984) Plasma concentrations in pregnancy. In: Shinagawa S, Sato T (eds) Antiepileptic drugs and pregnancy. Excerpta Medica, Amsterdam, pp 3–11

Ieiri I, Goto W, Hirata K et al (1995) The effect of 5-(p-hydroxyphenyl)-5-phenylhydantoin (p-HPPH) enantiomers, major metabolites of phenytoin on the occurrence of chronic-gingival hyperplasia: in vivo and in vitro study. Eur J Clin Pharmacol 49:51–56

Ishizaki T, Yokochi K, Chiba K, Tabuchi T, Wagatsuma T (1981) Placental transfer of anticonvulsants (phenobarbital, phenytoin valproic acid) and the elimination from neonates. Pediatr Pharmacol 1:291–303

Julien RM, Hollister RP (1975) Carbamazepine: mechanism of action. Adv Neurol 11:263–276

Kaaja E, Kaaja R, Matila R, Hiilesmaa V (2002) Enzyme-inducing antiepileptic drugs in pregnancy and the risk of bleeding in the neonate. Neurology 58:549–553

Kamali F, Thomas SH (1994) Effect of flow rate on saliva phenytoin concentrations: implications for therapeutic monitoring. Eur J Clin Pharmacol 46:565–567

Kan R, Masubuchi Y, Nikaido T, Yoshijima T, Ono T, Takahashi Y, Kumashiro H (1984) Antiepileptic drug trends during pregnancy. In: Shinagawa S, Sato T (eds) Antiepileptic drugs during pregnancy. Excerpta Medica, Amsterdam, pp 12–19

Kaneko S, Sato T, Suzuki K (1979) The levels of anticonvulsants in breast milk. Br J Clin Pharmacol 7:624–627

Kaneko S, Suzuki K, Sato T, Ogawa Y, Nomura Y (1982) The problem of antiepileptic medication in the neonatal period: is breast feeding advisable? In: Janz D, Bossi L, Dam M, Helge H, Richens A, Schmidt D (eds) Epilepsy, pregnancy, and the child. Raven, New York, pp 343–348

Kaneko S, Fukushima Y, Sato T, Ogawa Y, Nomura Y, Shinagawa S (1984) Breast feeding in epileptic mothers. In: Shinagawa S, Sato T (eds) Antiepileptic drugs and pregnancy. Excerpta Medica, Amsterdam, pp 38–45

Kapetanovic IM, Kupferberg HJ, Porter RJ, Theodore W, Schullmann E, Penry JK (1981) Mechanism of valproate-phenobarbital interaction in epileptic patients. Clin Pharmacol Ther 29:480–486

Karoly R, Lenkey N, Juhasz AO, Vizi ES, Mike A (2010) Fast- or slow-inactivated state preference of Na^+ channel inhibitors: a simulation and experimental study. PLoS Comp Biol 17:6. e1000818

Kesavan R, Narayan SK, Anithan C (2010) Influence of CYP2C9 and CYP2C19 genetic polymorphisms on phenytoin-induced neurological toxicity in Indian epileptic patients. Eur J Clin Pharmacol 66:689–696

Kluck RM, Cannell GR, Hooper WD, Eadie MJ, Dickinson R (1988) Disposition of phenytoin and phenobarbitone in the isolated perfused human placenta. Clin Exp Pharmacol Physiol 15:827–836

Kuo CC (1998) A common anticonvulsant binding site for phenytoin carbamazepine and lamotrigine in neuronal Na channels. Mol Pharmacol 54:712–721

Kutt H, Winters W, Kokenge R, McDowell F (1964) Diphenylhydantoin metabolism, blood levels, and toxicity. Arch Neurol 11:642–648

Lambie DG, Nanda RN, Johnson RH, Shakir RA (1976) Therapeutic and pharmacokinetic effects of increasing phenytoin in chronic epileptics on multiple drug therapy. Lancet 7:486–489

Lander CM, Eadie MJ (1991) Plasma concentrations of antiepileptic drugs during pregnancy. Epilepsia 32:257–264

Lander CM, Edwards VE, Eadie MJ, Tyrer JH (1977) Plasma anticonvulsant concentrations during pregnancy. Neurology 27:128–131

Lander CM, Smith MT, Chalk JB, DeWytt C, Symoniw P, Livingstone I, Eadie MJ (1984) Bioavailability and pharmacokinetics of phenytoin during pregnancy. Eur J Clin Pharmacol 27:105–110

Lecamwasam DS, Franklin C, Turner P (1975) Effect of phenobarbitone on hepatic drug metabolising enzymes and urinary D-glucaric acid excretion in man. Br J Clin Pharmacol 2:257–262

Levy RH, Pitlick WH, Troupin AS, Green JR, Neal JM (1975) Pharmacokinetics of carbamazepine in normal man. Clin Pharmacol Ther 17:657–668

Levy R, Mattson R, Meldrum BS, Perucca E (2002) Antiepileptic drugs, 5th edn. Lippincott Williams & Wilkins, Philadelphia

Lipkin GM, Fozzard HA (2010) Molecular model of anticonvulsant drug binding to the voltage-gated sodium channel inner pore. Mol Pharmacol 78:631–638

Loiseau P, Brachet Liermain A, Legroux M, Jogeix M (1977) Interet du dosage des anticonsulsivants dans le traitment des epilepsies. Nouv Presse Med 16:813–817

Loscher W (2007) Drug transporters in the epileptic brain. Epilepsia 48(Suppl 1):8–13

MacKichan JJ, Duffner PK, Cohen ME (1981) Salivary concentrations and plasma protein binding of carbamazepine and carbamazepine-10,11-epoxide in epileptic patients. Br J Clin Pharmacol 12:31–37

Majer RV, Green PJ (1987) Neonatal afibrinogenaemia due to sodium valproate. Br Med J 2:740–741

Mantegazza M, Curia G, Biagini G, Ragsdale DS, Avoli M (2010) Voltage-gated sodium channels as therapeutic targets in epilepsy and other neurological disorders. Lancet Neurol 9:413–424

Marangos PJ, Patel J, Smith KD, Post RM (1987) Adenosine antagonist properties of carbamazepine. Epilepsia 28:387–394

Mattson RH, Gallagher BB, Reynolds EH, Glass D (1973) Folate therapy in epilepsy. A controlled study. Arch Neurol 29:78–81

Mattson GF, Mattson RH, Cramer JA (1982) Interaction between valproic acid and carbamazepine: an in vitro study of protein binding. Ther Drug Monit 4:181–184

McKauge L, Tyrer JH, Eadie MJ (1981) Factors influencing simultaneous concentrations of carbamazepine and its epoxide in plasma. Ther Drug Monit 3:63–70

Melchior JC, Svensmark O, Trolle D (1967) Placental transfer of phenobarbitone in epileptic women, and elimination in newborns. Lancet 2:860–861

Meraw SJ, Sheridan PL (1998) Medically induced gingival hyperplasia. Mayo Clin Proc 73:1196–1199

Mirkin BL (1971) Diphenylhydantoin: placental transport, fetal localization, neonatal metabolism and possible teratogenic effect. J Pediatr 78:329–337

Monaco F, Piredda S, Mutani R, Mastropaolo C, Tondi M (1982) The free fraction of valproic acid in tears, saliva, and cerebrospinal fluid. Epilepsia 23:23–26

Morselli PL (1975) Carbamazepine: absorption, distribution and excretion. Adv Neurol 11:279–293

Morselli PL, Rizzo M, Garattini S (1971) Interaction between phenobarbital and diphenylhydantoin in animals and in epileptic patients. Proc N Y Acad Sci 179:88–107

Mygind KI, Dam M, Christiansen J (1976) Phenytoin and phenobarbitone plasma clearance during pregnancy. Acta Neurol Scand 54:160–166

Nakajima M, Sakata N, Ohashi N, Kume T, Yokoi T (2002) Involvement of multiple UDP-glucuronosyltransferase 1A isoforms in glucuronidation of 5-(4′-hydroxyphenyl)-5-phenylhydantoin in human liver microsomes. Drug Metab Dispos 30:1250–1256

Nation RL, Evans AM, Milne RW (1990) Pharmacokinetic drug interactions with phenytoin. Clin Pharmacokinet 18(37–60):131–150

Nau H, Helge H, Luck W (1984) Valproic acid in the perinatal period: decreased maternal serum protein binding results in fetal accumulation and neonatal displacement of the drug and some metabolites. J Pediatr 104:627–634

Neuvonen P (1979) Bioavailability of phenytoin: clinical, pharmacokinetic and therapeutic implications. Clin Pharmacokinet 4:91–103

Neuvonen PJ (1985) Bioavailability and central side effects of different carbamazepine tablets. Int J Clin Pharmacol Ther Toxicol 23:226–232

O'Brien TJ, Cascino GD, So EL, Hanna DR (1998) Incidence and clinical consequences of the purple glove syndrome in patients receiving intravenous phenytoin. Neurology 51:1034–1039

Omtzigt JGC, Los FJ, Grobbee DE et al (1992) The risk of spina bifida aperta after first-trimester exposure to valproate in a prenatal cohort. Neurology 42(Suppl 5):119–125

Painter MJ, Pippenger C, Carter G, Pitlick W (1977) Metabolism of phenobarbital and phenytoin by neonates with seizures. Neurology 27:370

Panesar S, Orr J, Burton R, Farrell K (1986) Effect of carbamazepine on valproic acid metabolism. Epilepsia 27:591

Patsalos PN (2013) Drug interactions with the newer antiepileptic drugs (AEDs) -Part 1: pharmacokinetic and pharmacodynamic interactions between AEDs. Clin Pharmacokinet 52:927–966

Patsalos PN, Perucca E (2003a) Clinically important drug interactions in epilepsy: general features and interactions between antiepileptic drugs. Lancet Neurol 2:347–356

Patsalos PN, Perucca E (2003b) Clinically important drug interactions in epilepsy: interactions between antiepileptic drugs and other drugs. Lancet Neurol 2:473–481

Patsalos PN, Berry DJ, Bourgeois BF et al (2008) Antiepileptic drugs – best practice guidelines for therapeutic drug monitoring: a position paper by the subcommission on therapeutic drug monitoring, I.L.A.E. Commission on Therapeutic Strategies. Epilepsia 49:1239–1276

Pennell PB (2003) Antiepileptic drug pharmacokinetics during pregnancy and lactation. Neurology 61(Suppl 2):S35–S42

Philbert A, Petersen B, Dam M (1985) Concentration of valproate during pregnancy in the newborn and in breast milk. Acta Neurol Scand 72:460–463

Pisani F, Fazio A, Oteri G, Ruello C, Gitto C, Russo F, Perucca E (1986) Sodium valproate and valproamide: differential interactions with carbamazepine in epileptic patients. Epilepsia 27:548–552

Pitlick W, Painter M, Pippenger C (1978) Phenobarbital pharmacokinetics in neonates. Clin Pharmacol Ther 23:346–350

Pynnonen S, Sillanpaa M (1975) Carbamazepine and mother's milk. Lancet 3:563

Qiao X, Sun G, Clare JJ, Werkman TR, Wadman WJ (2014) Properties of human brain sodium channel (alpha)-subunits expressed in HEK293 cells and their modulation by carbamazepine, phenytoin and lamotrigine. Br J Pharmacol 171:1054–1067

Ramsay RE, Strauss RG, Wilder BJ, Willmore LJ (1978) Status epilepticus in pregnancy: effect of phenytoin malabsorption on seizure control. Neurology 28:85–89

Rey E, D'Arthis P, DeLautre D, Duklac O, Aicardi J, Olive G (1979) Pharmacokinetics of carbamazepine in the neonate and in the child. Int J Clin Pharmacol Biopharm 17:90–96

Reynolds EH, Travers RD (1974) Serum anticonvulsant concentrations in epileptic patients with mental symptoms. A preliminary report. Br J Psychiatry 124:440–445

Richens A (1975) Discussion. In: Schneider H, Janz D, Gardner-Thorpe C, Meinardi H, Sherwin AL (eds) Clinical pharmacology of antiepileptic drugs. Springer, Berlin, pp 46–47

Rościszewska D, Buntner B, Guz I, Zawisza L (1986) Ovarian hormones, anticonvulsant drugs, and seizures during the menstrual cycle in women with epilepsy. J Neurol Neurosurg Psychiatry 49:47–51

Ruprah M, Perucca E, Richens A (1982) Serum protein binding of phenytoin in women: effect of pregnancy and oral contraceptives. In: Janz D, Dam M, Bossi B, Richens A, Helge H, Schmidt D (eds) Epilepsy, pregnancy and the child. Raven, New York, pp 115–120

Schmidt D, Einicke I, Haenel F (1986) The influence of seizure type on the efficacy of plasma concentrations of phenytoin, phenobarbital, and carbamazepine. Arch Neurol 43:263–265

Shavit G, Lerman P, Korczyn AD, Kivity S, Bechar M, Gitter S (1984) Phenytoin pharmacokinetics in catamenial epilepsy. Neurology 34:959–961

Sherwin AL, Lloynd JS, Bock GW, Sokolowski CD (1974) Effect of age, sex, obesity and pregnancy on plasma diphenylhydantoin levels. Epilepsia 15:507–521

Shorvon SD, Reynolds EH (1982) Anticonvulsant peripheral neuropathies. A clinical and electrophysiological study of patients on single drug treatment with phenytoin, carbamazepine, or barbiturates. J Neurol Neurosurg Psychiatry 47:621–626

Shorvon S, Perucca E, Engel JJ (2009) The treatment of epilepsy, 3rd edn. Wiley Blackwell, Oxford

Thomas EA, Petrou S (2013) Network-specific mechanisms may explain the paradoxical effects of carbamazepine and phenytoin. Epilepsia 54:1195–1202

Tomson T, Tybring G, Bertilsson L (1983) Single-dose kinetics and metabolism of carbamazepine-10,11-epoxide. Clin Pharmacol Ther 33:58–65

Tomson T, Landmark CJ, Battino D (2013) Antiepileptic drug treatment in pregnancy: changes in drug disposition and their clinical implications. Epilepsia 54:405–414

Travers RD, Reynolds EH, Gallagher BB (1972) Variations in response to anticonvulsants in a group of epileptic patients. Arch Neurol 27:29–33

Vakil SD, Critchley EMR, Phillips JC, Fahim Y, Haydock C, Cocks A, Dyer T (1976) The effect of sodium valproate (Epilim) on phenytoin and phenobarbitone blood levels. In: Legg NJ (ed) Clinical and pharmacological aspects of sodium valproate (Epilim) in the treatment of epilepsy. MCS Consultants, Tunbridge Wells, pp 75–77

Westenberg HGM, Van Der Kleijn E, Oei TT, De Zeeuw RA (1978) Kinetics of carbamazepine and carbamazepine-epoxide determined by use of plasma and saliva. Clin Pharmacol Ther 23:320–328

Wilder BJ, Willmore LJ, Bruni J, Villareal HJ (1978) Valproic acid: interaction with other anticonvulsant drugs. Neurology 28:892–896

Windorfer AJ, Sauer W (1977) Drug interactions during anticonvulsant therapy in childhood: diphenylhydantoin, primidone, phenobarbitone, clonazepam, nitrazepam, carbamazepine and dipropylacetate. Neuropediatrie 8:29–41

Yerby MS, Friel P, Miller DQ (1985) Carbamazepine protein binding and disposition in pregnancy. Ther Drug Monit 7:269–273

Yerby MS, Friel PN, McCormick K et al (1990) Pharmacokinetics of anticonvulsants in pregnancy: alterations in plasma protein binding. Epilepsy Res 5:223–228

Chapter 5
Commonly Used Newer Antiepileptic Drugs

Abstract Data are available in the literature for the clinical pharmacologies of three newer antiepileptic drugs which have achieved a moderate amount of use in pregnant women, viz. lamotrigine, topiramate and levetiracetam. There is more information available for the first of these drugs than for the other two. The clearance value for lamotrigine, which is almost fully biotransformed to glucuronides, is considerably increased during pregnancy, with the clearances of topiramate (eliminated by a mix of metabolism and renal excretion unchanged) and levetiracetam (eliminated mainly by renal excretion without prior metabolism) being less increased. Relatively little information is available concerning the dispositions of the three drugs in the neonate, though there are published data for maternal plasma to breast milk concentration ratios.

At the time of writing, several of the antiepileptic drugs that have been introduced into therapeutic practice in the past quarter of a century seem to have become used increasingly by pregnant women, with apparently satisfactory outcomes. The clinical pharmacologies of the three most commonly encountered of these agents are discussed below.

Lamotrigine

Lamotrigine was developed as an antiepileptic agent after it was noticed that use of high doses of the older antiepileptic drugs phenobarbitone and phenytoin was associated with reduced circulating folate concentrations. This knowledge suggested that lamotrigine, with a molecular structure resembling part of the folate molecule, might have antiepileptic effects by interfering with the actions of folate. This has proved not to be lamotrigine's mechanism of antiepileptic action. Nevertheless, the drug has been found effective in treating many of the commonly occurring varieties of epilepsy. Lamotrigine has a reasonably trouble-free adverse effect profile and, at least in more affluent countries, has come into rather extensive use both in treating epilepsy and in managing certain psychiatric disorders.

M.J. Eadie, F.J.E. Vajda, *Antiepileptic Drugs and Pregnancy: A Guide for Prescribers*, DOI 10.1007/978-3-319-21434-4_5

Chemistry

Lamotrigine [3,5-diamino-6-(2,3-dichlorophenyl)-1,2,4-triazine] is a white solid with a relatively poor aqueous solubility, a molecular weight of 256.09 and a pK value of 5.7. It is marketed in 5, 25, 50, 100 and 200 mg solid dosage forms.

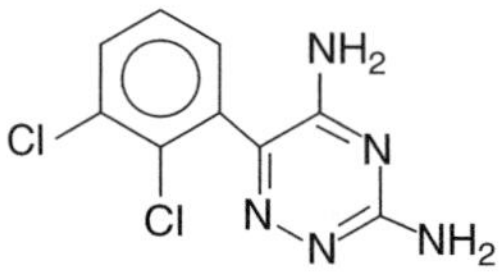

Pharmacodynamics

As mentioned above, lamotrigine does not act via folate-related mechanisms. Like phenytoin and carbamazepine, its antiepileptic effect is achieved by blocking voltage-, use- and frequency-dependent Na^+ ion channels in cell membranes. In doing this, lamotrigine in effect discriminates against the passage of rapid trains of axon impulses while interfering less with axon impulse transmission at more physiological frequencies. This mode of action reduces the release of neurotransmitters at axon terminals, particularly that of the excitatory molecule glutamate. Thus the drug's mechanism of action is hardly different from those of the other Na^+ channel-blocking antiepileptic agents phenytoin and carbamazepine. However, lamotrigine also has some inhibitory effects on voltage-activated Ca^{2+} currents and on K^+ conductances. The drug's action on Na^+ channels may explain its effectiveness in controlling focal epilepsies and the generalised convulsive seizures of genetic generalised epilepsy. However, the known biochemical mechanisms of action of the drug do not seem capable of explaining why it can also be effective against absence seizures and against some forms of myoclonic seizure (though there are reports that it can make the latter worse).

Pharmacokinetics

The pharmacokinetic parameters that are quoted below apply for lamotrigine when used as the sole antiepileptic agent. In clinical practice the drug is not infrequently prescribed in combination with other antiepileptic drugs. The various parameters may then have different values, as will be mentioned when the pharmacokinetic interactions that involve the drug are considered.

Absorption

Lamotrigine is nearly always administered by mouth and seems to have a virtually complete oral bioavailability. Peak plasma levels of the drug occur 1–3 h after intake.

Distribution

The drug has an apparent volume of distribution of around 1.2 or 1.3 L per kg, consistent with its being distributed throughout body water and also achieving some higher local concentration somewhere in body tissues. Lamotrigine's concentrations in the brain are calculated to be about 2.8 times of those in serum. Approximately 55 % of the lamotrigine in plasma is bound to proteins, a figure which correlates with the drug's concentration in cerebrospinal fluid (which averages 43 % of its plasma concentrations). Lamotrigine's concentration in saliva is also similar to its unbound concentration in plasma (Malone et al. 2006).

Elimination

Lamotrigine's elimination follows linear kinetics. Its half-life after an initial dose is approximately 33 h and in chronic use around 25 h. The drug's first-dose clearance is 0.026 L per kg per hour, but the value is higher when the drug is in continued use. This is not a particularly high clearance value and does not suggest that the drug undergoes any extensive pre-systemic metabolism. The clearance is higher in children, some 0.038 L per kg per hour. There is no evidence that lamotrigine induces its own metabolism to any significant extent, and it does not induce the cytochrome P450 drug-metabolising enzyme system.

Excretion Unchanged

Very little unmetabolised lamotrigine is excreted in urine. In view of its complete apparent oral bioavailability, the drug therefore appears to be eliminated almost exclusively by metabolism.

Metabolism

A little more than 3/4 of a lamotrigine dose is excreted in urine as a 2-N-glucuronide, with a small amount as a 5-N-glucuronide and with something less than 1 % as a 2-N-methyl derivative. The glucuronidations are catalysed by UDP glucuronosyl transferase 1A4 (Chen et al. 2009). In Gilbert's syndrome, with its decreased glucuronidation capacity, the clearance of lamotrigine is diminished. The glucuronide metabolites of lamotrigine appear to lack biological activity.

Clinical Pharmacokinetics

Lamotrigine concentrations can be monitored in plasma or serum or in saliva (Malone et al. 2006). There is a broad correlation between increasing plasma levels of the drug and increasing proportions of patients who achieve seizure control if they have types of epilepsy that normally respond to the drug. However the concentration range over which seizure control is achieved in the individual is quite wide. Early suggestions that the drug has a therapeutic range of 1–4 mg/L have been superseded by a proposed therapeutic set of values ranging between 1 and 15 mg/L. Patsalos et al. (2008) cited a range of 2.5–15 mg/L. Such a range is too wide to be helpful clinically in providing a preliminary indication that a therapeutically adequate dose of the drug has been prescribed. Nevertheless, the plasma lamotrigine concentration in the individual whose seizures are controlled provides a valuable indicator for guiding the future management of the seizure disorder in that particular patient, for instance, during pregnancy.

Interactions

The pharmacokinetic interactions in which lamotrigine is involved are mainly ones with agents that affect the glucuronidation of the drug, its main pathway of elimination.

Drugs which induce the capacity for glucuronidation, such as the older antiepileptic drugs phenobarbitone, phenytoin and carbamazepine and also rifampicin and lopinavir, may cause reduced lamotrigine plasma levels relative to the lamotrigine dose. As mentioned previously (Chap. 3), oestrogens may induce UDP-glucuronosyl transferases, and oestrogen-containing oral contraceptive use is associated with a tendency for plasma lamotrigine concentrations to be lower relative to the drug dose (Herzog et al. 2009; Wegner et al. 2009). This particularly is the case in the earlier parts of the menstrual cycle where the combined oral contraceptives provide oestrogen only. This same interaction with oestrogens contributes to the behaviour of plasma lamotrigine concentrations during the course of pregnancy.

Valproate inhibits the glucuronidation of lamotrigine and raises its plasma level relative to its dose. There have been reports that plasma lamotrigine levels may not fall during the course of pregnancy if valproate is also taken by the woman involved. Presumably, the effects of pregnancy and of the drug–drug interaction cancel each other. The magnitude of the interaction between valproate and lamotrigine in clinical practice is such that significantly lower than otherwise expected lamotrigine doses should be used if the drug is introduced into the treatment regimen of a patient already taking valproate.

Adverse Effects

Lamotrigine is not a particularly troublesome antiepileptic drug from the viewpoint of causing adverse effects.

Skin rashes may occur, nearly always quite early in the course of treatment. When the drug was first introduced into therapeutics, it was reported to cause a very fine, almost pinpoint, erythematous rash in the first few days of intake. If treatment with the drug was ceased and then resumed in lower dosage, this rash was reported not to recur. Sometimes rashes associated with the drug may be quite severe and even life-threatening, e.g. a Stevens–Johnson syndrome.

The drug does produce a degree of sedation which is dosage related and can be responsible for mental dulling, dizziness, blurred or double vision, drowsiness and ataxia of gait. Lamotrigine has a reputation for interfering less with sexual function than certain other antiepileptic agents.

Other adverse effects of the drug are uncommon.

Teratogenesis

The issue of lamotrigine-associated teratogenesis is discussed in Chap. 9.

Pregnancy

The Mother

While studying lamotrigine concentrations in breast milk and in the neonate, Rambeck et al. (1997) noticed that the drug's concentration in maternal plasma relative to the drug dose fell during pregnancy and rose again by the third postpartum week, necessitating a reduction in the lamotrigine dose at that stage. In the same year, Tomson et al. (1997) followed the relationship between the lamotrigine dose and the circulating concentration of the drug throughout pregnancy and the postnatal period, thus obtaining data on the course of the steady-state apparent clearance of the drug. Compared with the situation that applied five months after giving birth, by late pregnancy the apparent clearance of lamotrigine had increased by a factor of 3.6 and at term was 5.8 times higher than postpartum. Tran (2002) then reported that lamotrigine's clearance increased by 50 % during pregnancy. De Haan et al. (2004) later followed the relationship between circulating lamotrigine concentrations and drug dose during 12 pregnancies in women who took the drug in monotherapy. The ratio (i.e. the reciprocal of the steady-state apparent clearance) fell by about 40 % during pregnancy and quickly returned to its pre-pregnancy value after the baby was delivered. The ratio reached its trough in the period between 20 and 30 weeks of pregnancy and began to rise again in the final 10 weeks. Pennell et al. (2004) followed plasma lamotrigine levels monthly throughout pregnancy in 14 women and found the drug's apparent clearance increased (by more than 330 %) by the 32nd week of gestation and thereafter declined. Figure 5.1 shows the course of the apparent clearance of lamotrigine during and after pregnancy in one woman.

Thus, by about a decade after lamotrigine began to come into general clinical use, reasonably good evidence had become available that the clearance of the drug increased during human pregnancy.

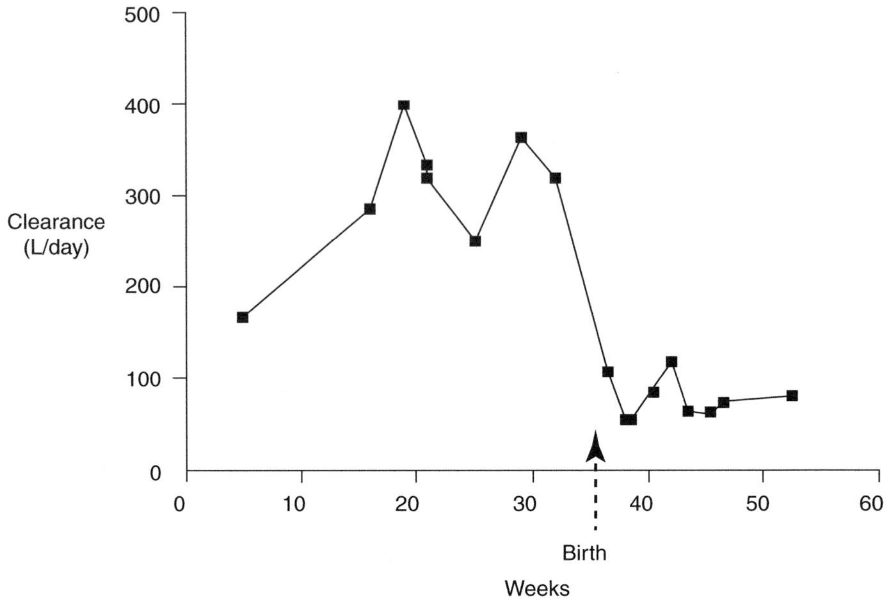

Fig. 5.1 The behaviour of the apparent clearance of lamotrigine during and after pregnancy in one woman

Subsequent studies have confirmed the existence of this increased clearance when the drug is used in pregnancy in the absence of potentially interacting co-medication. Petrenaite et al. (2005), in 11 pregnancies, described a 65 % clearance increase in the second trimester with the increase remaining at 65.8 % in the third trimester. These authors commented on the degree of variation in the increase in the individual women. Franco et al. (2008) found a mean increased clearance of 164 % by late pregnancy, and Pennell et al. (2008) in 53 pregnancies found that both the total clearance and the clearance of unbound lamotrigine were increased in all trimesters of pregnancy, the peak increases being 94 and 89 % respectively in the third trimester. Fotopoulou et al. (2009) cited a 197 % increase in the first trimester, a 236 % increase by the second trimester and a 248 % increase by the final trimester, with the clearance reverting to its baseline value by three weeks after giving birth. In 69 pregnancies in which lamotrigine was used in monotherapy, Reisinger et al. (2013) found the mean apparent clearance of the drug in L per day was first trimester, 1.64 ± 0.82 [0.068 L/h]; second trimester, 2.53 ± 1.47 [0.105 L/h]; and third trimester, 2.09 ± 1.01 [0.087 L/h], as compared with a value of 0.87 ± 0.42 [0.036 L/h] when not pregnant. Polepally et al. (2014), on the basis of a population pharmacokinetic analysis, found that two sets of pregnant women existed in relation to their capacities to eliminate lamotrigine. The smaller group had only a small increase in clearance; in the larger group, the clearance increase was roughly an order of magnitude greater. They did not determine the different clearance mechanisms that were involved.

Pennell et al. (2004) inferred that an increased renal excretion of the drug might be responsible for the drug's increased clearance during pregnancy. However, when Ohman et al. (2008) measured the ratio of the circulating concentrations of lamotrigine-2-N-glucuronide to lamotrigine in pregnancy and at 3 months postpartum, they found the ratio was 154 % higher during pregnancy. The subsequent evidence continues to be consistent with the maternal metabolism of lamotrigine being increased during pregnancy via enhanced glucuronidation. Reimers et al. (2011) found that the lamotrigine clearance was 118 % higher in the eighth month of pregnancy than in the second, and in the eighth month, the concentration ratio of lamotrigine-2N-glucuronide to lamotrigine in plasma was increased by 164 %. These workers also noted that, though plasma lamotrigine levels had begun to fall relative to drug dose in the second month of pregnancy, the plasma lamotrigine-2N-glucuronide to lamotrigine ratio was unchanged at that stage. They interpreted this finding in terms of plasma lamotrigine levels initially falling because of increased renal excretion of the drug, with the enhanced glucuronidation developing later. The increased glucuronidation of lamotrigine during pregnancy appears to correlate with the statement of Sabers (2008) that oestrogens induce UDP-glucuronosyl transferases and with the demonstration of Chen et al. (2009) that the enzyme induction is produced by 17-β-oestradiol.

The Foetus

In an ex vivo study, Myllynen et al. (2003) showed that lamotrigine crossed the perfused human placenta from the maternal to the foetal side readily and achieved a mean foetal–maternal ratio of 0.83 ± 0.41 at a maternal lamotrigine plasma concentration of 2.5 mg/L, and a ratio of 1.26 ± 0.20 at a maternal 10 mg/L plasma concentration of the drug.

Some measurements of the concentration of lamotrigine in umbilical cord venous blood, relative to the simultaneous concentration of the drug in maternal blood, are available. The values provide some indication of the likely concentrations of the drug to which the foetus would be exposed, at least in later pregnancy. Fotopoulou et al. (2009) found that the concentrations were virtually identical in maternal and umbilical vein blood. Kacirova et al. (2010) determined that the median infant to maternal plasma concentration ratio was 0.91 (range 0.40–1.38).

Breast Milk

There was interest in the concentration of lamotrigine in breast milk from a relatively early stage in the drug's use in clinical practice. Rambeck et al. (1997) found a milk to maternal serum mean ratio of 0.56 ± 0.11 while they followed the parameter over 145 days of breast feeding in one patient. Tomson et al. (1997) found the ratio was 0.6 at 2 weeks postpartum, when the baby's circulating lamotrigine concentration was 25 % of the maternal one. Ohman et al. (2000) cited the mean value for the ratio as

0.61 at a time when the baby's lamotrigine concentrations had a mean value of about 30 % of that of the mother. De Haan et al. (2004) quoted a 0.54 value for the ratio, though only three women were studied, Newport et al. (2008) a mean value of 0.41, Fotopoulou et al. (2009) one of 0.59 and Clark et al. (2013) one of 0.33. Davanzo et al. (2013) reported a wide range of values for the parameter (0.57–1.47).

The Neonate

As mentioned immediately above, during breast feeding the baby's circulating lamotrigine concentrations are about 25 % or 30 % of those in the mother, though Newport et al. (2008) cited a figure of 18.3 %. There is a report of an infant who became unacceptably sleepy while being breast fed by a mother who was taking lamotrigine. The baby, who had a circulating lamotrigine concentration of 4.87 mg/L, became alert again once breast feeding was ceased (Nordmo et al. 2009).

Published data for the elimination half-life of the drug in the neonate who is not breast fed have not been traced.

Topiramate

Topiramate's antiepileptic effectiveness was discovered after it was realised that the molecule, synthesised for a different purpose, possessed a degree of structural resemblance to that of acetazolamide, a drug that had some success in treating epilepsy but never became established in that role (Shank et al. 2000). Topiramate has proved a reasonably potent antiepileptic agent that has achieved moderately widespread use in recent years, at least in more affluent countries. The drug has subsequently found increasing employment in migraine prevention.

Chemistry

Chemically, topiramate is 2,3:4,5-bis-*O*-(1-methylethylidene)-α-D-fructopyranose sulphamate, a whitish monosaccharide derivative (MW 339.37, pKa value 8.61). It is moderately soluble in water and is marketed in solid dosage forms for oral use, mainly as tablets containing 25, 50, 100 and 200 mg of the active ingredient, and is also available as a sprinkle preparation.

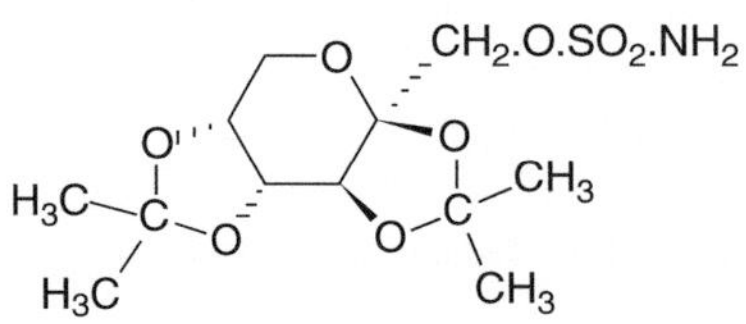

Pharmacodynamics

Topiramate has several known mechanism of action at the molecular level. The role that each of these mechanisms plays in its antiepileptic, migraine-preventing and other actions is unclear. The drug inhibits voltage-sensitive Na^+ and high-voltage-activated L-type Ca^{2+} ion channels, inhibits kainate-activated AMPA-type glutamate receptors and potentiates the actions of GABA in increasing Cl^- flux at GABA receptors. It also is a relatively weak carbonic anhydrase inhibitor, and as already mentioned, a rather more potent inhibitor, acetazolamide, had previously been used for treating some forms of childhood epilepsy. Any or all of these mechanisms of actions might achieve an antiepileptic effect. However, the drug's mechanism of action on Na^+ channels is not identical with that shared by phenytoin, carbamazepine and lamotrigine. The mechanism through which topiramate prevents migraine is currently unexplained.

Clinically, the drug is capable of controlling all varieties of focal (partial) epilepsy and the generalised convulsive seizures of idiopathic, i.e. genetic, generalised epilepsies. It is also useful in preventing the drop attacks of the Lennox–Gastaut syndrome but does not seem able to prevent absence seizures occurring.

Pharmacokinetics

The published pharmacokinetic information relating to topiramate is not particularly extensive. Garnett (2000) assembled the data available at his time of writing. Not a great deal has been added since.

Absorption

When given by mouth, topiramate seems to be reasonably fully absorbed. It has a calculated oral bioavailability fraction of 0.81–0.95. Peak plasma levels are attained some 2–4 h after oral intake of the drug.

Distribution

Topiramate has a somewhat limited distribution in the body, the value of its apparent volume of distribution being 0.6–0.8 L per kilogram, suggesting that the molecule is largely confined to body water without any particular concentration in tissues. Jovanovic et al. (2013) carried out population pharmacokinetic modelling on data from 78 patients treated with the drug, though in many instances the patients involved were also receiving other antiepileptic agents. These authors calculated that the apparent volume of distribution value for topiramate was 0.575 L per Kg.

Some 9–17 % of the topiramate in the circulation is bound to plasma proteins.

Elimination

The elimination kinetics of topiramate are linear.

In their population pharmacokinetic study, Jovanovic et al. (2013) found that topiramate had an elimination half-life of 20–30 h in the absence of potential enzyme-inducing agents and one of 10–15 h in their presence. Garnett (2000) cited a half-life value of 19–23 h.

The apparent clearance of the drug in the non-induced subject is 1.32–2.16 L per hour or 1.53 L per hour (Jovanovic et al. 2013). In those whose drug-metabolising enzymes are already induced, the clearance value may be perhaps twice as great. The renal clearance of the drug is 1.02–1.08 L per hour. This value suggests that, after glomerular filtration, the unmetabolised drug undergoes substantial reabsorption from renal tubular urine. Topiramate is a P-glycoprotein substrate, but it is not known whether this molecular transport mechanism is involved in the drug's renal handling. The apparent clearance of the drug from the body is higher in children aged over 6 months than in adults and decreases a little in the elderly. Because a substantial proportion of the topiramate dose is excreted in urine as the intact molecule, the drug's clearance might be expected to diminish if glomerular function is impaired.

Excretion Unchanged

When used in the absence of substances which induce drug-metabolising enzymes, some 60–70 % of a topiramate dose is excreted in urine without being metabolised. Garnett (2000) put the figure at 80 %. In the presence of enzyme-inducing substances, the proportion of the dose excreted unchanged decreases to about 40 %.

Metabolism

In the absence of CYP450 drug-metabolising enzyme induction, the majority of a topiramate dose is excreted intact in urine, but the remaining topiramate molecule in the body may undergo a rather extensive array of metabolic alterations. None of the metabolites possess biological activity. There are hydroxylated derivatives, products of hydrolysis, residues after the sulphamate moiety is split from the parent molecule, and glucuronide and sulphate conjugates. Quantitative data regarding these various biotransformation pathways are not available.

Clinical Pharmacokinetics

Topiramate plasma levels tend to be proportional to the drug dose ingested. A therapeutic range of plasma concentrations for the drug (5–20 mg/L) has been proposed (Patsalos et al. 2008). However, in clinical practice, topiramate dosages are nearly always adjusted on the basis of the clinical response and on the absence or presence of adverse effects that can be ascribed to the drug. Topiramate is commonly used in conjunction with other antiepileptic drugs when seizure disorders are being treated. In these circumstances, induction of topiramate metabolism may occur, shortening the drug's half-life so that twice-daily intake may become desirable to maintain relatively stable steady-state drug concentrations across the dosage interval.

Steady-state conditions should apply again 4–6 days after a topiramate dosage change.

Interactions

As mentioned above, drugs such as phenytoin and carbamazepine, which induce both CYP450 isoenzymes and UDP-glucuronosyl transferases, increase the clearance of topiramate and lower its plasma concentrations. The available information concerning the effects of valproate co-administration on topiramate concentrations is difficult to assess.

Topiramate does not appear to produce induction of the body's drug-metabolising enzymes though, at high drug doses, some induction of CYP2C19 may occur. This particular P450 isoenzyme is involved in phenytoin metabolism but accounts for only a very small proportion of the phenytoin dose. Therefore the induction is unlikely to have any significant consequence for plasma phenytoin concentrations. At topiramate doses above 200 mg a day, there is evidence that the drug can lower plasma concentrations of ethinyl oestradiol (Rosenfeld et al. 1997), though the study that demonstrated this was carried out in women co-medicated with valproate. This raises the possibility that topiramate may induce UDP-glucuronosyl transferase synthesis. If this induction did occur, its effect on ethinyl oestradiol could have implications for the efficacy of combined oral contraceptives.

Adverse Effects

Topiramate probably has a greater tendency to produce sedation than several other antiepileptic drugs in contemporary use. This sedation can lead to mental slowing, somnolence and impaired cognition and may limit the possibilities of prescribing effective antiepileptic dosages of the drug. Topiramate may produce a tendency to overbreathing, but patients are not likely to be significantly distressed by this. Like other carbonic anhydrase inhibitors, topiramate fairly frequently causes tingling around the lips and in the fingers. This side effect is rarely severe enough to cause patients to cease taking the drug once they know the origin of the symptom.

There have been occasional reports of the occurrence of renal calculi associated with the use of topiramate. Rather frequently, intake of the drug has been associated with some weight loss, a side effect that may not necessarily be unacceptable to patients.

Teratogenicity

The teratogenicity of the drug is discussed in Chap. 9.

Pregnancy

A few papers have been published that contain information on the pharmacokinetics of topiramate during human pregnancy.

The Mother

Westin et al. (2009) studied 15 pregnancies in 12 women taking topiramate, sometimes in conjunction with other antiepileptic drugs. In the first trimester, the mean plasma topiramate concentration to dose ratio was 0.0686 ± 0.0262, in the second trimester 0.0499 ± 0.0160 and in the third trimester 0.0476 ± 0.0213, the baseline non-pregnant ratio being 0.0752 ± 0.0240. (These values are reciprocals of steady-state apparent clearances.) It thus appears that there was a statistically significant increase in the clearance of the drug in the second and third trimesters of the pregnancies, with the increases probably beginning in the first trimester.

At much the same time, Ohman et al. (2009) followed the apparent clearances of topiramate throughout the course of 10 pregnancies, in not all of which the women were taking the drug in monotherapy. Outside pregnancy, the apparent clearance averaged 37.3 ± 15.9 L per day [1.55 L/h], in the first trimester 49.4 ± 29.4 L per day [2.06 L/h], in the second trimester 67.5 ± 23.4 L per day [2.81 L/h] and in the third trimester 65.1 ± 30.4 L per day [2.71 L/h]. Thus there was a mean increase in clearance during pregnancy of 71.8 %. Ohman et al. (2009) commented on the degree of variation in the increased clearances of topiramate in different women that was found in their study. The increased clearances in pregnancy occurred, irrespective of whether the women involved took topiramate in antiepileptic drug monotherapy or together with enzyme-inducing co-medications.

In both the above studies, the increase in clearance appeared to plateau in the last trimester of pregnancy. There was no clear indication as to how quickly the clearance returned to its normal value after pregnancy ended. As well, no information was provided concerning possible alterations in the pathways of metabolism of the drug during pregnancy. Ohman et al. (2009) did raise the possibility that pregnancy might impair the oral bioavailability of the drug and, through this means, increase its apparent clearance. However, they thought increased metabolism was a more likely explanation, though they had no direct evidence to support this interpretation.

The Foetus

Ohman et al. (2002) had earlier carried out some measurements of circulating topiramate concentrations in five mother–baby pairs shortly after delivery, again at 24, 48 and 72 h postpartum and also at 1 and 3 months after childbirth. At birth, the drug's concentrations in the maternal circulation (2.6–17 μM, i.e. approximately 0.9–5.8 mg/L) and in umbilical cord veins were virtually identical, suggesting that during pregnancy the drug crossed the placenta easily.

Breast Milk

The measurements of Ohman et al. (2002), referred to in the paragraph immediately above, showed that topiramate concentrations in breast milk averaged 86 % (67–100 %) of those in maternal plasma during the second and third months of breast feeding. Davanzo et al. (2013) quoted a similar figure for the parameter (86–110 %).

The Neonate

No information is available regarding the behaviour of topiramate concentrations in the neonate during breast feeding or after exposure to the drug ceases.

Levetiracetam

Levetiracetam first became available for therapeutic use in 1999 and relatively rapidly found a place as a major antiepileptic agent. It possesses certain advantages over previously available antiepileptic drugs.

Chemistry

Chemically, levetiracetam is (–) (S)-α ethyl-2-oxo-1-pyrrolidine-acetamide. The drug is supplied as the S-enantiomer only, not as the racemate, the R-enantiomer being biologically inactive. It is a water-soluble whitish material, molecular weight 170.1, and has a pKa value that cannot be determined accurately.

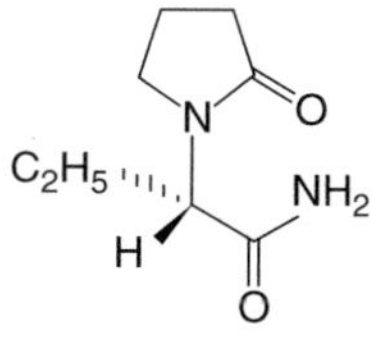

The drug is marketed in solid dosage forms in units containing 250, 500, 1000 and 2000 mg of active substance. Modified-release forms are available in some countries. It is also available as a solution for intravenous injection (100 mg per ml).

Pharmacodynamics

Unlike nearly all other marketed antiepileptic drugs, levetiracetam exerts no protective effects in the very commonly used experimental model, the maximum electroshock seizure, which has become virtually the standard screening test to detect antiepileptic activity. The drug is also ineffective experimentally in certain other commonly employed experimental seizure disorder models, though it is effective in others.

Levetiracetam's molecular mechanism of action is thought to be mediated through its binding to the synaptic vesicle protein SV2A. How this binding achieves the antiepileptic effect of the drug is not easily explained. Possibly the binding interferes with neurotransmitter release at axon terminals. The drug is displaced from its SV2A binding sites by the structurally analogous molecule piracetam and also by the antiepileptic agent ethosuximide. There is some tentative evidence that levetiracetam may act at N-type Ca^{2+} channels. However, it has no action on the T-type Ca^{2+} channels involved in the genesis of absence seizures, on Na^{+} channels or on the GABA-Cl^{-} mechanism, sites where other antiepileptic drugs exert their effects.

Despite these differences in mechanism of action, in clinical practice levetiracetam is effective in controlling all forms of focal (partial) epilepsy, whether or not the seizures become secondarily generalised. It is also useful in treating idiopathic, i.e. genetic, generalised epilepsies in which there are generalised convulsive or myoclonic seizures, but it does not seem useful in preventing absence seizures.

Pharmacokinetics

There is a reasonable amount of information available concerning the pharmacokinetics of the drug, which are linear.

Absorption

Levetiracetam is fully bioavailable after oral administration, with maximum plasma concentrations occurring from 0.5 to 2 h after intake, unless the drug is taken in a modified-release preparation.

Distribution

The value of the apparent volume distribution of levetiracetam is 0.5–0.7 L per kilogram. This value suggests that the drug is distributed through total body water but undergoes little or no selective tissue concentration. Less than 10 % of the drug in the circulation is bound to plasma proteins.

Elimination

The plasma half-life of levetiracetam is around 6–8 h. However, there is some evidence that the duration of the half-life of levetiracetam's biological activity may be longer, possibly because of the drug's more prolonged presence at its sites of action. Its clearance value is 0.06 L per kilogram per hour.

Excretion Unchanged

An average of 66 % of a levetiracetam dose is excreted in urine without being metabolised so that only a relative minority of the drug dose is eliminated by biotransformation. The value of the renal clearance of the drug (0.6 ml/min/kg [2.5 L/h]) suggests that the majority of the amount of drug that is filtered through the glomeruli is subsequently reabsorbed from tubular urine.

Metabolism

The main metabolic pathway of the drug involves hydrolysis of its amide moiety, forming the molecule's corresponding carboxylic acid derivative. This metabolite is biologically inactive and is excreted as such in urine. There are also minor oxidative metabolites which appear to account for less than 3 % of the drug dose.

Clinical Pharmacokinetics

Steady-state plasma lamotrigine concentrations appear to be dose proportional. A provisional therapeutic range for the drug of 12–46 mg/L has been suggested (Patsalos et al. 2008). In practice, the drug's dosage is nearly always adjusted in relation to the clinical response. However, knowledge of the plasma levetiracetam concentration at which a satisfactory clinical response applies in the individual can be valuable in the subsequent management of the seizure disorder in that person.

Interactions

Levetiracetam does not induce the isoenzymes of the CYP450 system or the various UPD-glucuronosyl transferases or epoxide hydrolase. Because of this, and because of its low plasma protein binding, it is unlikely that the drug would interact with co-administered drugs to alter their plasma concentrations relative to their dose.

However, the co-administration of drugs which induce the body's drug-metabolising enzyme mechanisms may cause an increase in levetiracetam clearance and produce a fall in its plasma concentration relative to dose.

Probenecid increases the clearance of the levetiracetam's carboxylic acid metabolite, but this is of no clinical consequence since the metabolite lacks biological activity.

Adverse Effects

Levetiracetam has a relatively trouble-free adverse effect profile compared with those of many other antiepileptic drugs. It does cause some sedation and, particularly at high dosage levels, patients may complain of somnolence, asthenia, fatigue and dizziness. Depression of mood may occur in some patients. Sometimes there may be disturbances of behaviour with irritability and, if the doses are high enough, some impairment of consciousness. Rashes from the drug are uncommon. There have been reports that its use may occasionally exacerbate seizure activity.

Teratogenicity

The question of the drug's teratogenicity is discussed in Chap. 9.

Pregnancy

The Mother

Tomson et al. (2007) studied 15 pregnancies in 14 women taking levetiracetam. They noted that the mothers' plasma concentrations of the drug in the third trimester of pregnancy were about 40 % of their subsequent baseline values after pregnancy. In the same year, Tomson and Battino (2007) provided data for five pregnancies in which apparent clearances of levetiracetam had been measured in each trimester of pregnancy and also some months after pregnancy. The clearances were expressed in the unfamiliar unit of mg per kg per μg per ml, without any measure of time being specified, though the values are probably per day ones. The values obtained were, respectively, 2.15 ± 0.72, 2.24 ± 0.45, 1.99 ± 0.75 and 1.29 ± 0.57 [there are too many uncertainties involved, e.g. as regards dosages and body weights, to justify calculating clearances in L/h units]. These values seem to suggest the presence of an increased clearance of the drug during pregnancy and also that the increase reaches its maximum in the second trimester. In a further paper in the same year, Tomson et al. (2007) stated that the clearance in pregnancy was 297 ± 147 ml per minute [17.8 ± 8.8 L/h] and after pregnancy 87 ± 40 ml per minute [5.2 ± 2.4 L/h].

Westin et al. (2008) quoted values for levetiracetam plasma concentrations divided by dose (i.e. reciprocals of clearances) from before pregnancy, throughout the trimesters of pregnancy and during the postpartum month, in 11 women. The values were: before pregnancy 0.043 ± 0.0 22, first trimester 0.026 ± 0.008, second trimester 0.022 ± 0.005, third trimester 0.021 ± 0.009, third to fifth postpartum day 0.029 ± 0.009, 2 weeks postpartum 0.031 ± 0.005 and 1 month postpartum 0.040 ± 0.018. Thus these workers found that levetiracetam clearance has already fallen in the first trimester, continued to fall in the second but fell only minimally further in the final trimester. The values began to return to their baseline ones within a few days of giving birth. Subsequently Lopez-Fraile et al. (2009), in a study involving five pregnant women, reported that the plasma level of levetiracetam, compared to its baseline value, fell by 47 % in the first trimester of pregnancy and by 62 % in the final trimester. Reisinger et al. (2013), in 15 pregnancies exposed to levetiracetam monotherapy, found that the apparent clearances of the drug increased from a mean baseline value of 1.09 ± 0.30 L per kg per day, through 2.16 ± 1.72 L per kg per day in the first trimester and 3.35 ± 2.60 L per kg per day in the second trimester to 2.15 ± 1.11 L per kg per day in the third trimester. Overall, the time courses of the clearance changes were reasonably similar in all the above studies.

There thus is reasonably convincing evidence that the clearance of levetiracetam is increased in pregnancy. None of the published investigations has provided evidence regarding the mechanisms involved in the increased clearances. Because levetiracetam is normally eliminated mainly by renal excretion as the unchanged substance, it has been suggested that the increased renal function of pregnancy may be responsible, but no actual renal clearance values appear to have been determined. Nor has levetiracetam metabolism been studied during pregnancy so that it is possible that the increased clearances of the drug may be partly due to high female sex hormone levels inducing the capacities of the drug's metabolic pathways during pregnancy.

The Foetus

Soon after childbirth, levetiracetam concentrations are similar in maternal and umbilical cord plasma (Tomson et al. 2007). Johanessen et al. (2005), in four mother–neonate pairs, found the cord venous to maternal plasma levetiracetam ratio was 1.14. Lopez-Fraile et al. (2009) cited a figure of 1.214 for this parameter. For practical purposes, it seems likely that, at least in later pregnancy, levetiracetam equilibrates across the placenta on a 1 to 1 concentration basis.

Breast Milk

Levetiracetam concentrations in breast milk have been reported to be similar to those in maternal plasma, where there is little protein binding of the drug (Johanessen et al. 2005). Tomson et al. (2007) quoted a milk to maternal plasma ratio of 1.05 (range 0.78–1.55).

The Neonate

Tomson et al. (2007) calculated that the elimination half-life of levetiracetam was about 18 h in neonates born to mothers who had been taking the drug during pregnancy. When the mother was breast feeding, the baby's plasma levetiracetam concentration was approximately 13 % of the simultaneous concentration in the mother's blood. Allegaert et al. (2006) cited a value of 16–18 h for the half-life in a pair of bottle-fed twins.

References

Allegaent K, Lewi L, Naulars G, Lagae L (2006) Levetiracetam pharmacokinetics in neonates at birth. Epilepsia 47:1068–1069

Chen H, Yang K, Choi S, Fischer JH, Jeong H (2009) Up-regulation of UDP-glucuronosyltransferase (UGT) 1A4 by 17beta-estradiol: a potential mechanism of increased lamotrigine elimination in pregnancy. Drug Metab Dispos 37:1841–1847

Clark CT, Klein AM, Perel JM, Helsel J, Wisner KL (2013) Lamotrigine dosing for pregnant patients with bipolar disorder. Am J Psychiatry 170:1240–1247

Davanzo R, Bo SD, Bua J, Copertino M, Zanelli E (2013) Antiepileptic drugs and breastfeeding. Ital J Pediatr 39:50

de Haan GJ, Edelbroek P, Segers J, Engelsman M, Lindhout D, Devile-Notschaele M, Augustin P (2004) Gestation-induced changes in lamotrigine pharmacokinetics: a monotherapy study. Neurology 63:571–573

Fotopoulou C, Kretz R, Bauer S, Schefold JC, Schmitz B, Dudenhausen JW, Henrich W (2009) Prospectively assessed changes in lamotrigine-concentration in women with epilepsy during pregnancy, lactation and the neonatal period. Epilepsy Res 85:60–64

Franco V, Mazzucchelli I, Gatti G, Specchio LM, Papantonio A, Ozkaynakci AE, Perucca E (2008) Changes in lamotrigine pharmacokinetics during pregnancy and the puerperium. Ther Drug Monit 30:544–547

Garnett WR (2000) Clinical pharmacology of topiramate: a review. Epilepsia 41(Suppl 1):S61–S65

Herzog AG, Blum AS, Farina EL et al (2009) Valproate and lamotrigine level variation with menstrual cycle phase and oral contraceptive use. Neurology 72:911–914

Johanessen SI, Helde G, Brodtkorb E (2005) Levetiracetam concentrations in serum and in breast milk at birth and during lactation. Epilepsia 46:775–777

Jovanovic M, Sokie D, Grabner I, Vovk T, Postran M, Vucicevic K, Miljkovic B (2013) Population pharmacokinetics of topiramate in adult patients with epilepsy using nonlinear mixed effects modelling. Eur J Pharm Sci 50:282–289

Kacirova I, Grundmann M, Brozmanova H (2010) Serum levels of lamotrigine during delivery in mothers and their infants. Epilepsy Res 91:161–165

Lopez-fraile IP, Cid AO, Juste AO, Modrego PJ (2009) Levetiracetam plasma level monitoring during pregnancy, delivery, and postpartum: clinical and outcome implications. Epilepsy Behav 15:372–375

Malone S, Addison R, Eadie MJ, Dickinson RG (2006) The monitoring of salivary lamotrigine concentrations. J Clin Neurosci 13:902–907

Myllynen PK, Pienimaki PK, Vahakangas KH (2003) Transplacental passage of lamotrigine in a human placental perfusion system in vitro and in maternal and cord blood in vivo. Eur J Clin Pharmacol 58:677–682

Newport DJ, Pennell PB, Calamaras MR et al (2008) Lamotrigine in breast milk and nursing infants: determination of exposure. Pediatrics 122:e223–231

Nordmo E, Aronsen L, Wasland K, Smabrekke L, Vorren S (2009) Severe apnea in an infant exposed to lamotrigine in breast milk. Ann Pharmacother 43:1893–1897

Ohman I, Vitols S, Tomson T (2000) Lamotrigine in pregnancy: pharmacokinetics during delivery, in the neonate, and during lactation. Epilepsia 41:709–713

Ohman I, Vitols S, Luef G, Soderfeldt B, Tomson T (2002) Topiramate kinetics during delivery, lactation, and the neonate: preliminary observations. Epilepsia 43:1157–1160

Ohman I, Beck O, Vitols S, Tomson T (2008) Plasma concentrations of lamotrigine and its 2-N-glucuronide metabolite during pregnancy in women with epilepsy. Epilepsia 49:1075–1080

Ohman I, Sabers A, de Flon P, Luef G, Tomson T (2009) Pharmacokinetics of topiramate during pregnancy. Epilepsy Res 87:124–129

Patsalos PN, Berry DJ, Bourgeois BF et al (2008) Antiepileptic drugs – best practice guidelines for therapeutic drug monitoring: a position paper by the subcommission on therapeutic drug monitoring, I.L.A.E. Commission on Therapeutic Strategies. Epilepsia 49:1239–1276

Pennell PB, Newport DJ, Stowe ZN, Heimers SL, Montgomery JQ, Henry TR (2004) The impact of pregnancy and childbirth on the metabolism of lamotrigine. Neurology 62:292–295

Pennell PB, Peng L, Newport DJ et al (2008) Lamotrigine in pregnancy: clearance, therapeutic drug monitoring, and seizure frequency. Neurology 70:2130–2136

Petrenaite V, Sabers A, Hansen-Schwartz J (2005) Individual changes in lamotrigine plasma concentrations during pregnancy. Epilepsy Res 65:185–188

Polepally AR, Pennell PB, Brundage RC et al (2014) Model-based lamotrigine clearance changes during pregnancy: clinical implication. Ann Clin Transl Neurol 1:99–106

Rambeck B, Kurlemann G, Stodieck SR, May TW, Jurgens U (1997) Concentrations of lamotrigine in a mother on lamotrigine treatment and her newborn child. Eur J Clin Pharmacol 51:481–484

Reimers A, Helge G, Brathen G, Brodkorb E (2011) Lamotrigine and its N2 glucuronide during pregnancy: the significance of renal clearance and oestradiol. Epilepsy Res 94:198–205

Reisinger TL, Newman M, Loring DW, Pennell PB, Meador KL (2013) Antiepileptic drug clearance and seizure frequency during pregnancy in women with epilepsy. Epilepsy Behav 29:13–18

Rosenfeld WE, Doose DE, Walker SA, Nayak RA (1997) Effect of topiramate on the pharmacokinetics of oral contraceptives containing norethindrone and ethinyl oestradiol in patients with epilepsy. Epilepsia 38:317–323

Sabers A (2008) Pharmacokinetic interactions between contraceptives and antiepileptic drugs. Seizure 17:141–144

Shank RP, Gardocki JF, Streeter AJ, Maryanoff BE (2000) An overview of the preclinical aspects of topiramate: pharmacology, pharmacokinetics, and mechanism of action. Epilepsia 41(Suppl 1):S3–S9

Tomson T, Battino D (2007) Pharmacokinetics and therapeutic drug monitoring of newer antiepileptic drugs during pregnancy and the puerperium. Clin Pharmacokinet 46:209–219

Tomson T, Ohman I, Vitols S (1997) Lamotrigine in pregnancy and lactation: a case report. Epilepsia 38:1039–1041

Tomson T, Palm R, Kallen K et al (2007) Pharmacokinetics of levetiracetam during pregnancy, delivery, in the neonatal period, and lactation. Epilepsia 48:1111–1116

Tran TA (2002) Lamotrigine clearance during pregnancy. Neurology 59:251–255

Wegner I, Edelbroek PM, Bulk S, Lindhout D (2009) Lamotrigine kinetics within the menstrual cycle, after menopause, and with oral contraception. Neurology 73:1388–1393

Westin AA, Reimers A, Heide G, Nakken KO, Brodtkorb E (2008) Serum concentration/dose ratio of levetiracetam before, during and after pregnancy. Seizure 17:192–198

Westin AA, Nakken KO, Johannessen SI, Reimers A, Lillestolen KM, Brodkorb E (2009) Serum concentration/dose ratio of topiramate during pregnancy. Epilepsia 50:480–485

Chapter 6
Antiepileptic Drugs Sometimes Used in Pregnancy

Abstract This chapter contains information concerning the dispositions of various antiepileptic drugs that have sometimes been used in pregnancy, in particular oxcarbazepine. The information concerning the effects of pregnancy on the pharmacokinetics of gabapentin, ethosuximide, vigabatrin, zonisamide and various benzodiazepines with antiepileptic properties is relatively scanty, though the available data do not suggest that there are significant departures from the principles set down in Chap. 3 in relation to the anticipated effects of pregnancy on drug disposition.

Some information is available concerning the dispositions during pregnancy of several antiepileptic drugs that are sometimes taken by contemporary pregnant women. Several of these drugs have been marketed for a number of years but their use is diminishing as time passes. Others are relatively new agents whose place in therapeutics is not yet well established. One, ethosuximide, has a long established but limited and specific place in treating a type of epileptic disorder that is not often encountered in pregnant women. The drugs are dealt with individually in this chapter, though in less detail than the more commonly used drugs considered in the previous two chapters. There is little useful information available in the literature concerning the dispositions in pregnancy of a few older antiepileptic drugs that may still be taken by a few pregnant women, e.g. sulthiame and felbamate. At the time of writing, there is virtually no relevant information for certain newer antiepileptic drugs such as lacosamide, perampanel and eslicarbazepine, which are beginning to play increasing roles in the treatment of epilepsy but do not yet appear to have become widely used in pregnancy.

Oxcarbazepine

Rather more information is available concerning the disposition in pregnancy of oxcarbazepine than that for the other drugs that are to be considered in this chapter. Oxcarbazepine has been available for a number of years and seems to have been rather extensively used in some European countries but less widely employed elsewhere. The drug has molecular structural and pharmacological similarities to carbamazepine.

Flesch (2004) has published a detailed account of the clinical pharmacology of the drug.

M.J. Eadie, F.J.E. Vajda, *Antiepileptic Drugs and Pregnancy: A Guide for Prescribers*, DOI 10.1007/978-3-319-21434-4_6

Chemistry

Oxcarbazepine (10,11-dihydro-10-oxo-5H-dibenz[b,f]azepine-5-carboxamide) is a white, poorly water-soluble material (molecular weight 252.3, pKa value 10.7), which is supplied for therapeutic purposes in 150, 300 and 600 mg solid dosage forms and in a 60 mg per ml suspension. Its molecular structural formula is shown in Fig. 4.6 in relation to that of carbamazepine.

Pharmacodynamics

In clinical use, oxcarbazepine in effect functions mainly as a prodrug for its pharmacologically active 10-hydroxy metabolite (whose name is often abbreviated to MHD, i.e. monohydroxy derivative, whose molecular formula also appears in Fig. 4.6). The mechanism of action of this substance is very similar to that of carbamazepine, viz. blocking voltage- and frequency-dependent Na^+ ion channels in neural cell membranes. The monohydroxy derivative of oxcarbazepine and carbamazepine itself both act at Ca^{2+} channels, but the actions of the two rather structurally similar molecules occur at different types of Ca^{2+} channel (Schmidt and Elger 2004). Oxcarbazepine is useful in controlling the seizures of the focal epilepsies and the generalised tonic–clonic convulsions of genetic generalised epilepsy, but the drug is not useful for preventing absence or myoclonic seizures.

Pharmacokinetics

The pharmacokinetics of oxcarbazepine is linear under the conditions that apply in human therapeutic use.

Absorption

Orally administered oxcarbazepine appears to be fully bioavailable.

Distribution

The apparent volume distribution of the drug was found to be 49 L, suggesting that it is probably distributed throughout body water. Some two-thirds of the oxcarbazepine in the circulation and 40 % of its monohydroxy metabolite are bound to plasma proteins.

Elimination

The plasma elimination half-life of oxcarbazepine is in the range 1.3–2.3 h, whereas the half-life of the monohydroxy derivative is 9.3 ± 1.8 h. The clearance value of the monohydroxy derivative is 91–122 ml per minute [5.46–7.32 L/h].

Excretion Unchanged

Less than 1 % of an oxcarbazepine dose appears in urine as the unmetabolised parent substance.

Metabolism

Oxcarbazepine is converted to its hydroxy metabolite by arylketone reductase enzymes in the cytosol; the majority of this metabolite is then conjugated with glucuronic acid before excretion in the urine. The monohydroxy derivative exist in two stereoisomeric forms, the [S]-enantiomer predominating. Both enantiomers are pharmacologically active. Part of the monohydroxy metabolite is converted to a biologically inactive dihydrodiol derivative that is subsequently excreted in urine mainly as a glucuronide conjugate. This same dihydrodiol metabolite is formed from carbamazepine via the epoxide hydrolase pathway that is involved in carbamazepine's biotransformation (see Fig. 4.6).

Clinical Pharmacokinetics

In human therapeutic use, plasma concentrations of the monohydroxy derivative of oxcarbazepine increase in proportion to the oxcarbazepine dose. Patsalos et al. (2008) proposed a plasma therapeutic range of 3–35 mg/L for this monohydroxy derivative.

Interactions

Neither oxcarbazepine nor its monohydroxy derivative induces the CYP450 enzyme system, though both substances inhibit the isoenzyme CYP2C19. The monohydroxy derivative does not alter circulating concentrations of phenytoin, carbamazepine or valproate. However, in the case of co-administered carbamazepine, it causes raised circulating concentrations of carbamazepine-10,11-epoxide. Oxcarbazepine administration may lower plasma concentrations of lamotrigine.

Co-administered phenytoin, carbamazepine and valproate will reduce circulating concentrations of oxcarbazepine's monohydroxy derivative.

Adverse Effects

Oxcarbazepine is less likely than carbamazepine to produce skin rashes and tends to cause less sedation at doses which produce similar degrees of antiepileptic effect. Unfortunately, the drug has a greater tendency to produce hyponatraemia, particularly early in the course of its use. This hyponatraemia may sometimes be severe enough to compromise seizure control.

Teratogenicity

The teratogenicity of the drug is considered in Chap. 9.

Pregnancy

The Mother

In five women, Mazzucchelli et al. (2006) found that, during pregnancy, plasma concentrations of the [S]-isomer of the monohydroxy derivative of oxcarbazepine fell relative to the oxcarbazepine dose. The plasma concentration of oxcarbazepine itself also fell. Christensen et al. (2006) followed the relationship between plasma monohydroxy derivative concentrations and the oxcarbazepine dose throughout nine pregnancies that occurred in seven women. They found that the relationship between the plasma metabolite concentrations and the drug dose decreased to 72 % of its pre-pregnancy value in the first trimester, to 74 % in the second and to 64 % in the third. They suggested that the increased clearance of the metabolite probably depended on increased formation and renal excretion of its glucuronide conjugate, though they did not prove that this was the case. Subsequently Petrenaite et al. (2009) carried out a rather similar study with a similar result, the ratio between plasma metabolite concentration and the drug dose falling by 26.2 % in the first trimester, by 36.5 % in the second and by 38.2 % in the third. In the following year, Wegner et al. (2010) also noted an increased clearance of the metabolite in two pregnancies. There thus seems consistent evidence that the drug and its major biologically active metabolite undergo increased clearances during pregnancy, though the details of the responsible mechanism have not been established.

The Foetus

In ex vivo perfusion experiments, Pienimäki et al. (1997) showed that oxcarbazepine was converted to its monohydroxy derivative in the human placenta. The monohydroxy derivative was not metabolised further in that organ. It appears that the drug probably equilibrates crosses the placenta, at least in late pregnancy. Myllynen et al. (2001) found that concentrations of oxcarbazepine and its monohydroxy and dihydrodiol derivatives were similar in maternal and umbilical cord serum shortly after birth. Measurable quantities of oxcarbazepine, its monohydroxy derivative and its dihydrodiol derivative were present in neonatal plasma shortly after birth.

Breast Milk

Breast milk concentrations of drug and its main metabolite are about half those in simultaneously collected maternal plasma. Davanzo et al. (2013) also cited the same 50 % figure.

The Neonate

It has not been possible to trace information about the elimination of the drug or its biologically active metabolite in the neonate.

Gabapentin

Gabapentin was synthesised in an attempt to produce a molecule with structural similarities to the inhibitory amino acid neurotransmitter γ-aminobutyrate (GABA) but with an increased lipophilicity that might permit it to cross the blood–brain barrier and in that organ mimic the effects of GABA. The drug has been marketed for some 20 years and has an established role as a moderately effective antiepileptic agent.

Chemistry

Gabapentin (1-aminomethyl-cyclohexyl-acetic acid) is a water-soluble white crystalline substance (molecular weight 171.34, pKa values 3.68 and 10.70). It is marketed in 100, 300, 400, 600 and 800 mg solid dosage forms and in a solution in a concentration of 50 mg per ml.

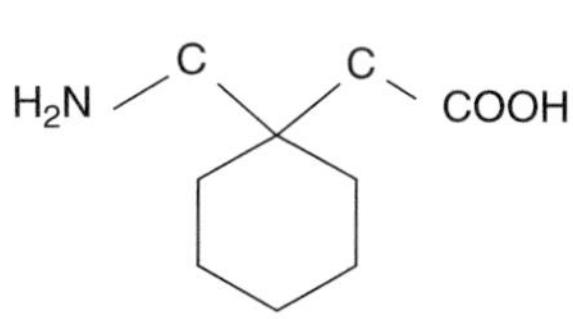

Pharmacodynamics

Despite the concept which led to the development of gabapentin, viz. the idea that it would reproduce the inhibitory neurotransmitter effects of GABA within the central nervous system, there is little convincing evidence that the drug acts through this mechanism. Instead, the drug appears to bind specifically to a protein which forms part of voltage-gated Ca^{2+} channels (Striano and Striano 2008), though exactly how this binding translates into an antiepileptic effect is not yet fully explained.

Clinically, the drug demonstrates efficacy against focal (partial) seizures. Its role in the treatment of genetic generalised tonic–clonic seizures is not well established and it appears ineffective in managing absence seizures. It has also found a use in treating neuropathic pain.

Pharmacokinetics

Absorption

Orally administered gabapentin is absorbed from the alimentary tract through the saturable active transport mechanism in the gut wall that is responsible for the uptake of L-amino acids. Because of its potentially saturable absorption, the oral bioavailability of the drug, which is around 60 % for a 300 mg dose, lessens with the increasing size of individual oral drug doses.

Distribution

Gabapentin does not bind to plasma proteins, has an apparent volume of distribution (approximately 0.9 L per kilogram) that is a little greater than the volume of total body water and enters the brain by active transport mediated by the L-amino acid uptake mechanism in the blood–brain barrier. The gabapentin concentration in CSF can be anywhere between 7 % and 35 % of its simultaneous concentration in plasma.

Elimination

The half-life of gabapentin is 5–7 h and the plasma clearance around 0.9 L per kilogram per hour. The half-life is inversely related to the creatinine clearance.

Excretion Unchanged

No metabolite of gabapentin has been found in human urine. Apparently the entire absorbed dose of the drug is excreted intact.

Metabolism

In humans, as mentioned immediately above, gabapentin forms no known biotransformation products.

Clinical Pharmacokinetics

Steady-state conditions should apply approximately 2 days after a gabapentin dosage change. The clearance of the drug tends to be inversely related to the efficiency of renal function.

Patsalos et al. (2008) proposed that the therapeutic range of plasma concentrations for the drug was between 2 and 20 mg/L.

Interactions

Since gabapentin is not metabolised in the human body, it does not interact with co-administered drugs, including antiepileptic agents, which are cleared from the human body by biotransformation. It also does not interact with the steroidal sex hormones contained in combined oral contraceptive pills (Eldon et al. 1998). Virtually no interactions involving the drug are known, though antacids containing aluminium or magnesium hydroxides may interfere with its absorption from the alimentary tract.

Adverse Effects

The main adverse effects of the drug include drowsiness and sometimes dizziness, unsteadiness, headache, and double vision. Gabapentin seems to have very few serious idiosyncratic unwanted effects.

Teratogenicity

The issue of gabapentin's teratogenicity is considered in Chap. 9.

Pregnancy

Relatively little information is available regarding the disposition of gabapentin in the mother and her foetus.

The Mother

No relevant data have been found in the literature.

The Foetus

At birth, Öhman et al. (2005) found that, in five mother–infant pairs, the average umbilical cord vein gabapentin concentration was 1.7 times (range 1.3–2.1) that in maternal plasma.

Breast Milk

Öhman et al. (2005) also found that, between 2 weeks and 3 months after childbirth, gabapentin concentrations were similar in maternal plasma and in breast milk. This is not surprising, because the drug is not bound to plasma proteins and probably simply equilibrates between the two fluids. Davanzo et al. (2013) stated that the milk concentration could be between 70 and 130 % of that in maternal plasma.

The Neonate

According to Öhman et al. (2005), in the breastfed baby, the plasma gabapentin concentration was approximately 12 % of that in the mother, with the drug's elimination half-life being 14 h.

Vigabatrin

Vigabatrin was developed with the strategic intention of raising brain concentrations of the inhibitory neurotransmitter GABA by inactivating the enzyme responsible for catalysing its catabolism, viz. GABA transaminase. For a time the drug seemed to offer very useful therapeutic benefits in treating focal epilepsies. However, the subsequent recognition that vigabatrin could be responsible for serious adverse effects involving vision has considerably limited the drug's use.

Chemistry

Vigabatrin (γ-vinyl-GABA) is a white, water-soluble material (molecular weight 129.16) which is supplied commercially as a mix of equal parts of the [S]- and [R]-stereoisomers, though only the former is biologically active. It is marketed in a 500 mg solid dosage form and as a powder.

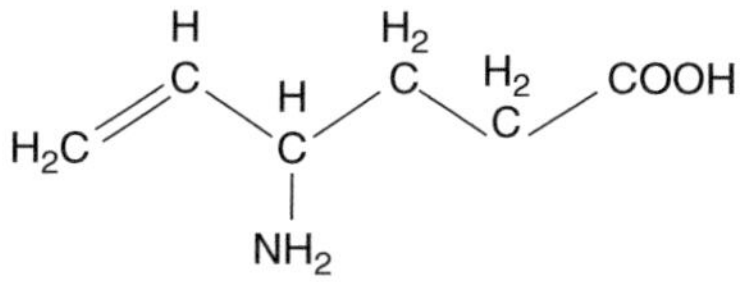

Pharmacodynamics

Vigabatrin is an irreversible inhibitor of the enzyme GABA transaminase. After a dose, the drug's action persists, irrespective of the presence of intact vigabatrin in biological fluids, until new transaminase is synthesised. The drug was being used with success in treating focal epilepsies and some varieties of genetic generalised epilepsies, until the frequency of the visual problems associated with the drug's use was recognised. At the present time, vigabatrin's use is largely confined to the treatment of myoclonic epilepsies in the very young, in particular infantile spasms.

Pharmacokinetics

Absorption

Based on urinary excretion data, the oral bioavailability of the [S]-enantiomer of vigabatrin appears to be at least 50 % and that of the biologically inactive [R]-enantiomer 65 % or greater.

Distribution

The apparent volume of distribution of [S]-vigabatrin is around 1.2 L per kg. The drug is not bound to plasma proteins. CSF concentrations of the racemic drug are about 10 % of those in plasma.

Elimination

In the doses formerly used in adults, the kinetics of vigabatrin are reported to be linear. The half-life is in the range 5–7 h, but because of the irreversible nature of the drug's mechanism of action, its biological half-life is considerably longer, basically being determined by the rate of new GABA transaminase synthesis.

Excretion Unchanged

The full absorbed dose of vigabatrin is excreted unchanged in urine.

Metabolism

The drug is not metabolised in humans.

Clinical Pharmacokinetics

No relevant data are available, except that Patsalos et al. (2008) considered that the therapeutic range of plasma concentrations of the drug was 0.8–34 mg/L.

Interactions

Relatively few pharmacokinetic interactions of vigabatrin are known. When the drug is taken by persons who are also taking phenytoin, there is a decline in plasma phenytoin levels after a delay of some weeks. The mechanism involved is not clear.

Adverse Effects

Vigabatrin is responsible for the relatively frequent occurrence of a delayed-onset and progressive concentric constriction of the periphery of the visual fields. This adverse effect has very seriously limited the use of an otherwise promising antiepileptic agent. Apart from this adverse effect, the drug seems to cause relatively few problems though fatigue, drowsiness, dizziness, mood changes, depression and psychosis have been reported.

Teratogenicity

The available information concerning the teratogenicity of the drug is mentioned in Chap. 9.

Pregnancy

The Mother

Challier et al. (1992) found that the human placenta took up S(+)-vigabatrin in preference to the R(−) enantiomer and that no metabolism of the drug occurred in placental tissue. These authors suggested that the drug might have a stereospecific uptake mechanism which is situated on the maternal side of the placental barrier.

The Foetus

With measurements being made at different times after drug intake, Tran et al. (1998) observed in one of two newborn mother–infant pairs that the ratio of foetal to maternal concentrations of R(−) vigabatrin was 0.068 and that for the S(+) enantiomer 0.16. For the other mother–infant pair, the ratios were 1.39 and 0.91, respectively.

Breast Milk

Vigabatrin concentrations in breast milk were lower than those simultaneously present in maternal plasma (Tran et al. 1998). The transfer of the [S]-enantiomer into milk was slower than the transfer of the [R]-enantiomer.

The Neonate

No relevant data have been found in the available literature.

Ethosuximide

Ethosuximide has been in use since 1958 as an agent with specific efficacy in treating absence seizures. Not a great deal of information is available about the drug's disposition in pregnancy, probably because childbearing often is delayed in affluent societies until after the age in which absence seizures still occur.

Chemistry

Ethosuximide (2-ethyl-2methylsuccinimide) is a white crystalline water-soluble material (molecular weight 141.2, pKa value 9.3). It is marketed in 250 mg capsules and in a syrup formulation for younger children.

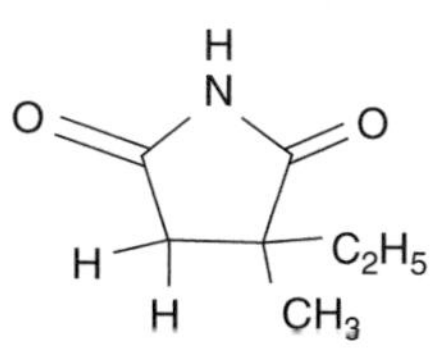

Pharmacodynamics

The action of ethosuximide is mediated through its binding to 'T'-type Ca^{2+} channels in the thalamus. Inactivation of these channels interrupts circuits connecting the thalamus to the frontal lobes and thereby prevents absences. The drug is not effective in other epileptic syndromes.

Pharmacokinetics

The pharmacokinetics of ethosuximide appears to be linear at therapeutic dosages.

Absorption

It is believed that oral doses of the drug are reasonably fully absorbed, though it has been difficult to find actual measured values of its oral bioavailability.

Distribution

Several groups of workers have estimated that the mean value of the apparent volume of distribution of the drug is close to 0.7 L per kilogram, suggesting that the drug is distributed throughout body water. Ethosuximide is not bound to plasma proteins and its concentrations in cerebrospinal fluid and in saliva are close to its plasma ones.

Elimination

A number of measurements of the elimination half-life of ethosuximide have been published, the majority of the values being in the 52–56 h range. Published values for the apparent clearance of the drug have averaged between 0.010 and 0.016 L per kilogram per hour.

Excretion Unchanged

About 20 % of an ethosuximide dose is excreted unchanged in urine.

Metabolism

The drug is oxidised to a number of hydroxy or keto derivatives, the main one being 2-(1-hydroxyethyl)-2-methylsuccinimide.

Clinical Pharmacokinetics

Steady-state plasma ethosuximide concentrations increase in proportion to drug dose, at least up to plasma drug concentrations of around 100 mg per ml. There is some evidence of a departure from linearity at higher plasma ethosuximide concentrations (Eadie et al. 1977). A consensus has developed that plasma ethosuximide concentrations in the range of 40–100 mg/L seem to offer the best prospects of controlling absence seizures while avoiding unacceptable adverse effects.

Interactions

There is an old, subsequently unconfirmed, report that ethosuximide co-administration may raise plasma phenytoin concentrations in humans (Frantzen et al. 1967).

Carbamazepine and primidone, if taken in conjunction with ethosuximide, tend to lower the plasma levels of the latter. There is a report of ethosuximide intoxication following the addition of isoniazid to existing ethosuximide therapy (van Wieringen and Vrijlandt 1983).

Adverse Effects

Excessive ethosuximide doses produced tiredness, headache and feelings of dysequilibrium. Idiosyncratic unwanted effects include skin rashes and a lupus erythematosus-type syndrome, but these are uncommon.

Teratogenesis

Information regarding the teratogenic potential of ethosuximide is to be found in Chap. 9.

Pregnancy

The Mother

Kuhnz et al. (1984) noted a slight decrease in the clearance of ethosuximide during two of three pregnancies treated with the drug. Their mean value of the clearance was 0.014 L per kilogram per hour, which is not appreciably different from the value which applies for non-pregnant adults cited above. Tomson et al. (1990)

measured the clearances of ethosuximide before pregnancy and in each trimester of 6 pregnancies. However, in some of these pregnancies, other antiepileptic drugs were being taken. There was no definite change in the drug's clearance at any stage. Later Tomson and Villén (1994) noted little change in plasma ethosuximide concentrations during the course of three pregnancies in two women. In these women the concentration relationship between the enantiomeric metabolites of the drug remained unchanged throughout.

The Foetus

Rane and Tunell (1981) found that, during several months of breastfeeding, the plasma ethosuximide concentrations in the infant of a mother taking the drug averaged 24 % of those in the mother's plasma. Kuhnz et al. (1984) described a plasma ethosuximide concentration ratio of 0.7–1.0 between the foetus and the mother.

Breast Milk

Rane and Tunell (1981) followed the milk to maternal plasma ethosuximide concentration ratio throughout one woman's 4 1/2-month period of breastfeeding. The ratio over this period had an average value of 0.8–1.0. Kuhnz et al. (1984) found that breast milk concentrations of ethosuximide averaged 86 % of those in the mother's plasma. Davanzo et al. (2013) put the figure for this parameter at 94 %.

The Neonate

In one neonate, Koup et al. (1978) measured the elimination half-life of ethosuximide as 41.3 h. Kuhnz et al. (1984) found the half-lives of the drug in three neonates were 32, 37 and 38 h, respectively, in their first few days of extrauterine life. All these values are lower than those that apply in adults.

Clonazepam

Several benzodiazepine derivatives have been used as antiepileptic agents since this class of drug became available some two-thirds of the way through the twentieth century. Only clonazepam is discussed here. There are many pharmacological similarities between the various 1,4-benzodiazepines, but clonazepam was the member of that drug family that was marketed in particular for epilepsy, though it has subsequently found other uses.

A 1,5-benzodiazepine, clobazam, has also found some use in managing epilepsy in pregnant women, but in the great majority of instances, it has been employed in conjunction with other antiepileptic drugs. It has not been possible to trace reports of the effects of pregnancy on aspects of its clinical pharmacology. There appear to be no reports suggesting that it may harm the foetus.

Chemistry

Clonazepam (7-nitro-5-(2-chlorophenyl)-1,3-dihydro-2H-1,4 benzodiazepine-2-one) is one of a number of 1,4-benzodiazepines that have been synthesised. It is a yellowish-white crystalline substance (molecular weight 315.72; pKa values 1.5 and 10.5).

The drug is supplied for therapeutic use as 0.5 and 2 mg tablets, as an oral solution and as an injection for intramuscular or intravenous administration.

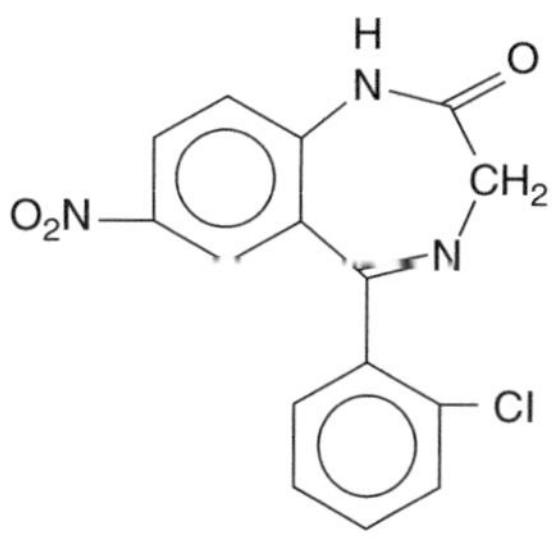

Pharmacodynamics

Like other 1,4-benzodiazepines, clonazepam acts at a molecular level by binding to specific sites on brain $GABA_A$ receptors. The binding facilitates Cl^- ion entry into neurons, resulting in their becoming hyperpolarised. Clonazepam may also temporarily raise brain serotonin concentrations, an effect which could play a part in the anti-myoclonic actions of the drug.

These molecular actions appear capable of accounting for the drug's ability to control the convulsive seizures of both focal (secondarily generalised) and genetic generalised epilepsies and also myoclonic seizures. Clonazepam may help relieve the pain of trigeminal neuralgia and the orbicularis oculi contractions of blepharospasm. The drug also appears to be finding a use in providing symptomatic relief for vertigo.

Pharmacokinetics

The kinetics of clonazepam are linear over the concentration range likely to be encountered in human therapy.

Absorption

The absorption of orally administered clonazepam appears to be virtually complete. Peak plasma levels occur within 3 h of intake.

Distribution

Published values for the apparent volume distribution of clonazepam have usually been around 2–3 L per kilogram, suggesting that the drug is accumulated within body tissues.

In the adult some 80 % or 86 % of the drug in plasma is protein bound.

Elimination

A number of measurements of the elimination half-life of clonazepam have produced values mainly in the range 22–36 h, though both higher and lower figures have been obtained in some studies. Apparent clearance values have been around 0.09 ± 0.05 L per kilogram per hour (Eadie et al. 1977).

Excretion Unchanged

Virtually no clonazepam is excreted in urine unmetabolised.

Metabolism

Clonazepam is biotransformed into a number of metabolites, either by reduction of the nitro group on positions 7 of the benzene ring or by oxidation at the 3 position on the diazepine moiety. As far as is known, the metabolites lack biological activity.

Clinical Pharmacokinetics

With regular intake, steady-state conditions for clonazepam should apply 5–8 days after a dosage change. In the treated population, there appears to be relatively little correlation between the drug's concentration in plasma and its biological effects, though this lack of correlation does not necessarily apply in the individual.

Patsalos et al. (2008) considered that the therapeutic range of plasma concentrations for the drug lay between 0.02 and 0.07 mg/L.

Interactions

Some rather contradictory data have been published in relation to a possible interaction between clonazepam and phenytoin. Different authors have shown that plasma phenytoin levels may be reduced or increased, if clonazepam is added to phenytoin therapy. The drug does not appear to alter plasma phenobarbitone, primidone or carbamazepine levels.

Phenytoin or phenobarbitone co-administration may lower plasma clonazepam levels.

Adverse Effects

Clonazepam may cause dose-related drowsiness and ataxia, while some patients taking the drug become aggressive. A degree of tolerance to sedation from the drug can develop. If continuous treatment with clonazepam is ceased abruptly, withdrawal seizures may occur. Idiopathic toxicity is rare. The drug may cause some increase in salivary and bronchial secretions.

Teratogenicity

The teratogenicity of the drug is considered in Chap. 9.

Pregnancy

The Mother

In seven women, Tomson et al. (1990) investigated the relationship between plasma clonazepam concentrations and drug dose before pregnancy and in all three trimesters of pregnancy. Before pregnancy the mean clearance rate was 0.1219 ± 0.0820 L per minute [7.32 L/h], in the first trimester 0.128 ± 0.884 L per minute [7.68 L/h], in the second trimester 0.1336 ± 0. 0857 L per minute [8.02 L/h] and in the third trimester 0.1432 ± 0.0818 L per minute [8.58 L/h]. These numbers reflect a statistically significant increase in the drug's clearance during pregnancy.

The Foetus

In a breastfed infant, Rane and Tunell (1981) found that the plasma clonazepam concentration was approximately 24 % of that simultaneously present in maternal plasma.

Breast Milk

Rane and Tunell (1981) calculated that the milk concentration of clonazepam averaged around 80 % of its simultaneous maternal plasma concentration during the course of four and a half months of breastfeeding in the one infant.

The Neonate

In the neonate, Pacifi et al. (1984) found that the proportion of unbound clonazepam in plasma (17.3 ± 0.7 %) was a little higher than in the adult (13.9 ± 0.2 %). In neonates who had previously been treated with phenobarbitone because of neonatal seizures and who had subsequently been injected with clonazepam, but had not been exposed to the drug during pregnancy, André et al. (1986) obtained elimination half-life values for the benzodiazepine that ranged between 20 and 43 h. Such figures may not necessarily apply in neonates exposed to clonazepam throughout pregnancy and who were not breastfed afterwards.

Zonisamide

Zonisamide was developed in Japan and had been in use there for some time before it began to be marketed in Europe (from 2007 onwards).

Chemistry

The drug is a benzisoxazole derivative (1,2-benzisoxazole-3-methanesulphonamide) with a molecular weight of 212.2. It is a white crystalline material (pKa value 9.7) which is supplied in solid dosage forms containing 25, 50 and 100 mg of active substance.

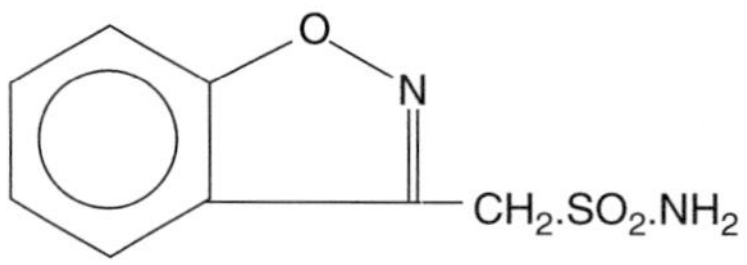

Pharmacodynamics

At the molecular level, zonisamide appears to act by blocking voltage- and use-dependent Na^+ ion channels in cell membranes. It also exerts some effects through inactivating voltage-gated T-type Ca^{2+} channels, by binding to the

GABA–benzodiazepine receptor complex and by raising brain GABA, dopamine and serotonin concentrations. As well, the drug is a carbonic anhydrase inhibitor.

Pharmacokinetics

Sills and Brodie (2007) have published an account of the drug's pharmacokinetics.

Absorption

The drug's oral bioavailability is thought to be close to 100 %.

Distribution

The apparent volume of distribution of zonisamide is in the range 1.1–1.8 L per kilogram. Some 40–50 % of zonisamide in plasma is protein bound. The drug accumulates in red blood cells.

Elimination

The elimination half-life of zonisamide is relatively long, some 50–70 h, when it is used in the absence of enzyme-inducing antiepileptic agents. The drug's apparent clearance is between 0.010 and 0.020 L per kilogram per hour, i.e. 0.7 L per hour.

Excretion Unchanged

Some 15–30 % of a zonisamide dose is excreted in urine without being metabolised. Thus the drug appears to be eliminated mainly by virtue of biotransformation.

Metabolism

About 50 % of a zonisamide dose undergoes reduction catalysed by CYP3A4 and 20 % by acetylation. Most of the remainder of a zonisamide dose is cleared by direct glucuronidation.

Clinical Pharmacology

Some studies have suggested that steady-state plasma zonisamide levels show disproportionately great increases relative to the size of dosage increases.

Patsalos et al. (2008) considered that the drug's therapeutic range in plasma was 10–40 mg per L.

Interactions

Zonisamide does not induce or inhibit the liver microsomal enzymes involved in drug metabolism. Consequently it does not alter steady-state concentrations of phenytoin, carbamazepine, valproate or lamotrigine when added to existing therapy with these drugs.

On the other hand, co-administered drugs which induce CYP3A4 such as phenytoin, carbamazepine and phenobarbitone increase the clearance of zonisamide.

Adverse Effects

The drug causes drowsiness and dizziness and sometimes headache, nausea or loss of appetite, confusion, irritability and agitation. Occasionally double vision and ataxia occur. These unwanted effects tend to be dose related.

Zonisamide intake may also be responsible for the formation of renal calculi.

Teratogenicity

The question of the drug's capacity to produce foetal malformations is considered in Chap. 9.

Pregnancy

The available details of the pharmacokinetics of zonisamide during pregnancy are rather sparse.

The Mother

There is one report of an increased clearance of zonisamide during pregnancy in one woman who was taking no other antiepileptic drug (Oles and Bell 2008). These authors' conclusion as to the increased clearance depended on a solitary measurement of the drug's plasma concentration at 27 weeks of gestation.

The Foetus

No data are available.

Breast Milk

Davanzo et al. (2013) reported that breast milk zonisamide concentrations were 93 % of maternal plasma ones.

The Neonate

In two neonates, Kawada et al. (2002) determined that the elimination half lives of zonisamide were 109 and 61 h, respectively.

References

André M, Boutroy MJ, Dubruc C et al (1986) Clonazepam pharmacokinetics and therapeutic efficacy in neonatal seizures. Eur J Clin Pharmacol 30:585–589

Challier JC, Rey E, Bintein T, Olive G (1992) Passage of S(+) and R(−) γ-vinyl-GABA across the human isolated perfused placenta. Br J Clin Pharmacol 34:139–143

Christensen J, Sabers A, Sidenius P (2006) Oxcarbazepine concentrations during pregnancy: a retrospective study in patients with epilepsy. Neurology 67:1497–1499

Davanzo R, Bo SD, Bua J, Copertino M, Zanelli E (2013) Antiepileptic drugs and breastfeeding. Ital J Pediatr 39:50

Eadie MJ, Tyrer JH, Smith GA, McKauge L (1977) Pharmacokinetics of drugs used for petit mal absence epilepsy. Clin Exp Neurol 14:172–183

Eldon MA, Underwood BA, Randinitis EJ, Sedman AJ (1998) Gabapentin does not interact with a contraceptive regimen of norethindrone acetate and ethinyl estradiol. Neurology 50:1146–1148

Flesch G (2004) Overview of the clinical pharmacokinetics of oxcarbazepine. Clin Drug Invest 24:185–203

Frantzen E, Hansen JM, Hansen OE, Kristensen M (1967) Phenytoin (Dilantin[R]) intoxication. Acta Neurol Scand 43:440–446

Kawada K, Itoh S, Kusaka T, Isobe K, Ishii M (2002) Pharmacokinetics of zonisamide in perinatal period. Brain Dev 24:95–97

Koup R, Rose JQ, Cohen ME (1978) Ethosuximide pharmacokinetics in a pregnant patient and her newborn. Epilepsia 19:535–539

Kuhnz W, Koch S, Jakob S, Hartmann A, Helge H, Nau H (1984) Ethosuximide in epileptic women during pregnancy and lactation period. Placental transfer, serum concentrations in nursed infants and clinical status. Br J Clin Pharmacol 18:671–677

Mazzucchelli I, Onat FY, Ozaka C et al (2006) Changes in the disposition of oxcarbazepine and its metabolites during pregnancy and the puerperium. Epilepsia 47:504–509

Myllynen P, Pienimäki P, Jouppila P, Vähäkangas K (2001) Transplacental passage of oxcarbazepine and its metabolites in vivo. Epilepsia 42:1482–1485

Öhman I, Vitols S, Tomson T (2005) Pharmacokinetics of gabapentin during delivery, in the neonatal period, and lactation: does a fetal accumulation occur during pregnancy? Epilepsia 46:1621–1624

Oles KS, Bell WL (2008) Zonisamide concentrations during pregnancy. Ann Pharmacother 42:1139–1141

Pacifi GM, Taddeucci-Brunelli G, Rane A (1984) Clonazepam serum protein binding during development. Clin Pharmacol Ther 35:354–359

Patsalos PN, Berry DJ, Bourgeois BF et al (2008) Antiepileptic drugs - best practice guidelines for therapeutic drug monitoring: a position paper by the subcommission on therapeutic drug monitoring, I.L.A.E. Commission on Therapeutic Strategies. Epilepsia 49:1239–1276

Petrenaite V, Sabers A, Hansen-Schwartz J (2009) Seizure deterioration in women treated with oxcarbazepine during pregnancy. Epilepsy Res 84:245–249

Pienimäki P, Lampela E, Hakkola J, Arvela P, Raunio H, Vähäkangas K (1997) Pharmacokinetics of oxcarbazepine and carbamazepine in human placenta. Epilepsia 38:309–316

Rane A, Tunell R (1981) Ethosuximide in human milk and in plasma of a mother and her nursed infant. Br J Clin Pharmacol 12:855–858

Schmidt D, Elger CE (2004) What is the evidence that oxcarbazepine and carbamazepine are distinctly different antiepileptic drugs? Epilepsy Behav 55:627–635

Sills GJ, Brodie MJ (2007) Pharmacokinetics and drug interactions with zonisamide. Epilepsia 48:435–441

Striano P, Striano S (2008) Gabapentin: a Ca^{2+} channel α-2-δ ligand far beyond epilepsy. Drugs Today 44:353–368

Tomson T, Villén T (1994) Ethosuximide enantiomers in pregnancy and lactation. Ther Drug Monit 16:621–623

Tomson T, Lindbom U, Hasselström J (1990) Plasma concentrations of ethosuximide and clonazepam during pregnancy. J Epilepsy 3:91–95

Tran A, O'Mahoney T, Rey E, Mai J, Mumford JP, Olive G (1998) Vigabatrin: placental transfer in vivo and excretion into breast milk of the enantiomers. Br J Clin Pharmacol 45:409–411

van Wieringen A, Vrijlandt CM (1983) Ethosuximide intoxication caused by interaction with isoniazid. Neurology 33:1227–1228

Wegner I, Edelsbroek P, de Haan G-J, Lindhout D, Sander JW (2010) Drug monitoring of lamotrigine and oxcarbazepine combinations during pregnancy. Epilepsia 51:2500–2502

Part II
Antiepileptic Drugs and the Foetus

Chapter 7
Antiepileptic Drugs, Epileptic Seizures and the Foetus

Abstract This chapter deals with two main issues, viz. the possible effects of pregnancy on the course of maternal epileptic seizure disorders and the effects of seizure disorders on pregnant women and their foetuses.

The little information that is available suggests that pregnancy tends to increase the risk of loss of seizure control in women whose epilepsy is untreated. The interpretation of the more extensive literature concerning antiepileptic drug-treated epilepsy in pregnancy is confounded by the effect of pregnancy in tending to decrease circulating concentrations of antiepileptic drugs relative to drug dose. It appears that, in the majority of instances, seizure control does not deteriorate during antiepileptic drug-treated pregnancy but that, if seizure control changes, it is more likely to worsen than to improve. However, when attention has been given to maintaining satisfactory pre-pregnancy circulating concentrations of antiepileptic drugs throughout pregnancy, the impaired seizure control seems to be avoided.

There is little published evidence of maternal injury from epileptic seizures during pregnancy or of significantly increased pregnancy complications such as spontaneous abortion or stillbirth, though neonates born to women taking antiepileptic drugs tend to be a little premature, smaller and of lower birth weight for gestation age than would be expected. Seizures during pregnancy do not seem to be a significant cause of foetal damage.

If epileptic seizures ceased occurring during human pregnancy, as migraine attacks often do, there would be relatively little justification for the existence of the present book. Unfortunately seizures do occur in pregnant women. Therefore certain possibilities need to be considered: (1) Does the physiological state of pregnancy in its own right temporarily or permanently modify the course of seizure disorders? (2) Does the altered disposition of antiepileptic drugs during pregnancy (see Chap. 3) affect the occurrence of seizures? (3) Does having epilepsy, and in particular experiencing epileptic seizures during pregnancy, influence the course of pregnancy or affect the well-being of the foetus?

M.J. Eadie, F.J.E. Vajda, *Antiepileptic Drugs and Pregnancy: A Guide for Prescribers*, DOI 10.1007/978-3-319-21434-4_7

Effects of Pregnancy on Seizure Disorders

Catamenial Epilepsy

The entity of catamenial epilepsy reflects the fact that, at least in some women, epileptic seizures tend to be experienced at particular stages of the menstrual cycle. The circulating steroidal sex hormone changes that take place during the ovulatory menstrual cycle are a forerunner to those hormonal changes that occur in the earlier weeks of pregnancy. Therefore what happens to seizure occurrence across the menstrual cycle may be seen to provide a possible precedent to the behaviour of seizure disorders during pregnancy.

Depending on how the term 'catamenial epilepsy' is defined, it appears that one-third to one-half of women with epilepsy may have this disorder, in which seizures show a proclivity to occur at mid-cycle or around the time of menstruation. Herkes et al. (1993) used measurements of the course of daily salivary progesterone concentrations throughout the menstrual cycle to define if, and when, catamenial seizures occurred. They studied 20 menstrual cycles (12 ovulatory and 8 anovulatory) in 11 women with catamenial epilepsy who were not using oral contraceptives. In the ovulatory cycles, there were statistically significant increases in seizure frequency at the onset of the rise in progesterone concentrations at mid-cycle and also increases in seizures premenstrually, but in anovulatory cycles, there were only premenstrual increases. Allowing for some possible time lag in hormonal effects, this behaviour of seizure occurrence appears to correlate in a general way with the knowledge that oestrogens increase the excitability of the brain and therefore the chance of having seizures, while progestogens decrease it (Morrell 2002). The decreased cerebral excitability known to be associated with progesterone intake may be mediated mainly by the non-hormonally active progesterone metabolite allopregnanolone which acts at $GABA_A$ receptors. However, additional factors may bear on the situation.

It is possible that concurrent antiepileptic drug therapy in women with epilepsy may alter sex hormone concentrations during the menstrual cycle. As mentioned in Chap. 2, the so-called 'inducing' antiepileptic drugs not only increase the activities of CYP isoenzymes, including CYP3A4, but also that of UDP-glucuronosyl transferases which catalyse the metabolism of oestrogens and progestogens (Reddy 2010). Possibly such enzyme induction could cause reduced circulating concentrations of the steroidal sex hormones and by doing this influence the tendency to catamenial patterns of seizure occurrence. We have not traced investigations that have studied this possibility in detail.

Another relevant possibility is that the hormonal changes of the menstrual cycle may alter circulating concentration of antiepileptic drugs in a cyclic pattern and that this alteration may influence the timing of seizure occurrence during the cycle. Some information is available concerning antiepileptic drug clearance changes across the menstrual cycle. In some women there appears to be a tendency for plasma phenytoin levels to fall, relative to drug dose, around the time of menstruation

(Rosciszewska et al. 1986). In keeping with this observation, Shavit et al. (1984) showed that the clearance of phenytoin tended to be higher at the time of menstruation than at mid-interval and that the elimination half-life of the drug was a little shorter premenstrually. Wegner et al. (2010) measured plasma lamotrigine concentrations every second day across the menstrual cycle in 7 women who were not taking oral contraceptives and found no statistically significant change in lamotrigine clearance. Also in women who were not using oral contraceptives, Herzog (2009) found a nonstatistically significant 31.3 % decrease in circulating lamotrigine levels and an 8.3 % decrease in valproate ones, in the mid-luteal phase as compared with the mid-follicular phase of the menstrual cycle. Both of these groups of workers also studied women taking oral contraceptives. In these women, clearances of the antiepileptic drugs concerned were statistically significantly increased in the stage of the cycle when synthetic hormone intake was present.

Overall, the above data suggest that during the menstrual cycle, variation in plasma concentration of antiepileptic drugs relative to drug dose and physiological or iatrogenically produced sex hormonal level changes may both contribute to the catamenial occurrence of epileptic seizures. Is this experience consonant with what happens in women with epilepsy during their pregnancies?

Seizure Occurrence Rates in Pregnancy

At first sight, it might seem simple enough to determine whether pregnancy in its own right altered the rate of occurrence of epileptic seizures. In practice, attempts to settle the matter have been confounded by the possible effects of the antiepileptic drug therapy that is usually taken during pregnancy by women with epilepsy.

The first at least modestly effective antiepileptic agents began to come into use after 1857 when Locock's comments about the effectiveness of potassium bromide in 'hysterical' epilepsy appeared in the medical press (Eadie 2012). The effects of these comments were soon afterwards reinforced by Wilks (1861) who, unaware of Locock's comments, published a report of the drug's effectiveness in a small series of patients with epilepsy. Over the subsequent century and a half, further agents possessing greater antiepileptic efficacies became available and were then used extensively. As a result, at least in Western societies, for very many years there has been almost no experience of the natural history of untreated epilepsy. Attempts have been made to remedy this deficiency in knowledge of the course of the untreated disorder by studying the natural history of epilepsy in societies where drug treatments are unavailable or are too expensive for widespread use. Unfortunately, in those societies the aetiologies of epilepsy may be different from those in Western societies, and medical records, if available, are less likely to be adequate for later study. If one were to attempt to ascertain the course of untreated, or ineffectively treated, epilepsy in Western societies before the introduction of potassium bromide in the mid-nineteenth century, there would again be problems. Prior to that time, relatively few statistical data concerning epilepsy had been published, and the clinical spectrum of the disorder then diagnosed as 'epilepsy' was considerably less extensive than it now is. In the latter half of the nineteenth century, it was rather widely held that epilepsy was a disease in its own right, one with no detectable pathological basis, though Gowers (1881) in his monograph seemed to accept that such epilepsy could also be due to inactive, though not to active, brain pathology. Hence epileptic seizures attributed to a recognised cause were often not included in the epilepsy statistics at the time when no effective therapy was available. Herpin's posthumous monograph, which described the wealth of epileptic aura and minor seizure phenomena, appeared before 1870 (Herpin 1867), but it received little notice until near the end of the century. Consequently, focal epilepsies which did not culminate in convulsing also tended not to be included in epilepsy statistics until well after potentially effective antiepileptic drug therapy in the form of potassium bromide was available. Therefore the few available statistics concerning seizure frequency that were collected prior to 1850 usually applied to generalised convulsive seizures that had no recognised underlying pathological cause. Such data do not easily equate with what is today considered to be epilepsy.

The above matters and the evidence that plasma levels of many antiepileptic drug levels fall, relative to dose, during pregnancy (Chaps. 3, 4, 5 and 6) need to be kept in mind when considering what is known about the reported behaviour of epileptic seizure disorders during pregnancy.

Nineteenth-century monographs on epilepsy do contain some statements concerning the course of seizure disorders during pregnancy. For the most part, these statements seem to have been based not on quantitative data but on individual authors' impressions or on memories of particular instances, e.g. of a woman with previously active epilepsy who became seizure-free while pregnant. The account of Raoul Béraud in a University of Paris MD thesis in 1884 is probably the first to contain useful statistics. In his series of 31 pregnancies, seizures became more frequent in 26 % and less frequent in 48 % and were unaltered in frequency in the remaining 26 %. Béraud concluded that (1) pregnancy did not cause epilepsy or modify the pattern of an individual's seizures and that (2) the influence of pregnancy on epilepsy did not extend beyond the duration of pregnancy. He stated that epilepsy did not predispose to eclampsia and that maternal bromide intake was not harmful to the foetus. This latter item of information suggests that not all of his collection of pregnancies had been untreated.

Knight and Rhind (1975) studied 153 pregnancies in 59 women with epilepsy. Seizure frequency increased during pregnancy in 45.2 % and decreased in 4.8 % and was unchanged in the remainder. A few years later, Schmidt (1982) summarised the numerical data concerning the effects of pregnancy on seizure frequency that could be found in the available literature published during the preceding century. In total, he found record of 2165 pregnancies in women with epilepsy. Seizures had become more frequent in 24.1 % of these pregnancies and less frequent in 22.7 % and were unaltered in frequency in 53.2 %. He recognised that different authors had employed different criteria for determining seizure improvement or worsening. Possibly because of this, he did not pursue his analysis in greater detail. The individual 28 data sets that he analysed contained substantially different numbers of pregnancies. Seizure numbers were in fact increased in pregnancy in 16 of the data sets and decreased in 10. All the series dated from times when antiepileptic drug therapy was available, but it was only at the end of the time period that Schmidt surveyed that the possible implications of altered antiepileptic drug disposition during pregnancy began to be appreciated.

In the following year, Schmidt et al. (1983) reported on their monitoring of the course of 136 pregnancies in 122 women with epilepsy. In 37 %, the number of seizures increased during pregnancy or the puerperium, and in 13 % the number decreased. In half of their pregnancies, the rate of seizure occurrence was unaltered. Otani (1985) found that 27 % of a series of 125 women with epilepsy were poorly compliant with antiepileptic drug therapy during pregnancy. The seizure frequency was unaltered in 80 % of the remaining women, increased in 16 % and decreased in 4 %. Bardy (1987) compared seizure numbers in the pre-pregnancy year, during pregnancy and in the three postnatal months, in 140 women with epilepsy. Seizure numbers increased during pregnancy in 32 % and decreased in 14 %. Gjerde et al. (1988), on the other hand, found no statistically significant difference in seizure occurrence rates before and during pregnancy.

Sabers and Dam (1990) analysed the literature reports of seizure occurrence during pregnancy that had been published between 1884 and 1987. This data set must have largely coincided with that of Schmidt (1982) referred to immediately above. Sabers and Dam subdivided their material into three time periods, viz. 1884–1937, 1938–1970 and 1971–1987. They showed that the proportions of pregnancies in which seizure frequency was unchanged increased from 26 %, through 47 % to 58 % over these periods, that the proportions of pregnancies with increased seizures fell from 42 % through 35 % to 28 % and that the proportions with decreased seizures fell from 32 % through 18 % to 14 %. Thus in all three time periods, seizure frequency increased in pregnancy more often than it decreased. Tanganelli and Regesta (1992) found seizure frequency unchanged in nearly 80 % of pregnancies in their women with epilepsy.

In the past quarter of a century, further case series have been published whose findings are increasingly relevant to the current clinical situation regarding epilepsy. For instance, Chen et al. (2009) remarked on a statistically significant increase in seizures in 1016 pregnancies in Taiwanese women, and Yerby (2008) stated that, in the literature, seizures had increased in one-quarter to one-third of the pregnancies of women with epilepsy. Further, the increase was unrelated to the seizure type that was present.

More recently, there has been an increasing trend to report results of seizure disorder behaviour during pregnancy in terms of whether pregnancy was or was not seizure-free, rather than in terms of alterations in the numbers of seizure that occurred. This all or nothing criterion has become increasingly significant in relation to the life situations of women with epilepsy when loss of seizure control increasingly limits the sufferer's lifestyle, particularly in relation to vehicle driving. The EURAP Study Group (2006) reported that 58.3 % of 1956 pregnancies in their pregnancy registry had been seizure free. Mawer et al. (2010) found that 50 % of their series of 277 pregnancies in women with epilepsy were seizure-free throughout pregnancy. Battino et al. (2013) subsequently indicated that 66.6 % of 3806 pregnancies in the EURAP registry that had been treated with carbamazepine, phenobarbitone, valproate or lamotrigine monotherapy had remained seizure-free throughout pregnancy. Women with genetic generalised epilepsies were more likely than women with focal epilepsies to experience seizure-free pregnancies (73.6 % as compared with 59.5 %). Seizure control had worsened during pregnancy in 15.8 % of the EURAP pregnancies. It was noted that the pregnancies managed with lamotrigine monotherapy were less likely to be seizure-free than the remaining treated pregnancies. Reisinger et al. (2013) found that, in 115 pregnancies in 95 women with epilepsy, seizures were more likely to occur during pregnancy if the epilepsy involved was a focal one.

Some Australian Pregnancy Register data are probably included in the above EURAP data, but the amount is unknown. The Australian Register has continued to accumulate pregnancies since the time of the Battino et al. (2013) analysis. Of 1592 antiepileptic drug-treated pregnancies in the Australian Register by the end of 2013, some 53.5 % had been seizure-free throughout pregnancy. In 692 of these 1592 Australian pregnancies, the women involved had suffered seizures in their pre-pregnancy year, whereas in the remaining 900 the women (56.5 %) had been free from seizures for at least a year before becoming pregnant. Of those with active seizure disorders in the pre-pregnancy year, 78.9 % continued to have seizures during pregnancy. Of the 900 who were seizure-free for at least a year before pregnancy, only 21.7 % experienced seizures during pregnancy. Generalised convulsive seizures are more likely to be remembered than more minor epileptic manifestations. In the Australian Register, 258 of the 1592 pregnancies were associated with generalised convulsive seizures in the pre-pregnancy year, but 298 had such seizures during the shorter nine-month duration of pregnancy (16.2 % versus 18.7 %).

Of the pregnancies in the Australian Register, 785 had occurred in women with focal epilepsies and 669 in women with genetic generalised epilepsies (the seizure disorder type being uncertain in the remainder). Seizures of some type had occurred in the pre-pregnancy year in 49.9 % of the pregnancies in women with focal epilepsies and in 53.6 % during pregnancy. In these same women, generalised convulsive seizures had occurred in 28.2 % during the pre-pregnancy year but in 17.1 % during the shorter nine-month period of pregnancy. As to the pregnancies of women with genetic generalised epilepsies, the rate of occurrence of any type of seizure was 37.1 % during the pre-pregnancy year and 39.6 % during pregnancy. Generalised convulsive seizures had occurred in 18.4 % of the pregnancies in this idiopathic/genetic generalised epilepsy subset during the year prior to pregnancy and in 19.9 % during the nine months of pregnancy. Thus, in a series of pregnancies managed by what one would hope, but could not guarantee, was contemporary good therapeutic practice, there still appeared to be a tendency for decreased complete seizure disorder control during antiepileptic drug-treated pregnancy. Nevertheless, more than half of all pregnancies remained totally seizure-free throughout.

Factors Influencing Seizure Occurrence During Pregnancy

The above data suggest that the types of seizure disorder present in a very considerable majority of treated women probably were not significant factors in determining whether or not seizure control deteriorated during pregnancy. In contrast, the overall activity of the seizure disorders in the year before pregnancy appeared to have a significant effect on seizure freedom rates during pregnancy.

In the Australian Register data then available, Vajda et al. (2008) analysed the likelihood of seizures occurring during pregnancy in relation to the duration of seizure freedom prior to pregnancy. The outcome is summarised in Fig. 7.1, which contains data subsequent to the 2008 publication. There appeared to be a substantially lower risk of seizures recurring during pregnancy if there had been 18 months seizure freedom before pregnancy. Longer periods of seizure freedom than this offered almost negligible further advantages. As a general guide, 1 year seizure freedom before pregnancy probably would offer the best compromise between the disadvantage arising from experiencing seizures in pregnancy and the disadvantages from delaying pregnancy for extended periods to minimise the risk of seizures occurring during pregnancy. In the year after the publication of Vajda et al. (2008), Harden et al. (2009) reached a basically similar conclusion but in relation to a 9-month seizure-free interval before pregnancy. Thomas et al. (2012), in a study of 1297 pregnancies, commented that seizures in the pre-pregnancy month increased the risk of further seizures occurring during pregnancy.

Cangetti et al. (2014) drew attention to a further factor of prognostic relevance. They obtained evidence that having had a past history of seizures predominantly in

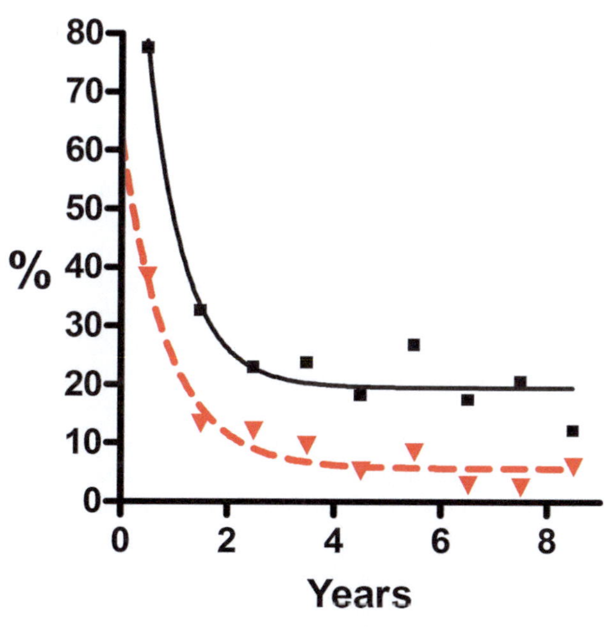

Fig. 7.1 Rates of occurrence during pregnancy for any seizures (*continuous line*) and for generalised convulsive seizures (*broken line*), related to duration of seizure freedom prior to pregnancy

the peri-menstrual few days, or in addition at the approximate time of ovulation, increased the chances of a woman experiencing a pregnancy without seizures or with reduced numbers of seizures.

From the recent literature, it appears that a majority of women with antiepileptic drug-treated epilepsy will remain seizure-free throughout their pregnancies if contemporary optimal therapeutic management practices are followed. Unfortunately, a tendency exists for some women's apparently fully controlled seizure disorders to relapse during pregnancy or for their seizures to become more frequent. There are several possible explanations for this seizure disorder worsening. Despite existing knowledge of the increased eliminations of many antiepileptic drugs during pregnancy, it is possible that antiepileptic drug dosages have not always been adjusted appropriately during pregnancy to counter the effects of falling circulating drug concentrations. This fall may have been responsible for seizures continuing to occur in 47 % of the pregnant women in the series of Schmidt et al. (1983), as at the time of that study, the importance of maintaining pre-pregnancy plasma concentration of antiepileptic drugs during pregnancy was not as widely appreciated as it now is. Accidental or deliberate noncompliance with recommended antiepileptic drug dosages is another possibility. There is some published evidence, as well as anecdotal data, indicating that noncompliance with prescribed antiepileptic drug therapy does sometimes occur during pregnancy in women with epilepsy (Schmidt et al. 1983). The latter authors also suggested that sleep deprivation in pregnancy could impair seizure control. There is the further possibility that in some women impaired seizure disorder control in pregnancy may be due to the state of being pregnant itself, by altering the intrinsic activity, or the nature, of the underlying epileptogenic process.

Seizures During Pregnancy in Women with Untreated Epilepsies

The data discussed above have been derived from pregnancies in which a substantial proportion of the women involved probably were treated with antiepileptic drugs. Are contemporary data available from women with untreated epilepsy that could clarify the effects of pregnancy on seizure control in the absence of the confounding effects of drug treatment?

In the published material summarised in the review of Schmidt (1982), there was one series of 108 pregnancies that were not treated with antiepileptic drugs. In this series, seizures increased in pregnancy in 22 %, decreased in 39 % and remained unaltered in frequency in the remaining 39 %. This report came from a University of Heidelberg dissertation (Fuchs 1965) which we have been unable to access.

The Australian Pregnancy Register at the end of 2013 contained record of 148 pregnancies in which women with epilepsy were not taking antiepileptic drugs when pregnancy commenced. In 58.1 % of these 148 pregnancies, the women involved either had never taken antiepileptic drugs or had not taken them for many months prior to pregnancy. In the remaining 41.9 % of the untreated pregnancies, the women involved had ceased drug intake shortly before becoming pregnant, probably with the intention of becoming pregnant. Of this latter group, 56.1 % had resumed antiepileptic drug intake by later pregnancy. In exactly half of the 148 pregnancies, the women involved had experienced seizures in the pre-pregnancy year. During pregnancy, seizures occurred in 56.1 % of the pregnant women, a not statistically significant change from the 50 % of seizure-affected women in the pre-pregnancy year. Unfortunately, comparing seizure occurrences in the 9-month period of pregnancy with those in the preceding 12 months may have biased the comparison against showing a significant increase in women with loss of seizure control during pregnancy. The 148 pregnancies contained 12 in which the women concerned had resumed antiepileptic drug intake before the end of pregnancy, though they remained free of seizures throughout pregnancy. Since the resumption of treatment in these 12 pregnancies may have prevented seizures that would otherwise have occurred, the 12 were excluded from further consideration. When that was done, seizures had occurred in the pre-pregnancy year in 52.2 % of those untreated during pregnancy, but in 61.0 % during pregnancy, a statistically significant increase despite the possible consequences of the two different time periods being compared. In their pre-pregnancy years, 20.6 % of these women suffered generalised convulsive seizures, while in pregnancy 26.5 % suffered such seizures, a nonstatistically significant increase.

In the whole Australian data set, there were 39 pregnancies in which the woman involved had not taken antiepileptic drugs for many months or years prior to pregnancy and had been seizure-free for at least 1 year before pregnancy. In this subset with seemingly stable inactive epilepsy, 35.9 % developed seizures of some type during pregnancy ($P<0.01$) and generalised convulsive seizures in 15.4 % ($P<0.05$).

Based on this experience, it seems that pregnancy in its own right may sometimes increase the activity of the processes underlying epileptogenesis. Simply ensuring patient compliance with therapy and maintaining circulating concentrations of antiepileptic drugs at values similar to those which prevailed before pregnancy may therefore not always suffice to prevent deterioration in seizure control during pregnancy. It is conceivable that in some women the threshold circulating concentrations of antiepileptic drugs during pregnancy that are needed to prevent seizure occurrence may be higher than in the same women when not pregnant. At present, it is impossible to know whether this is the case. However, in the current state of uncertainty regarding this matter, there may be an argument for attempting to maintain circulating plasma concentrations of antiepileptic drugs at higher levels than were necessary for seizure control before pregnancy, so long as these higher concentrations do not cause undesirable consequences for pregnant women and their foetuses. It may take considerable time to accumulate the data necessary to decide whether this suggestion is warranted.

Effects of Altered Antiepileptic Drug Disposition in Pregnancy on Seizure Occurrence

Enough clinical experience has accumulated to make it generally accepted that the proportion of patients whose seizures are controlled by a particular antiepileptic drug will probably increase as the plasma concentrations of the drug increase, at least up to a certain concentration level. This belief is the basis of the idea of the 'therapeutic range' for the drug. Values for that parameter for the individual antiepileptic drugs are cited in Chaps. 4, 5 and 6. There seems every reason to assume that a similar consideration regarding seizure control would apply during pregnancy. Therefore the known increases in antiepileptic drug clearance in pregnancy would be likely to be associated with decreased seizure control during pregnancy unless drug doses were increased to compensate for the expected decreases in circulating drug concentrations. Clinical experience seems to be in keeping with this expectation. However, there is relatively little published data that actually demonstrates its validity. Most of the relevant published material relates to lamotrigine, for which Pennell et al. (2008) and Sabers and Petrenaite (2009) provided evidence that seizure control in pregnancy was better when attempts were made to adjust dosage of the drug to compensate for the fall in plasma lamotrigine concentrations that occurs in pregnancy. Subsequently Pirie et al. (2013) traced further literature reports that were in accord with this experience.

Despite the relative paucity of specific studies concerning the matter, there seems little reason to question the clinical wisdom that reduced plasma concentrations of antiepileptic drugs during pregnancy are likely to correlate with decreased seizure disorder control.

Effects of Epilepsy, and Experiencing Seizures, on Pregnant Women and Their Foetuses

It seems reasonably widely accepted that contemporary antiepileptic drug therapy fails to fully control seizure disorders in perhaps 30 % of those treated in the general population. Despite the best contemporary therapeutic efforts, there probably also is a treatment failure rate of 30–50 % in the pregnancies in women with epilepsy. Continuing seizures, particularly in those living in more complex and technologically sophisticated societies, clearly constitute a significant source of handicap and of limitation in the quality of life. But do they confer additional physical disadvantages on pregnant women? Do seizures in pregnancy affect the course of pregnancy adversely or otherwise harm foetuses?

In a good deal of the literature that appears potentially relevant to this matter, the authors have not distinguished clearly between the effects of having actually suffered seizures during pregnancy and the effects of suffering from a seizure disorder, usually a drug-treated one, and also being pregnant.

Physical Disadvantages for Pregnant Women

There seems to be no suggestion in the literature that the occasional physical injuries brought about by, or occurring during, epileptic seizures in the general population do not also occur in pregnant women with epilepsy. Little has been published concerning whether the increased laxity of the ligaments and muscles that develops during normal pregnancy alters the hazard of bony or ligamentous injury caused by the violence of generalised convulsive seizures. As Battino and Tomson (2007) mentioned, it has generally been assumed that uncontrolled generalised convulsive seizures constitute a hazard for the mother, but actual published evidence that supports this assertion is not easily found. Published data exist for pregnancy complications in women with epilepsy (Teramo and Hillesmaa 1982), but pregnancy complications and complications attributable to seizures are not necessarily identical. There seems to be almost an unwritten consensus that the effects of epileptic seizures on the pregnant woman will not differ from those that apply to her in her nonreproductive state, except in so far as the contents of her reproductive organs are concerned.

In perhaps surprising contrast to the relatively undisturbed general physical health situations of most pregnant women with epilepsy, Edey et al. (2013) noted that in the United Kingdom official statistics for the year 2004, there was a tenfold increased mortality associated with pregnancy in women with epilepsy. Eleven of the 14 fatalities that had been reported were instances of sudden unexplained maternal death. Nine of the 14 deaths had occurred during pregnancy and the other five postnatally. Presumably most of the foetuses that these women carried were lost. Such events might easily be too rare to ever be encountered by the individual clinician or even by institutions that manage the pregnancies of substantial numbers of epileptic women. They also might not be recognised in data from the pregnancies that find their way into pregnancy registers. It is clearly important that this finding of increased mortality be confirmed in other large-scale studies.

No actual evidence is available that the maternal deaths mentioned immediately above were due to seizures. Nevertheless, the finding should encourage efforts to achieve full seizure control during pregnancy, because the data currently available suggest that sudden unexplained death in persons with epilepsy is often related to failure of seizure control, sometimes apparently consequent on failure to take prescribed antiepileptic medication.

Altered Course of Pregnancy

There have been very occasional reports of pregnancy complications such as premature labour, antepartum haemorrhage and placental abruption that have taken place in a close time relationship to the occurrence a convulsive seizure. This association might suggest that the violence of the seizure caused the complication. However, most studies have failed to find statistical evidence consistent with seizures actually being responsible for pregnancy complications, in that the complication rates have not been higher in the pregnancies of women with epilepsy, some of whom would be expected to have experienced seizures during pregnancy, than in the pregnancies of women who do not have epilepsy.

For instance, in Heidelberg Janz and Fuchs (1964) studied 426 pregnancies in women with epilepsy, employing data obtained retrospectively. No antiepileptic drug therapy was taken in 130 of these pregnancies, and one would have expected that seizures would have occurred in some of this subgroup. However, the authors reported that miscarriages and stillbirths occurred in 12.1 % of the antiepileptic drug-treated pregnancies but in 7 % of the untreated ones. The incidences of other complications of pregnancy such as premature or post-mature birth also were not greater than the average incidences for the population and as well were similar for both the treated and the untreated pregnancies. These authors gave the impression that their findings would not have been regarded as unusual if they had been obtained in a population of pregnant women who did not have seizure disorders. Speidel and Meadow (1972), in a study described further in Chap. 8, encountered similar rates of miscarriage, preterm birth and low birth weight offspring in their antiepileptic drug-treated pregnancies and in control pregnancies in women who did not have epilepsy.

Annegers et al. (1988) compared the rates of occurrence of certain pregnancy complications in women with epilepsy and in the non-epileptic wives of men with epilepsy. The gestation age-adjusted rate ratio for spontaneous abortion was not increased (0.80: 95 % confidence interval 0.45, 1.40). The cumulative risk of spontaneous abortion (18 %) for antiepileptic drug-exposed pregnancies was similar to the risk reported in non-epilepsy populations. In contrast, Schupf and Ottman (1997) found an increased hazard of spontaneous abortion in the pregnancies of women with focal-onset epilepsies which had commenced before the age of 21 years.

Bech et al. (2014) observed no increased risk of spontaneous abortion in the records of almost one million pregnancies in Danish women with antiepileptic drug-treated epilepsy. Curiously, there was a 12 % increase in the spontaneous abortion risk in women taking these drugs for indications other than epilepsy.

Richmond et al. (2004) and Katz et al. (2006) both found that the number of stillbirths among the pregnancies of adequately treated women with epilepsy was similar to that for the general population. They considered that there was no persuasive evidence for a heightened risk of obstetrical complications such as pre-eclampsia, premature birth or placental abruption in the pregnancies of women with epilepsy. However, Katz et al. (2006) also noted that a statistically significantly higher proportion of women with epilepsy had their babies delivered by Caesarean section. Thomas et al. (2009) compared the maternal pregnancy complications in women in an Indian pregnancy register with those occurring in non-epileptic women in a teaching hospital. These authors' interpretation was that there was no significant increase in complications in the pregnancies of women with epilepsy. In fact they reported a higher incidence of spontaneous abortions (4.2 % compared with 2.38 %) and of anaemia (0.62 % versus 0.22 %) in their women with epilepsy. In contrast, medical terminations of pregnancy, gestational diabetes, pregnancy-related hypertension, antepartum haemorrhage and postpartum haemorrhage were all more frequent in the control population (but the women in that population may have been admitted to hospital because their pregnancies either were complicated ones or were ones in which complications were feared).

In contrast, in at least two studies, there seem to have been increased complication rates in the pregnancies of women with epilepsy, though that does necessarily mean that seizures were responsible for the complications. When Borthen et al. (2011) in Bergen, Norway, compared the outcomes of 205 pregnancies in women with epilepsy with those in 205 control pregnancies, they found an increased risk of severe pre-eclampsia and of early pregnancy bleeding in the epilepsy-affected women. Borthen and Gilhus (2012) subsequently stated that pre-eclampsia, gestational hypertension, bleeding during pregnancy, induced labour and Caesarean section were found more often in pregnant women with epilepsy than in other pregnant women. Excessive postpartum bleeding was also more frequent in the women with epilepsy. It seems possible that the inductions of labour and the Caesarean sections reflected personal therapeutic policy rather than were consequences of epilepsy altering the course of pregnancy.

Unlike the majority of the above studies, in which there was little or no persuasive evidence of increased epilepsy-related hazards during pregnancy, Rauchenzaue et al. (2013)) did note an association between experiencing one or more generalised tonic–clonic seizures during pregnancy and giving birth to offspring with a lower gestation age, an increased incidence of prematurity and, in males, a lower birth weight.

Overall, the available literature suggests that, if epilepsy in pregnancy is managed in a manner consistent with optimal present-day standards, there probably is little heightened risk of pregnancy complications. Hence any risk due to actually suffering seizures during pregnancy appears to be, for practical purposes, small enough to be negligible in the individual woman. This is in keeping with the experience resulting from analysis of the recorded pregnancy complications in 1731 pregnancies in the Australian Pregnancy Register at the end of 2013. Of these pregnancies, 63 were associated with spontaneous abortions or stillbirths. Seizures of some type occurred in 36.5 % of pregnancies which ended in spontaneous abortion or stillbirth but in 47.6 % of the pregnancies that result in live births. In regard to generalised convulsive seizures, the corresponding figures were 12.7 and 29.9 %. The relative risk of spontaneous abortion or stillbirth was actually statistically significantly lower in pregnancies in which generalised convulsive seizures had occurred. However, it should be pointed out that, if there were spontaneous abortions that occurred at early stages of pregnancy, due either to lethal foetal malformation or other circumstances brought about by seizures, the associated pregnancies were unlikely to have been in existence long enough to have been reported to the Register. It is impossible to know whether there could have been enough such pregnancies to actually increase the spontaneous abortion risk so that it exceeded the risk associated with not having seizures.

Effects on the Foetus

It might be anticipated that the violent physical activity entailed in a generalised convulsive seizure in a pregnant woman, and the associated circulatory alterations and hypoxia, could damage the foetus she was carrying. Yerby (2008) took the view that generalised tonic–clonic seizures increased the risk of hypoxaemia, acidosis and injury from birth trauma and also the likelihood of stillbirth but then stated that such events rarely arose as consequences of seizures. There has been a report of foetal heart slowing during a maternal convulsive seizure (Teramo et al. 1979), and there have also been suggestions that foetal malformation may result from intrauterine hypoxia. But have these predictions been borne out in clinical practice?

Foetal Physical Development

Most communications dealing with pregnancies in women with epilepsy, the great majority of whom were taking antiepileptic drugs during the pregnancies, have reported that the offspring tended to be a little premature, of lower than expected birth weight and small for gestational age (e.g. Veiby et al. 2009; Lin et al. 2009; Pennell et al. 2012) and to have slightly smaller head circumferences than normal (though the circumferences reached normal values for age after 2 years). In contrast to such reports, McPherson et al. (2013) furnished statistics for 410 pregnancies in women with seizure disorders, compared with 47,118 pregnancies in non-epileptic women. These authors found that there was no increased risk of intrauterine growth retardation, stillbirth, pre-eclampsia or preterm delivery in the pregnancies of the women with epilepsy. In the records of all Danish pregnancies between 1997 and 2008, Kilic et al. (2014) detected no association between preterm birth and antiepileptic drug-treated seizure disorders but found an association between the two if the mothers had been taking these drugs for conditions other than epilepsy. Artama et al. (2013), in their analysis of Finnish national data, noted an excess of infant deaths in foetuses exposed to antiepileptic drugs during pregnancy. Barroso et al. (2014) also found an excess of neonatal deaths from pregnancies exposed to antiepileptic drugs (mainly phenobarbitone). As for pregnancy complications, there seems little convincing published evidence that the occurrence of seizures during pregnancy has significant consequences for the overall physical status of the foetus at term.

Foetal Malformations

There has been speculation as to whether maternal generalised convulsive seizures in early pregnancy may cause foetal malformation, perhaps as a result of foetal tissue injury from the hypoxia or acidosis produced by the convulsing. However, there again appears to be little or no published evidence demonstrating that maternal seizures are actually responsible for foetal malformations in humans. In the Australian Pregnancy Register data for pregnancies that resulted in foetal malformations, such malformations occurred in 50.9 % of the 114 seizure-affected pregnancies and in 47.4 % of the seizure-free ones. The relative risk of 1.074 was not statistically significant. The corresponding figures were 29.8 and 29.9 %, if only generalised convulsive seizures were considered, the relative risk then being 0.999. Considering only seizures of any type that occurred early in pregnancy, the more critical time in connexion with organogenesis, the corresponding figures became 40.4 and 35.0 % (relative risk 1.513) and for generalised convulsive seizures 23.7 and 23.2 % (relative risk 1.020). Thus in the Australian data, there was no statistically significant evidence that having seizures during pregnancy, and in particular seizures in earlier pregnancy, increased the hazard of giving birth to foetuses with malformations.

On the basis of the above data, it would seem that pregnancy, when managed to what would appear to be a contemporaneously appropriate standard, is probably associated with a risk of worsening seizure control and possibly a small chance of sudden unexplained maternal and foetal death (if the recently available British data are confirmed). However, seizures that occur during pregnancy are unlikely to add significantly to the risk of experiencing pregnancy complications or other important adverse consequences for the mother or her foetus. The matter of antiepileptic drug-related foetal malformations is discussed at some length in the next two chapters.

Seizure Disorders in the Offspring

There is evidence that unprovoked seizure disorders are statistically significantly more common in the offspring of mothers with epilepsy, as compared with the offspring of fathers with epilepsy (Ottman et al. 1988). The basis for the difference is unexplained, not being accounted for by seizure disorder aetiology or maternal use of antiepileptic drugs.

References

Annegers JF, Baumgartner KB, Hauser WA, Kurland LT (1988) Epilepsy, antiepileptic drugs, and the risk of spontaneous abortion. Epilepsia 29:451–458

Artama M, Gissler M, Malm L, Rilvanen A, the Drug and Pregnancy Group (2013) Effect of maternal epilepsy and antiepileptic drugs during pregnancy on personal health of offspring: national retrospective cohort study in Finland. Drug Saf 36:359–369

Bardy AH (1987) Incidence of seizures during pregnancy, labor and the puerperium in epileptic women: a prospective study. Acta Neurol Scand 75:356–360

Barroso FV, Araujo Júnior E, Guazelli CA, Santana EF, Rolo LC, Martins MD, Moron AF (2014) Perinatal outcomes from the use of antiepileptic drugs during pregnancy: a case–control study. J Matern Fetal Neonatal Med 10:1–6

Battino D, Tomson T (2007) Management of epilepsy during pregnancy. Drugs 67:2727–2746

Battino D, Tomson T, Bonizzoni E et al (2013) Seizure control and treatment changes in pregnancy: observations from the EURAP epilepsy pregnancy registry. Epilepsia 54:1621–1627

Bech BH, Kjaersgaard MI, Pedersen HS et al (2014) Use of antiepileptic drugs during pregnancy and risk of spontaneous abortion and stillbirth: population based cohort study. Br Med J 349:g5159

Béraud R (1884) De l'épilepsie dans ses rapports avec la grossesse et l'accouchment bromuration pendant la grossesse. Delahays et Lecrosnier, Paris

Borthen I, Gilhus NE (2012) Pregnancy complications in patients with epilepsy. Curr Opin Obstet Gynecol 24:78–83

Borthen I, Eide MG, Dalveit AK, Gilhus NE (2011) Obstetric outcome in women with epilepsy: a hospital-based, retrospective study. Br J Obstet Gynaecol 118:956–965
Cangetti C, Lattanzi S, Foschi N, Provincili L, Silvestrini M (2014) Seizure course during pregnancy in catamenial epilepsy. Neurology 83:339–344
Chen Y, Chiou HY, Lin HC, Lin HL (2009) Effect of seizures during gestation on pregnancy outcomes in women with epilepsy. Arch Neurol 66:979–984
Eadie MJ (2012) Potassium bromide and Sir Charles Locock. J R Coll Physicians Edinb 42:274–279
Edey S, Moran N, Nashef L (2013) SUDEP and epilepsy-related mortality in pregnancy. Epilepsia 55:72–74
Fuchs U (1965) Epilepsie und Schwangerschaft. Inaugural Dissertation. Heidelberg. Cited by Schmidt D (1982) *loc cit*
Gjerde IO, Strandjord RE, Ulstein M (1988) The course of epilepsy during pregnancy: a study of 78 cases. Acta Neurol Scand 78:198–205
Gowers WR (1881) Epilepsy and other chronic convulsive disorders, 1st edn. J & A Churchill, London
Harden C, Hopp J, Ting TY et al (2009) Management issues for women with epilepsy - Focus on pregnancy (an evidence-based review): 1. Obstetrical complications and change in seizure frequency. Epilepsia 50:1229–1236
Herkes GK, Eadie MJ, Sharbrough F, Moyes T (1993) Patterns of seizure occurrence in catamenial epilepsy. Epilepsy Res 15:47–52
Herpin T (1867) Des accès incomplets d'épilepsie. Ballière, Paris
Herzog AG (2009) Hormone therapies. Progesterone. Neurotherap 6:383–391
Janz D, Fuchs U (1964) Are anti-epileptic drugs harmful when given during pregnancy? Ger Med Mon 9:20–22
Katz O, Levy A, Wiznitzner A, Sheiner E (2006) Pregnancy and perinatal outcome in epileptic women: a population-based study. J Matern Fetal Neonatal Med 19:21–25
Kilic D, Pedersen H, Kjaersgaard MI et al (2014) Birth outcomes after prenatal exposure to antiepileptic drugs - A population-based study. Epilepsia 55:1714–1721
Knight AH, Rhind EG (1975) Epilepsy and pregnancy: a study of 153 pregnancies in 59 patients. Epilepsia 16:99–110
Lin HL, Chen YH, Lin HC, Lin HC (2009) No increase in adverse pregnancy outcomes for women receiving antiepileptic drugs. J Neurol 256:1742–1749
Mawer G, Briggs M, Baker GA et al (2010) Pregnancy with epilepsy: obstetric and neonatal outcome of a controlled study. Seizure 19:112–119
McPherson JA, Harper LM, Odibo AO, Roehl KA, Cahill AG (2013) Maternal seizure disorder and risk of adverse pregnancy outcomes. Am J Obstet Gynecol 208:378.e1–378.e5
Morrell MJ (2002) Epilepsy in women. Am Fam Physician 66:1489–1494
Otani K (1985) Risk factors for the increased seizure frequency during pregnancy and puerperium. Folia Psychiatr Neurol Jpn 39:33–41
Ottman R, Annegers JF, Hauser WA, Kurland LT (1988) Higher risk of seizures in offspring of mothers than of fathers with epilepsy. Am J Hum Genet 43:257–264
Pennell PB, Peng L, Newport DJ et al (2008) Lamotrigine in pregnancy: clearance, therapeutic drug monitoring, and seizure frequency. Neurology 70:2130–2136
Pennell PB, Klein AM, Browning N et al (2012) Differential effects of antiepileptic drugs on neonatal outcomes. Epilepsy Behav 24:449–456
Pirie DAJ, Wattar BHA, Pirie AM et al (2013) Effect of monitoring strategies on seizures in pregnant women on lamotrigine: a meta-analysis. Eur J Obstet Gynecol Reprod Biol 172:26–31
Rauchenzaue M, Ehrensberger M, Prieschl M et al (2013) Generalised tonic clonic seizures and antiepileptic drugs during pregnancy: a matter of importance for the baby? J Neurol 260:484–488
Reddy DS (2010) Clinical pharmacokinetic interactions between antiepileptic drugs and hormonal contraceptives. Expert Rev Clin Pharmacol 3:183–192

Reisinger TL, Newman M, Loring DW, Pennell PB, Meador KJ (2013) Antiepileptic drug clearance and seizure frequency during pregnancy in women with epilepsy. Epilepsy Behav 29:13–18

Richmond JR, Krishnamoorthy P, Andermann E, Benjamin A (2004) Epilepsy and pregnancy: an obstetric perspective. Am J Obstet Gynecol 190:371–379

Rosciszewska D, Buntner B, Guz I, Zawiaza L (1986) Ovarian hormones, anticonvulsant drugs, and seizures during the menstrual cycle in women with epilepsy. J Neurol Neurosurg Psychiatry 49:47–51

Sabers A, Dam M (1990) Pregnancy, delivery and puerperium. In: Gram L, Dam M (eds) Comprehensive epileptology. Raven Press, New York, pp 299–307

Sabers A, Petrenaite V (2009) Seizure frequency in pregnant women treated with lamotrigine monotherapy. Epilepsia 50:2163–2166

Schmidt D (1982) The effect of pregnancy on the natural history of epilepsy: review of the literature. In: Janz D, Bossi L, Dam M, Helge H, Richens A, Schmidt D (eds) Epilepsy, pregnancy, and the child. Raven, New York, pp 3–14

Schmidt D, Canger R, Avanzini G et al (1983) Change in seizure frequency in pregnant epileptic women. J Neurol Neurosurg Psychiatry 46:751–755

Schupf N, Ottman R (1997) Reproduction among individuals with idiopathic/cryptogenic epilepsy: risk factors for spontaneous abortion. Epilepsia 38:824–829

Shavit AG, Lermann P, Korczyn AD, Kivity S, Bechar M, Gitter S (1984) Phenytoin pharmacokinetics in catamenial epilepsy. Neurology 34:959–961

Speidel BD, Meadow SR (1972) Maternal epilepsy and abnormalities of the fetus and newborn. Lancet 2:839–843

Tanganelli P, Regesta G (1992) Epilepsy, pregnancy, and major birth anomalies; an obstetric perspective. Neurology 42:89–98

Teramo K, Hillesmaa VK (1982) Pregnancy and fetal complications in epileptic pregnancies: review of the literature. In: Janz D, Bossi L, Dam M, Helge H, Richens A, Schmidt D (eds) Epilepsy, pregnancy and the child. Raven, New York, pp 53–59

Teramo K, Hillesmaa VK, Bardy A, Saarikoski S (1979) Fetal heart rate during a maternal grand mal epileptic seizure. J Perinat Med 7:3–6

The EURAP Study Group (2006) Seizure control and treatment in pregnancy. Observations from the EURAP Epilepsy Pregnancy Registry. Neurology 66:354–360

Thomas SV, Sindhu K, Ajaykumar B, Sulekha Devi PB, Sujamol J (2009) Maternal and obstetric outcome of women with epilepsy. Seizure 18:63–66

Thomas SV, Syam U, Devi JS (2012) Predictors of seizures during pregnancy in women with epilepsy. Epilepsia 53:e85–e88

Vajda FJE, Hirchcock A, Graham J, O'Brien T, Lander C, Eadie M (2008) Seizure control in antiepileptic drug-treated pregnancy. Epilepsia 49:172–175

Veiby G, Daltveit AK, Engelsen BA, Gilhus NE (2009) Pregnancy, delivery, and outcome for the child in maternal epilepsy. Epilepsia 50:30–39

Wegner I, Edelsbroek P, de Haan G-J, Lindhout D, Sander JW (2010) Drug monitoring of lamotrigine and oxcarbazepine combinations during pregnancy. Epilepsia 51:2500–2502

Wilks S (1861) Bromide and iodide of potassium in epilepsy. Med Times Gaz ii:635–636

Yerby MS (2008) Pregnancy and the mother with epilepsy. In: Pedley TA, Engel J (eds) Epilepsy. A comprehensive textbook. Wolters Kluwer Lippincott Williams & Wilkins, Philadelphia, pp 2067–2074

Chapter 8
Antiepileptic Drugs and Foetal Malformations: A Possible Class Effect

Abstract About 50 years ago, reports began to appear suggesting that there was an association between taking antiepileptic drugs during pregnancy and the development of foetal malformations. The occurrence of such malformations is relatively uncommon, and it has taken time and the accumulation of moderately sized data collections before the following information has emerged, viz.

(i) The tendency of the drugs to be associated with foetal malformation is not a class effect that involves all antiepileptic drugs. Among the more widely used agents is a property of certain drugs, particularly valproate but also to a lesser extent topiramate, probably phenobarbitone and possibly carbamazepine.
(ii) The risk of foetal malformation associated with valproate is dose dependent.
(iii) The teratogenesis associated with individual antiepileptic drugs is not limited to the production of one or two particular patterns of malformation but involves an increased risk of many different types of malformation, though there is some evidence that there is a degree of dose specificity between valproate and a particular pattern of malformation, viz. spina bifida.
(iv) The reported increased hazard of malformations occurring when antiepileptic drugs are combined depends on the presence of a teratogenic substance such as valproate in the combinations, and on its dosage.
(v) If the use of valproate is not involved and if there is no history of foetal malformation in previous offspring, the hazard of foetal malformation from an antiepileptic drug-exposed pregnancy is not likely to be statistically significantly higher than the risk in pregnancy in the general population.

The thalidomide tragedy of the late 1950s made both the medical profession and the general public aware that taking therapeutic drugs during pregnancy could cause foetal abnormalities. Not long afterwards, the first publication appeared that assessed this possibility in relation to the antiepileptic drugs then in use.

M.J. Eadie, F.J.E. Vajda, *Antiepileptic Drugs and Pregnancy: A Guide for Prescribers*, DOI 10.1007/978-3-319-21434-4_8

Early Observations

In January 1964, Janz and Fuchs published a study based on a questionnaire sent to 325 women who had attended the epilepsy outpatient clinic of the Department of Neurology of the University of Heidelberg during the previous eight years. The women were asked about all of their pregnancies during that period. The published paper contained data on 426 pregnancies in 246 women. In 262 of the pregnancies, hydantoin or barbiturate antiepileptic drugs had been taken continuously through pregnancy, in another 34, the regularity of drug intake was uncertain, and in 130, the pregnancies were in untreated women, whether or not they had experienced seizures. Among the 348 live births, there were five instances of congenital abnormalities (1.4 %), comprising three instances of hare lip or cleft palate (one associated with an anal fistula), one instance of congenital heart disease and one of torticollis. The malformation rate was 2.2 % in the pregnancies exposed to the drugs and 0 % in the drug-unexposed pregnancies in women with epilepsy. On the basis of these results, Janz and Fuchs considered that the malformations were unlikely to have been due to the antiepileptic drug treatment. The subsequent literature has generally accepted their interpretation.

Six years later, Meadow (1970), from Guy's Hospital in London, warned that there might be an association between pregnancy in women with epilepsy and the occurrence of cleft palate and cleft lip in their offspring. Unexpectedly, he had encountered six instances of the combination, prompting him to write in the medical press seeking further accounts of such an association. By 1970, he had accumulated accounts of 32 such instances, in only one of which cleft palate was the sole abnormality. All the affected children had been exposed to antiepileptic drugs during pregnancy. The drugs involved were phenobarbitone, primidone, phenytoin and troxidone. On the basis of an expected cleft palate rate of 1.2 per 1000 births in the general population, Meadow calculated that 2.5 babies per year with the abnormality should have been born to women with epilepsy, whereas the rate based on his own limited series was 4.0 per 1000 per year. He did not claim that there was a causal relationship between pregnancy, antiepileptic drug intake and facial clefts, but suggested that there was need for a larger-scale investigation of the possibility.

By the time the outcome of this proposed investigation was published (Speidel and Meadow 1972), further evidence suggesting the existence of such an association had already appeared. Elshove and Van Eck (1971) studied 65 live births to mothers treated with antiepileptic drugs throughout pregnancy and reported a total foetal malformation rate of 154 per 1000, a cleft lip and/or cleft palate rate of 77 per 1000 and a congenital heart abnormality rate of 30 per 1000. In their control population of 12,051 births, the corresponding figures were 19 per 1000, 2.7 per 1000 and 0 per 1000, respectively. Watson and Spellacy (1971) had found an overall foetal malformation rate of 59 per 1000 in the live births of 51 women taking antiepileptic drugs throughout pregnancy. There were no instances of facial clefts, but there was a 20 per 1000 rate for congenital heart abnormalities. Their control population of 50 pregnancies contained no malformations of any type. South (1972) reported on the outcome of antiepileptic drug-exposed pregnancies in 23 women and, for comparison, the outcome in the pregnancies of 99 women who were not taking antiepileptic drugs. There was an overall foetal malformation rate of 90 per 1000, all being instances of facial clefts, in the drug-exposed pregnancies, but no abnormalities in the drug-unexposed pregnancies.

Speidel and Meadow (1972) had investigated the records of the pregnancies of 186 women with epilepsy drawn from hospitals in the English Midlands and, as a comparison group, had utilised the records of the pregnancies of 180 women without epilepsy. There was a 4.66 % major congenital abnormality rate in 365 antiepileptic drug-exposed pregnancies, a 0 % rate in 62 pregnancies in women with epilepsy who did not take the drugs and a 1.45 % rate in 483 normal control pregnancies. In contrast to the known Birmingham City foetal malformation rate of 26.7 per 1000 pregnancies, the comparable malformation rate in pregnancies exposed to antiepileptic drugs was 51.6 per 1000. The main drugs involved were phenytoin, phenobarbitone and primidone. There was no single predominant pattern of malformation associated with any drug, but the authors thought that there was a recognisable pattern of abnormalities in the affected offspring. In its complete form, this pattern comprised facial malformations, cleft lip and palate, trigonocephaly or microcephaly, and various minor changes including hypertelorism, low-set ears, short neck, low hairline, bilateral single transverse palmar creases, minor peripheral skeletal abnormalities and, in some instances, mental subnormality. Neural tube defects were not identified as part of the syndrome. Unlike the situation that applied for thalidomide, where the drug appeared responsible for a single type of foetal malformation, the association between the antiepileptic drugs then in use and foetal malformation appeared to involve a variety of different abnormalities. In a given individual, these might occur singly or in combination. Speidel and Meadow noted that no single antiepileptic drug seemed more closely associated with malformations than the others. They considered that the cause of the malformations might be (i) inherited factors, (ii) the drug used, which might be acting by virtue of reducing circulating folate concentrations, and (iii) the occurrence of convulsions in pregnancy (though they did not think that the latter provided a sufficient explanation).

The paper of Speidel and Meadow (1972) was followed by the publication of further studies, all showing increased foetal malformation rates associated with in utero exposure to the main antiepileptic substances then in use, viz. phenytoin and phenobarbitone (the latter also being a metabolic product of primidone).

At this time, the oxazolidinedione derivative troxidone (trimethadione) was still employed in treating absence seizures, though it and its congener paramethadione were disappearing from use, being supplanted by succinimide derivatives, particularly ethosuximide. The departure from the market of troxidone may have been hastened by the publication of reports of a pattern of foetal facial malformations associated with its use (German et al. 1970; Rischbieth 1979). Ethosuximide had been introduced into human therapeutics in 1958 but, probably because absence seizures have often ceased occurring by the age when women in Western societies undertake pregnancy, has never featured to any considerable extent in the records of associations between antiepileptic drugs and foetal malformations.

Annegers et al. (1974) and Janz (1975) reviewed the then existing literature, with the former authors adding to it a series of pregnancies in women with epilepsy drawn from Mayo Clinic records. They reported that 10 foetal malformations had occurred among 141 pregnancies in women with epilepsy taking antiepileptic drugs, mainly phenobarbitone and phenytoin. There was only one abnormality in 56 pregnancies not exposed to these drugs in women with epilepsy and no abnormalities in the offspring of 61 women from the epilepsy subset in whom the pregnancies had occurred before the women developed epilepsy (and therefore before they took antiepileptic drugs). Annegers et al. concluded from their own data and the literature material that there probably was an association between antiepileptic drug therapy in pregnancy and the development of foetal malformations. They pointed out that, if antiepileptic drugs acted as teratogens, they might be expected to cause a specific type of foetal malformation or a small number of types of malformation. If they acted as mutagens, they might be expected to be associated with an extensive variety of malformations. Further, such malformations would also be expected to affect the offspring of fathers with antiepileptic drug-treated seizure disorders. Meyer (1973) and Shapiro et al. (1976) obtained some evidence that the latter might be the case, whereas Annegers et al. (1974) and Annegers et al. (1982) considered that they had failed to find such evidence in their material. However, Janz (1982) pointed out that Annegers et al. had actually found a malformation rate in the offspring of epileptic fathers that was intermediate between the rate for the offspring of women with antiepileptic drug-treated epilepsy and that for the offspring of women with epilepsy not exposed to antiepileptic drugs in pregnancy. This particular issue has tended to be bypassed in the subsequent literature, possibly because of the sensitivities and other difficulties that might be involved in ascertaining the identities and then obtaining the health and reproductive records of the relevant biological fathers.

Annegers et al. (1974) also drew attention to certain limitations of the data that were available for their study. One of the major ones was the problem attendant on the small numbers of foetal malformations on which they had to base their conclusions. They calculated that if the foetal malformation rate in the pregnancies of women with epilepsy was the same as that in the general population, there would be only one malformed foetus born per 1000 pregnant women with epilepsy. There were other limitations, later reviewed by Källén (2005), but these can be discussed below in relation to the attempts to remedy the problems that may arise in investigating what are relatively uncommon events.

Limitations and Attempted Remedies

Subsequently, attempts have been made to collect larger numbers of pregnancies in women with epilepsy with the intention of overcoming the limitations inherent in studying comparatively rare events and, in addition, to try to ensure that the types of seizure disorder that are involved in the studies are representative of epilepsy in the wider community. In a professional life time, no individual medical practitioner or local group of practitioners is likely to be able to amass sufficient numbers of pregnancies in women with epilepsy to possess enough material for useful analysis. Therefore, investigators have sometimes availed themselves of data already collected in the records of large hospitals or in official governmental data bases. Alternatively, special pregnancy registers have sometimes been set up.

Retrospective Analyses of Hospital Records

Retrospective analyses of data retrieved from hospital records may have various limitations, because of the ways in which the data that they contain have been compiled. Nevertheless, they have sometimes yielded useful information. Details of individual patient records have often been set down by different people, sometimes in difficult-to-decipher handwriting. Though at the times of their creation these records may have been adequate for the purposes of the institutions that have housed them, they may prove to lack desired details relevant to particular teratogenicity issues that have subsequently become important. They also may not contain information that extends beyond the course of the patient's immediate periods of contact with the institution in question.

Use of Governmental Data Bases

Governmental data collections are likely to contain information on large numbers of pregnancies where there has been no antiepileptic drug exposure, and they often possess information on the pregnancies of women with epilepsy. They may, or may not, contain information on whether the epilepsy was treated, or not treated, during pregnancy. If they do not hold this information, in some countries, it has still been possible to link their contents with the contents of separate databases that contain national or regional information on drug prescriptions. The pregnancy and prescription data in such datasets will be retrospective and have probably been recorded without those collecting the data seeking specifically for the most appropriate information for evaluating the role of the drugs in producing foetal malformations. Also, such data collections are usually based on assessment of the offspring shortly after birth and hence may fail to include malformations that are not detected until later in infancy or childhood. The collections also may not contain information on therapeutic abortions, so that they may tend to exclude the most severe foetal malformations such as neural tube defects. Further, prescription of a drug, or the dispensing of such a prescription, does not necessarily mean that the drug has been taken during pregnancy.

Use of Pregnancy Registers (Registries)

Ethical Considerations

Pregnancy registers (or registries, as they are sometimes termed) are intended to prospectively collect information about the relative teratogenicities of antiepileptic drugs. They are in essence observational studies that do not interfere with the actual existing managements of individual participants, so that no issue of unethical or doubtfully ethical experimentation on humans arises. They provide the best available practical and ethical alternative to the randomised, placebo-controlled studies which would in other circumstances be preferable to obtain strictly evidence-based results, but which would probably be judged ethically unacceptable if proposed in relation to pregnant women.

Actual Registers

The register model of prospectively collecting pregnancy-related information that was established initially by Holmes in the USA was followed by the establishment of reasonably similar registers in several countries. Details of some of these registers have subsequently been reported (Beghi et al. 2001; Vajda et al. 2007). In 1999, Ettore Beghi convened a meeting that established collaboration between registers which had sufficiently similar features to enable their joining an international register called EURAP. Beghi (2012) summarised the situation concerning pregnancy registers as follows:

> Pregnancy registries have been activated by collaborative groups of physicians in Europe (EURAP), North America (NAREP), Australia and India (the latter two recently merged into EURAP), to enroll a large number of exposed women to be monitored prospectively with standardized methods, and by three pharmaceutical companies marketing lamotrigine, gabapentin and vigabatrin, as part of their post-marketing surveillance…… the implementation of a common database with information from the existing registries may provide valuable information in a shorter time period.

The European International Registry (EURAP) was established following the meeting convened by Beghi (above). After 15 years of existence, this registry involves over 45 countries worldwide. Collaboration between it and additional registers continues to be explored. Individual collaborating registers may still choose to publish their own data, derived from a smaller database, but also feed the information into EURAP.

As one example of a register's content, the protocol for inclusion in the Australian Register of Antiepileptic Drugs in Pregnancy involves interviews with women with informed consent at their time of enrolment, at 28 weeks of pregnancy, soon after delivery and at 12 months postnatally. Information on general medical, social, epileptic seizure and treatment history, past pregnancies and outcomes, non-epilepsy-related medications and events is recorded, and access to patients' medical records is obtained. Data are kept in a computerised database for subsequent analysis.

Other registers include the North American Epilepsy and Pregnancy Registry, the UK Epilepsy and Pregnancy Register, the Swedish Register, the Finnish National Drug Prescription Registry and the Danish Register. The main contemporary pharmaceutical company registers are the Prospective International Lamotrigine Registry and the Pregnancy Registry maintained by UCB to monitor levetiracetam.

There are differences between the registers. EURAP contains no internal control group of untreated women with epilepsy and endeavours to compare drugs and their effects on the foetus with each other. From the outset, the Australian Register has included antiepileptic drug-untreated women with epilepsy, comprising about ten per cent of the total, and also has attempted to recruit women receiving antiepileptic drugs for non-epileptic indications, such as pain or bipolar illness. The US Registry employs historical control groups. Although no single specific control group is ideal, the availability of sufficient numbers of women with untreated epilepsy probably represents the most appropriate comparator.

In the earlier days of the existence of such registers, Meador (2008a) commented that

> The registries have different data collection timing (e.g. malformations at birth *versus* at 1 year), some lack of information about the mothers as well as a lack of follow up, which restricts usefulness of registry data. In addition, each of the individual registries has weaknesses ranging from missing data on key variables to low numbers.

In more recently developed registers, some of these criticisms from an earlier time have been addressed, at least to an extent. Even so, such registers, in which enrolment necessarily is voluntary, are likely to capture only a minority of the women with epilepsy in the community and, unless they draw on very large populations, probably will not accumulate sufficient pregnancy numbers for useful analysis in data collection periods of less than several years. Over such periods, therapeutic practice may change, possibly confounding interpretations. As well, women with epilepsy who are prepared to enrol their pregnancies may not necessarily be representative of women with epilepsy in the wider community. For instance, despite its best efforts over its period of existence, the Australian Pregnancy Register appears to have been able to collect only some 8.7 % of the pregnancies calculated to have occurred nationwide in women with epilepsy (Vajda et al. 2014). Registers are likely to prove more suitable for detecting differences between women with treated and untreated epilepsies in pregnancy (if sufficient numbers of the latter become available) and in comparing the effects of individual epileptic drugs, than in comparing malformation rates between women with epilepsy and those in other pregnant women in the general community.

The approaches to obtaining sufficient pregnancy numbers mentioned above have other limitations. Because of their information-collecting and information-recording methods, as already noted, hospital records may not always contain relevant data from the foetal malformation point of view, official institutional databases tend to sacrifice data quality to achieve inclusiveness, while registers tend to sacrifice comprehensiveness for the advantage of relevance to the issue at hand.

One issue in relation to the various registers that does not seem to have received much discussion is the possibility that the material some of them contain may have been derived from pregnancies that have already been the subject of literature reports. Conceivably the same individual pregnancy may have been included more than once in the literature, without the replication of data being identifiable. This may lead to the impression that more information is available than is really the case.

Other Issues of Methodology

Malformation Rate Comparisons

Different studies have employed a variety of comparison data sets in assessing the significances of malformation rate values, e.g. known or expected malformation rates for the whole population or for particular and preferably matched population subsets, or malformation rates in siblings that were not exposed to antiepileptic drugs in utero (Dolk and McElhattan 2002). As already mentioned, probably the most satisfactory comparator would be the malformation rate in the offspring of women with untreated epilepsy. Unfortunately, the number of untreated pregnancies in women with epilepsy has usually proved to be substantially smaller than the number of antiepileptic drug-treated ones, generally about 10 % or 15 % of their number, though in the early series of Janz and Fuchs (1964), approximately one-third of all the pregnancies studied were not exposed to antiepileptic drugs. As noted above, the corresponding figure for the most recent analysis of the Australian Pregnancy Register was 8.7 % (Vajda et al. 2014). Little seems to have been published investigating whether such untreated pregnancies differ in important aspects from antiepileptic drug-treated ones, apart from the material in the paper of Vajda et al. (2008). This paper analysed the data from 68 pregnancies that were untreated in at least first trimester compared with the data from the remaining 709 simultaneously collected but drug-treated pregnancies in women with epilepsy then included in the Australian Pregnancy Register. More than 50 parameters were studied. The only statistically significant differences were that the untreated pregnancy group contained higher proportions of first pregnancies, pregnancies with seizures in the pre-pregnancy year, pregnancies that had been referred to the Register by neurologists and babies with slightly higher head circumferences at birth and slightly higher APGAR scores five minutes after delivery. There also were fewer pregnancies with postpartum seizures. Foetal malformations tended to be less frequent in the drug-unexposed pregnancies. Apart from the matter of taking or not taking antiepileptic drug treatment, the increased proportion of referrals from neurologists in the untreated group seemed to be the only difference that might suggest that the groups compared did not come from the same population. This difference in referral source raised the possibility that the epilepsies in the untreated group may have been managed by more skilled professionals. There were no significant differences in respect of family histories of birth defects in previous generations or in older siblings or pregnancies culminating in stillbirth. There also were no differences in preconception folate use or folate use in pregnancy, in illness in pregnancy or in smoking or alcohol intake in early pregnancy. Focal epilepsies were a little less frequent in the untreated group and generalised epilepsies more frequent, but the differences were not statistically significant. Seizure occurrence rates in earlier pregnancy were similar in the two groups. Overall, the untreated control and treated pregnancy groups may not have proved to be perfectly matched, but apart from the matter of antiepileptic drug intake, there did not seem to be any obvious difference between them that would have been expected to produce sizeably different foetal malformation rates. In 62 % of the pregnancies in the untreated group, antiepileptic drugs that had been taken previously had been withdrawn within a few months of the beginning of pregnancy. This suggests that the women who had done this had planned to be drug free in at least earlier pregnancy. There is published evidence that some women with epilepsy in the United Kingdom choose to adopt such a policy (Man et al. 2012).

There is also the related question of the denominator against which malformation rates are expressed. Often it has been live births, but doing this omits intrauterine deaths and stillbirths which may be due to antiepileptic drugs and also excludes therapeutic abortions which have been carried out because of detected major foetal malformation. The ideal denominator, conceptions, is impractical because of the difficulty in obtaining accurate data for spontaneous abortions, especially ones that occur early in pregnancy. Malformation rates have sometimes been expressed relative to the number of pregnancies studied, raising the question of how the data from multiple offspring from a single pregnancy have been handled. If the malformation rates are expressed relative to numbers of live offspring, pregnancies yielding multiple offspring will be counted more than once. Some of the differences in foetal malformation rates, and in types of malformation, recorded in different studies in the literature probably arise from such differences in the denominators used in the rate calculations.

Data Collection

Because of difficulty in agreeing when minor anatomical aberrations or unusual physical appearances would warrant the designation of 'malformation', investigators have often restricted themselves to the statistics of major congenital malformations. Even then, the boundaries between what is designated 'major' and what is considered 'minor' may be somewhat elastic. Mothers of newborn infants may not consider 'minor' what a medical observer does, and mothers are often the primary source of register information. In various studies, there have been differences between the time points when the presence or absence of malformations has been determined. The cut-off could be immediately after birth or, more commonly, during the postnatal few days, but sometimes has been after the first three months of postnatal life (e.g. in the North American Registry for some of the studies in which it has been utilised) or, in the case of the Australian Register of Pregnancies in women with epilepsy, at the end of the first year of postnatal life. This time factor may also contribute to differences between the results of the published analyses of data based on different registers. It is much less likely to apply for differences in findings between various studies based on analysis of retrospective data drawn from large institutional or national databanks, though these studies are likely to underestimate true malformation occurrence rates, particular rates of minor malformations, because their data are usually collected close to the time of birth, a stage at which less severe malformations may not have been noticed. Vajda et al. (2007) examined the effect of the time after birth in determining the presence of malformations in the Australian Pregnancy Register material. Approximately 21 % of the malformations that were ultimately included, based on the data available one year after the end of pregnancy, would have escaped inclusion if only assessment during the postnatal period had been used. Moreover, there were also pregnancies which could not be traced one year after birth. Had these been included, and assuming they would have had similar malformation rates to those offspring who had been followed to the end of the postnatal year, as many as 29 % of all offspring with malformations might have been missed in assessments made close to childbirth. Admittedly, a considerable majority of the late recognised malformations in the Australian Register were relatively minor, mainly genitourinary, cardiac and cranial ones, and changes in the appearances of the digits. Battino and Tomson (2007) observed that 40 % more malformations were found with an extended postnatal follow-up than would have been detected at birth.

The larger data sets that have become available in recent times that relate foetal outcomes in women with epilepsy to antiepileptic drug exposure during pregnancy fall into several types, viz. (i) Large scale, often whole pregnant female population data, almost always assembled retrospectively for the relevant age group over a designated period of time. Their data can provide indications of the malformation risk relative to that for the general population, but the roles of antiepileptic drug therapy in the situation may be difficult to define because therapy-related information is deficient. (ii) Usually smaller-sized malformation rate data collections from pregnant women with antiepileptic drug-treated epilepsy compared with matched and simultaneously collected data from pregnant women not taking antiepileptic drugs, at least during the first trimester of pregnancy, the time when foetal malformations probably develop. If the untreated women have epilepsy, this type of material permits the effects of pregnancy itself to be distinguished from the effects of the administered antiepileptic drugs, a matter of some scientific interest. (iii) Smaller-scale studies comparing malformation rates associated with individual antiepileptic drugs. In the latter type of study, the comparator employed usually is the antiepileptic drug associated with the lowest malformation rate, which it is assumed will not be less than the rate for the general population of pregnant women. Such information may identify increase malformation rates associated with a drug other than the comparator one. (iv) Small-scale studies in which malformation rates associated with particular drugs are investigated, and where, if any comparator is available, it is likely to be an assumed malformation rate for the general population (generally around 2–3 %).

Studies based on larger data sets form the background for much of the more useful information concerning antiepileptic drug teratogenesis that has become available in the past two decades, though small-scale studies continue to appear in the medical press.

More Recent Large-Scale Data

Samrén et al. (1997) pooled the data of five prospective and previously published studies from different European centres (totalling 1221 children exposed to antiepileptic drugs during pregnancy and 158 unexposed control pregnancies). There were regional differences between the data from the sites of the original individual studies, but overall there was a 2.3 times increased risk of malformation in the in utero antiepileptic drug-exposed children compared with healthy control children. Olafsson et al. (1998) employed Icelandic birth data for all women with active epilepsy over a 19-year period to calculate a foetal malformation rate of 3.3 per 1000 pregnancies. There was a 2.7 times increased major congenital malformation rate in the women taking antiepileptic drugs as compared with that in the general population. Kaneko et al. (1999) recorded a 9 % incidence of congenital malformations in 983 infants born in Japan, Italy and Canada to mothers treated with antiepileptic drugs during pregnancy, compared with an incidence of 3.1 % in the offspring of pregnancies without drug exposure. Canger et al. (1999) described a 9.7 % malformation rate (5.3 % structurally severe ones) in the pregnancies of 442 women with antiepileptic drug-treated epilepsy, as compared with no abnormalities in the 25 pregnancies in women with epilepsy who had not taken antiepileptic drugs. Holmes et al. (2001) reported a 20.6 % malformation rate in 223 infants who had been exposed to antiepileptic drug monotherapy during pregnancy, compared with an 8.5 % rate in 508 control infants (odds ratio 2.8; 95 % C.I. = 1.1, 5.1). The malformation risk was still higher (28.0 %) if antiepileptic drug polytherapy was involved. There was no increased hazard of malformation in 93 infants whose mothers, despite having epilepsy, did not take antiepileptic drugs during pregnancy. Kaaja et al. (2003) obtained a major malformation rate of 3.8 % from 740 pregnancies exposed to antiepileptic drugs in women with epilepsy, and one of 0.8 % from 239 antiepileptic drug-untreated pregnancies in women with seizure disorders. Thus, within half a decade spanning the end of the twentieth century, despite some variation in the figures, considerable evidence accumulated suggesting that antiepileptic drug exposure during pregnancy was associated with a heightened risk of foetal malformation. Nevertheless, further publications continued to appear.

Fried et al. (2004) employed meta-analysis to explore the question of the foetal malformation hazard in women with untreated epilepsy relative to that in non-epileptic healthy pregnant control women. After allowing for the effects of publication bias, they concluded that the malformation rate in the offspring of women with untreated epilepsy appeared virtually identical with that in the controls (odds ratio 0.99; 95 % C.I. = 0.49, 2.01). However, the offspring of women with epilepsy that was treated with antiepileptic drugs during pregnancy had a higher malformation rate compared with that of the untreated pregnancies in the women with epilepsy (odds ratio 3.26; 95 % C.I. = 2.15, 4.93). Wide et al. (2004) compared the foetal malformation rate in 1256 antiepileptic drug in utero exposed infants with that in 582,656 infants who were included in the Swedish Medical Birth Registry. In the comparison, the odds ratio for producing a malformed infant in the antiepileptic drug-exposed group was 1.86 (95 % C.I. = 1.42, 2.44). It was noticed in this study that malformations appeared to be more frequent if there had been intrauterine exposure to carbamazepine. Artama et al. (2005) analysed Finnish national collection data and found a congenital malformation rate among the offspring of women taking antiepileptic medication that exceeded the rate in the offspring of untreated women (4.6 % *versus* 2.8 %: $P=0.02$). Morrow et al. (2006), in the United Kingdom Epilepsy and Pregnancy Register data available at the time, calculated an overall major congenital malformation rate for antiepileptic drug-exposed pregnancies of 4.2 %. The rate for pregnancies in women with epilepsy where antiepileptic drugs had not been taken during pregnancy was only a little lower (3.5 %), though the number of such pregnancies was quite small (239) compared with the more than 3000 antiepileptic drug-exposed pregnancies.

In a review, Perucca (2005) assembled the data from these various publications with their generally similar outcomes, and Meador et al. (2008b) proceeded to publish a systematic review and meta-analysis that again attempted to determine the incidence of congenital malformation associated with antiepileptic drug exposure during pregnancy. In their analysis, the latter authors included 59 studies which embraced data from 65,503 pregnancies in women with epilepsy and 1,817,024 pregnancies in healthy women. They calculated that the incidence of births with congenitally malformed offspring in women with epilepsy (7.08 %) was higher than the incidence in healthy women (2.28 %).

There have been subsequent studies that have provided further malformation rate data (e.g. Hernandez-Diaz et al. 2012; Tomson and Battino 2012), but from the information already available, there was already almost overwhelming evidence that exposure to antiepileptic drugs during pregnancy probably doubled or trebled the hazard of a woman giving birth to a baby with some form of congenital malformation. In a significant proportion of instances, multiple malformations occurred in the same affected infant.

Factors Relevant to Foetal Malformation Rates

Information has become available concerning certain factors relevant to the relationships between the antiepileptic drugs and foetal malformations. For instance, the study of Cassina et al. (2013) reported what seemed a potentially very significant observation. There was a foetal malformation rate of 7.7 % in the offspring of 337 women with antiepileptic drug-treated epilepsy, one of 3.9 % in women taking antiepileptic drugs for disorders other than epilepsy, and one of 3.1 % in 803 women who did not have epilepsy. The similarity of the findings in the latter two groups and the higher malformation rate in pregnancies of women with treated epilepsy might suggest that it was having epilepsy rather than being treated for epilepsy that determined whether foetal malformations occurred. Unfortunately, in this study, antiepileptic drug doses were lower in the women taking the drugs for indications other than epilepsy as compared with women with epilepsy, and information to be discussed immediately below shows that foetal malformation rates may correlate with antiepileptic drug dosage.

Relationships Between Drug Dosage and Malformation Rates

The finding of a statistically significant difference ($P<0.05$) between foetal malformation rates for women with treated and with untreated epilepsy suggests that the presence of an apparent association between in utero exposure to an antiepileptic drug and the occurrence of a foetal malformation is more than a matter of chance. If the frequency of occurrence of foetal malformations was shown to be related to the dosage or to the maternal biological fluid concentration of a drug taken throughout pregnancy, the probability of a causal relationship between the two would be increased. This risk–dose relationship criterion has been utilised increasingly to assess possible causal relationships as larger pregnancy data collections have become available. Based on the common clinical experience that epileptic seizure control correlates better with plasma drug concentrations than with drug dosage, biological fluid drug concentrations might be expected to provide stronger evidence than the drug dosage can. However, there is the practical issue of determining the critical drug concentration at the time when the teratogenic process begins. Even if that time were known, the logistical difficulties in obtaining the fluid sample at the appropriate moment might prove almost prohibitive. A few data are available that permit correlation of malformation occurrence with concentrations of antiepileptic drug in plasma, but the measurements have often been made either at doubtfully appropriate times, e.g. at term, or at some stage when the malformation process probably was already underway. Therefore, correlation between malformation risk and the prescribed drug dosage taken during the expected period of maldevelopment usually proves to be the more practicable approach. In such correlations, malformation rates have sometimes been related to a series of drug dosage bands. Alternatively, regressions for malformation risk on dosage have been calculated.

The first such attempted correlation, employing regression, seems to have been that of Kaneko et al. (1999) carried out in relation to valproate. The regression approach has subsequently been used on several occasions in analysing the data in the Australian Pregnancy Register, mainly in relation to valproate but also for other antiepileptic agents. Figure 8.1 show logistic regressions for foetal malformation rate on drug dose for several antiepileptic drugs. None of the regressions, except that for valproate, is statistically significant Figure 8.2.

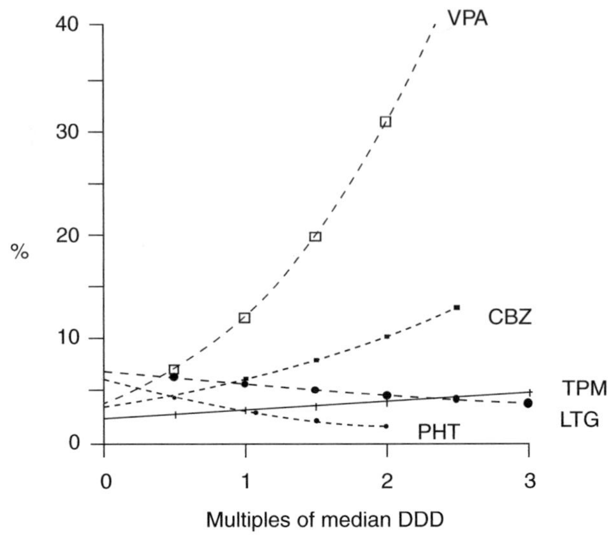

Fig. 8.1 Logistic regressions for foetal malformation rate on drug dose for several antiepileptic drugs. To bring the drug doses to some common basis, because their numerical values in terms of weight of active ingredient differ considerably, the doses are expressed as submultiples, or multiples, for each drug's WHO-defined daily dose (phenytoin *PHT*, lamotrigine *LTG* and topiramate *TPM*, each 300 mg/day; carbamazepine *CBZ* 1000 mg/day; levetiracetam *LEV* and valproate *VPA*, both 1500 mg/day). Only the regression for valproate is statistically significant (based on Australian Pregnancy Register data as of 2012)

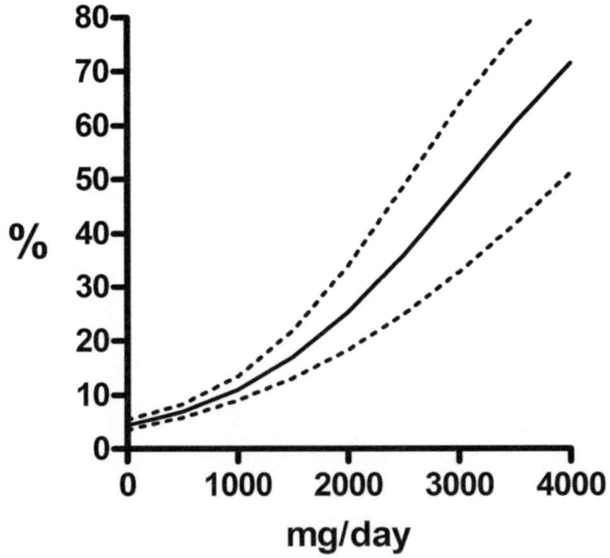

Fig. 8.2 Logistic regression for foetal malformation risk on valproate dose in mg/day (*continuous line*), with the 95 % confidence limits of the regression line (*broken lines*)

Antiepileptic Drug Polytherapy

In some of the early studies referred to above, a substantial proportion of the pregnancies were exposed to more than one antiepileptic drug simultaneously, most often to the combination of phenytoin and phenobarbitone. The effects of the individual agent in causing foetal malformation were difficult to isolate. As time passed, two events occurred more or less simultaneously and appear to have considerably reduced the extent of use of antiepileptic drug polypharmacy in women with epilepsy. First, the application of plasma antiepileptic drug concentration measurement showed that an individual agent had often been used in potentially inadequate dosage before a second antiepileptic drug was added to treatment. This knowledge resulted in advocacy for employing, whenever possible, antiepileptic drug monotherapy in appropriate dosage (Shorvon and Reynolds 1977). Second, statistical analyses of various case series rather consistently showed higher foetal malformation rates if pregnant women with epilepsy had been treated with more than one antiepileptic drug simultaneously (Nakane et al. 1980; Kaneko et al. 1992; Lindhout and Omtzigt 1992; Samrén et al.. 1997; Morrow et al. 2006). This knowledge also led to endeavours to avoid using antiepileptic drug combinations in women who were considering pregnancy. Consequently, the more recent series correlating foetal malformations with drug treatment usually contain only around 20 % of pregnancies that have been managed with antiepileptic drug combinations. The role of the individual agents in antiepileptic drug monotherapy data is easily recognised, though statistical techniques such as multivariate regression can separate mathematically the contributions of the individual agents used in polypharmacy.

Somewhat ironically, the published evidence that has more recently become available appears to show that it is not so much the combination of any two or more antiepileptic drugs that is responsible for the apparently higher foetal malformation rate associated with antiepileptic drug polypharmacy, but the presence of valproate in any antiepileptic drug combination. Artama et al. (2005) made that observation, almost in passing, but it tended to go unnoticed. Valproate carries a distinctly greater teratogenic hazard than the other available antiepileptic drugs (see Chap. 9). An analysis by Vajda et al. (2010) of the Australian Pregnancy Register data found that, while the relative risk of malformation associated with antiepileptic drug polytherapy was greater than 1.0 in 11 series drawn from the literature and was above 0.9 in the remaining three series, in the Australian data the relative risk was only 0.68. In the latter data, once instances of polytherapy which involved valproate were excluded, the malformation risk became similar for antiepileptic drug monotherapy and polytherapy. Interestingly, the malformation risk was lower relative to valproate dose when that drug was used in polytherapy than in monotherapy (Fig. 8.3). Logistic regression analysis of the Australian data suggested that combining valproate with other antiepileptic drugs might have diminished the hazard that valproate held for foetal development. Soon afterwards, Holmes et al. (2011) studied the outcomes of antiepileptic drug polytherapy that involved carbamazepine or lamotrigine and also concluded that it was not antiepileptic drug polytherapy per se

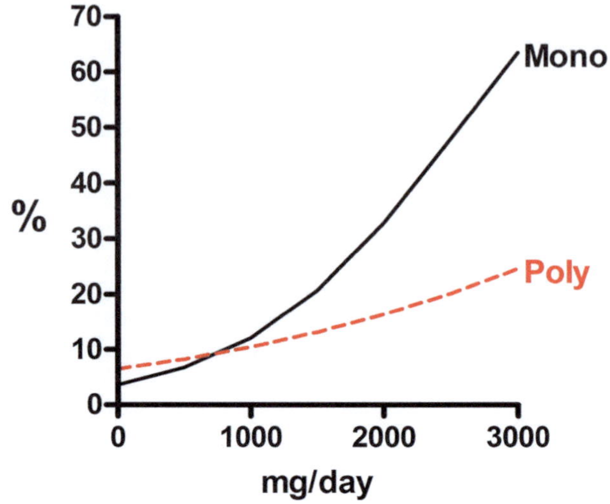

Fig. 8.3 Logistic regressions for foetal malformation risk on valproate (VPA) dose associated with the drug's use in monotherapy (*continuous line*) and polytherapy (*broken line*) (based on Australian Pregnancy Register data as of December 2014)

that increases the teratogenicity risk but the presence of valproate in the drug combinations. Mawer et al. (2010), a little earlier, had made a similar observation in material from a smaller case series.

An investigation of the data of the Australian Pregnancy Register as of the end of December 2014, as yet unpublished, has shown that the presence of topiramate in an antiepileptic drug combination is also associated with an increased risk of foetal malformation.

Genetic Influences

It is well enough known that certain types of foetal malformation, e.g. cleft palate and cleft lip, may be inherited. Particularly when some types of epilepsy are inherited, the question arises as to what role genetic factors may play in the occurrence of the foetal malformations that appear to be associated with exposure to antiepileptic drugs in utero. A certain amount of evidence exists that a genetic influence sometimes may be important. In the same issue of the journal *Epilepsia*, in 2013, two papers appeared reporting quite similar conclusions. Campbell et al. (2013) followed 1534 pregnancies in 719 women with epilepsy from the United Kingdom Register. They found that, if the first child born to a woman with epilepsy had a foetal malformation, there was a 16.8 % risk that a further child she had would also be born malformed, in contrast to the 9.8 % risk if the first child had not been malformed. There was a trend for the risk to be higher if valproate was the antiepileptic drug involved (21.9 %, relative risk = 1.47; 95 % C.I. = 0.68, 3.20) or if topiramate was involved (50 %: relative risk = 4.50; 95 % C.I. = 0.97, 20.82). There was no increased risk in relation to maternal use of other antiepileptic drugs. In the other paper, Vajda et al. (2013a)) studied the outcome of 2637 pregnancies in 1243 women with epilepsy from the Australian Register. Some of these pregnancies had occurred before women were enrolled in the Register. If a malformation or malformations had occurred in the first child born after recruitment into the Register, and the woman concerned continued to take the same epileptic drug in subsequent pregnancies, there was a 35.7 % risk of malformation in the subsequent pregnancy, compared with a 3.1 % risk if the initial pregnancy had produced an offspring that was not malformed (odds ratio 17.6; 95 % C.I. = 4.5, 68.7). If the woman was taking valproate, the risks of malformation in subsequent pregnancies were even higher, being 57.2 % as compared with 7.0 % (odds ratio 17.8; 95 % C.I. = 2.7, 119.1). There was no statistically significant increased risk in relation to maternal intake of antiepileptic drugs other than valproate. Veiby et al. (2014) noted a marked increase in the malformation risk for siblings if one child had a valproate-associated foetal malformation (42.9 % compared with 6.7 %: odds ratio 10.4; 95 % C.I. = 2.3, 46.7). It was also observed that the types of foetal malformation in the affected siblings in the two pregnancies usually were different. These reports suggest that genetic factors may play an appreciable role in the occurrence of antiepileptic drug-associated foetal malformations. However, in contrast to these findings, in 246 women with epilepsy, Begum et al. (2013) failed to find an increased risk of malformation in the subsequent pregnancy if there had been a malformation in an earlier pregnancy. The overall malformation rate in their study was 8.5 % in the first pregnancy, and 8.9 % in the second.

Antiepileptic Drugs and Specific Malformations

Despite the repeated observation that the use of antiepileptic drugs in human pregnancy is not associated with the occurrence of any particular foetal malformation, as larger data sets became available for study, some investigators continued to seek relationships between particular drugs and particular malformations.

Werler et al. (2011) found evidence in the US National Birth Defects Prevention Study data that there were drug-specific increased risks for valproate and the occurrence of neural tube defects and hyopospadias and for carbamazepine and neural tube defects. In the Australian Register data, Vajda et al. (2013b) failed to find any statistically significant association between valproate and hypospadias but did find one between the drug and spina bifida, facial clefts and malformations of skull bones, the digits and the heart and great vessels. They also found statistically significant associations between carbamazepine and renal tract abnormalities and topiramate and hypospadias and brain structural abnormalities. Thus far, there do not appear to be other published evidences of specificity between antiepileptic drugs and any particular malformation.

The Possible Role of Folate

Folate deficiency during pregnancy is associated with reduced neurogenesis and increased apoptosis in foetal mouse brains (Craciunescu et al. 2004). In pregnant women in general, as distinct from women with epilepsy, it has been recognised for some time that there is an association between maternal folate deficiency and the occurrence of neural tube defects. Blom et al. (2011) have provided a detailed review of the issue of folic acid physiology and its possible role in minimising antiepileptic drug-related teratogenicity, while Rothenberg et al. (2004) reported the finding of autoantibodies to folate receptors in women with pregnancies complicated by neural tube defects.

Champel et al. (1999) cited earlier literature showing that folic acid supplementation taken by the mother for at least a month before conception, in doses between 0.4 mg and 1 mg per day, decreased the incidence of a first neural tube defect occurring in her offspring. Even if a woman had already given birth to a baby with a neural tube defect, so that she or her partner might carry a genetic tendency for such defects, the supplementation still reduced the risk of her subsequent babies having neural tube defects. A controlled prevention trial from China, involving hundreds of thousands of women from normal populations, demonstrated the beneficial effects of folic acid in preventing neural tube defects (Berry et al. 1999). The British Medical Research Council trial (Anonymous 1991), a secondary prevention study which included women who had previously given birth to an infant with a neural tube defect, or who had a first degree relative with a child with a neural tube defect, found that intake of folic acid 4 mg per day was associated with a marked protective effect.

When reports began to appear of the occurrence of neural tube defects in association with antiepileptic drug exposure during pregnancy, it was already known that intake of both phenobarbitone and phenytoin, the most widely used antiepileptic drugs at the time, caused reduced plasma folate concentrations. In fact, Hiilesmaa et al. (1983) had shown that there was an inverse relationship between plasma folate concentrations and plasma concentrations of phenytoin and phenobarbitone. Understandably, this information, taken in conjunction with the reported benefits of preconception supplemental folic acid intake in reducing the incidence of neural tube defects in the offspring of women who for the most part did not have epilepsy, led to speculation that the antiepileptic agents produced malformations through causing maternal, and presumably foetal, folic acid depletion. Folic acid supplementation then became rather widely recommended for women with antiepileptic drug-treated epilepsy who intended to become pregnant, with the folic acid intake continuing into pregnancy. Thus, the American Academy of Neurology advocated administration of folate, 0.4 to 5 mg daily, to all pregnant women of child-bearing age, the intake commencing prior to conception. EURAP regarded three months of folic acid intake as a minimal period prior to conception to achieve possible benefit. Betts and Fox (1999) and Kaaja et al. (2003) did provide some evidence that the risk for major congenital malformations in the offspring of women with epilepsy was possibly decreased by folic acid supplementation. However, a number of authors such as Lindhout and Omtzigt (1992) and Champel et al. (1999) pointed out that, at their times of writing, there was no convincing evidence that such folic acid administration reduced the incidence of foetal malformations associated with antiepileptic drug exposure. Further, folic acid status during pregnancy has not been proven to impact on foetal neurodevelopment (Tamura et al. 2005), though Meador et al. (2007) were able to suggest a number of possible mechanisms through which folate deficiency might affect foetal development. Yerby (2003) noted at his time of writing that there was a general professional acceptance of the need for folic acid supplementation in pregnant women with epilepsy, but questioned whether it was useful. No writer seems to have queried whether it might actually be harmful.

Then Morrow et al. (2009) reported a 3.9 % (95 % C.I. = 3.1 %, 4.9 %) foetal major congenital malformation rate and a 0.4 % (95 % C.I. = 0.2 %, 0.8 %) neural tube defect rate in 1935 pregnancies where preconception folic acid supplementation had been instituted. In contrast, in 2375 pregnancies in which folic acid had been taken only during pregnancy, or in 550 pregnancies in which it had not been taken, the major congenital abnormality rate was 2.2 % (95 % C.I. = 1.7 %, 2.9 %), and the neural tube defect rate 0.34 % (95 % C.I. = 0.2 %, 0.7 %). Both the latter rates were lower than the malformation rates that applied when there had been preconception folate intake. Since that publication, it seems to have become increasingly accepted in the literature that dietary folic acid supplementation is unlikely to help prevent antiepileptic drug-associated foetal malformations. That is not to say that low-dose folate supplementation in preparation for, and during, pregnancy is unnecessary in other circumstances, but simply that it is unlikely to reduce the foetal malformation hazard in women with epilepsy who are treated with antiepileptic drugs, and particularly with valproate. Thus, Wyszynski et al. (2005) reported that 149 valproate-exposed women (all taking folic acid supplementation in a daily dose range of range of 0.4–5 mg during the first trimester of pregnancy) gave birth to 16 children with neural tube defects (10.7 %; 95 % C.I=6.3 %, 16.9 %). The prevalence of the defects in the internal comparison group was 2.9 % (95 % C.I. = 2.0 %, 4.1 %; O.R. 4.0, 95 % C.I. =2.1, 7.4; $P<0.001$). Jentink et al. (2010) analysed case control data from a population-based registry of congenital malformations (EUROCAT – Northern Netherlands). The risk for spina bifida was decreased with folate use in pregnancies not exposed to antiepileptic drugs as compared with controls (odds ratio 0.5; 95 % C.I. = 0.3, 0.7), but not in valproate-exposed pregnancies (odds ratio 1.0; 95 % C.I. = 0.1,7.6). Based on the data of the EURAP database, Tomson et al. (2011) stated that folate supplementation was associated with a greater risk of major congenital malformations. However, there authors went on to point out that this particular finding may have been influenced by confounding by indication, because women at greater risk were more likely to have taken folate.

It thus seems far from clear that folic acid supplementation is of benefit in reducing the incidence of foetal malformations in the offspring of antiepileptic drug-treated women with epilepsy. Nevertheless, it continues to be generally recommended that women with or without epilepsy should take at least 0.4 mg folic acid daily prior to and during pregnancy (Harden et al. 2009).

Foetal Malformations: An Antiepileptic Drug Class Effect?

While the present chapter has discussed general aspects of the relationships between antiepileptic drug exposure in utero and the development of foetal malformations, some of the information that it contains will have suggested that not all the currently available antiepileptic drugs have the same tendency to be associated with reports of teratogenesis. However, the next chapter goes into this matter explicitly, in relation to the individual drugs that are commonly taken by pregnant women with epilepsy.

References

Annegers JF, Elveback LR, Hauser WA, Kurland LT (1974) Do anticonvulsants have a teratogenic effect? Arch Neurol 31:364–373

Annegers JF, Hauser WA, Anderson VE, Kurland LT (1982) The risks of seizure disorders among relatives of patients with childhood onset epilepsy. Neurology 32:174–179

Anonymous (1991) Prevention of neural tube defects: results of the Medical Research Council Vitamin Study. MRC Vitamin Study Research Group. Lancet 338:131–137

Artama M, Auvinen A, Raudaskoski T, Isojarvi I, Isojarvi J (2005) Antiepileptic drug use of women with epilepsy and congenital malformations in the offspring. Neurology 64:1874–1878

Battino D, Tomson T (2007) Management of epilepsy during pregnancy. Drugs 67:2727–2746

Beghi E (2012) Randomised controlled monotherapy trials: which comparators to use? Epileptic Disord 14:235–241

Beghi E, Annegers JF, Collaborative Group for the Pregnancy Registries in Epilepsy (2001) Pregnancy registries in epilepsy. Epilepsia 42:1422–1425

Begum S, Sarma SP, Thomas SV (2013) Malformation in index pregnancy in women with epilepsy is not followed by recurrence in subsequent pregnancy. Epilepsia 54:e163–e167

Berry RJ, Li Z, Erickson JD et al (1999) Prevention of neural-tube defects with folic acid in China. China-U.S. Collaborative Project for Neural Tube Defect Prevention. N Engl J Med 341:1485–1490. Erratum in N Engl J Med (1999); 341:1864

Betts T, Fox C (1999) Proactive pre-conception counselling for women with epilepsy – is it effective? Seizure 8:322–327

Blom HJ, Shaw GM, den Heijer MS, Finnell RH (2011) Neural tube defects and folate; case far from closed. Nat Rev Neurosci 7:724–731

Campbell E, Devenney E, Morrow J et al (2013) Recurrence risk of congenital malformations in infants exposed to antiepileptic drugs in utero. Epilepsia 54:165–171

Canger R, Battino D, Canevini MP et al (1999) Malformations in offspring of women with epilepsy: a prospective study. Epilepsia 40:1231–1236

Cassina M, Dilaghi A, Di Gianantonio B et al (2013) Pregnancy outcome in women exposed to antiepileptic drugs: teratogenic role of maternal epilepsy and its pharmacologic treatment. Reprod Toxicol 39:50–57

Champel V, Radal M, Moulin-Vallez M, Jonville-Béra AP, Autret-Leca E (1999) Should folic acid be given to women treated with valproic acid and/or carbamazepine? Folic acid and pregnancy in epilepsy. Rev Neurol Paris 155:220–224

Craciunescu CN, Brown EC, Mar MH, Albright CD, Nadeau MR, Zeisel SH (2004) Folic acid deficiency during late gestation decreases progenitor cell proliferation and increases apoptosis. J Nutr 134:162–166

Dolk H, McElhattan P (2002) Assessing epidemiological evidence for the teratogenic effect of anticonvulsant medications. J Med Genet 39:243–245

Elshove J, van Eck JH (1971) Congenital abnormalities, cleft lip and cleft palate in particular, in children of epileptic mothers. Ned Tijdschr Geneeskd 115:1371–1375

Fried S, Kozer E, Nulman I, Einarson TR, Koren G (2004) Malformation rates in children of women with untreated epilepsy. Drug Saf 27:197–202

German J, Kowal A, Ehlers KH (1970) Trimethadione and human teratogenesis. Teratology 3:349–362

Harden CL, Pennell PB, Koppel BS et al (2009) Management issues for women with epilepsy – focus on pregnancy (an evidence-based review): III. Vitamin K, folic acid, blood levels, and breast-feeding: Report of the Quality Standards Subcommittee and Therapeutics and Technology Assessment Subcommittee of the American Academy of Neurology and the American Epilepsy Society. Epilepsia 50:1247–1255

Hernandez-Diaz S, Smith CR, Shen A et al (2012) Comparative study of antiepileptic drugs during pregnancy. Neurology 78:1692–1699

Hiilesmaa VK, Teramo K, Grandstrom M, Bardy AH (1983) Serum folate concentrations during pregnancy in women with epilepsy: relation to concentration, of antiepileptic drugs, number of seizures, and fetal outcome. Br Med J (Clin Res Ed) 287:577–579

Holmes LB, Harvey GA, Coull BA, Huntington KB, Khoshbin S, Hayes AM, Ryan LM (2001) The teratogenicity of antiepileptic drugs. N Engl J Med 344:1132–1138

Holmes LB, Mittendorf R, Shen A, Smith CR, Hernandez-Diaz S (2011) Fetal effects of anticonvulsant polytherapies. Arch Neurol 68:1275–1281

Janz D (1975) The teratogenic risk of antiepileptic drugs. Epilepsia 16:159–169

Janz D (1982) Antiepileptic drugs and pregnancy: altered utilization patterns and teratogenesis. Epilepsia 23(Suppl 1):S53–S63

Janz D, Fuchs U (1964) Are anti-epileptic drugs harmful when given during pregnancy? Ger Med Mon 9:20–22

Jentink J, Bakker MK, Nijenhuis CM, Wilffert B, de Jong-van den Berg LT (2010) Does folic acid use decrease the risk for spina bifida after in utero exposure to valproic acid? Pharmacoepidemiol Drug Saf 19:803–807

Kaaja E, Kaaja R, Hiilesmaa V (2003) Major malformations in offspring of women with epilepsy. Neurology 60:575–579

Kallen BAJ (2005) Methodological guidelines in the epidemiological study of the teratogenesis of drugs. Congenit Anom (Kyoto) 45:44–51

Kaneko S, Utami K, Kondo T et al (1992) Malformations in infants of mothers with epilepsy receiving antiepileptic drugs. Neurology 42(Suppl 5):68–74

Kaneko S, Battino D, Andermann E et al (1999) Congenital malformations due to antiepileptic drugs. Epilepsy Res 33:145–158

Lindhout D, Omtzigt JG (1992) Pregnancy and the risk of teratogenicity. Epilepsia 33(Suppl 4):S41–S48

Man S, Petersen I, Thompson M, Nazareth I (2012) Antiepileptic drugs during pregnancy in primary care: a UK population study. PLoS One 7, e52339

Mawer G, Briggs M, Baker GA et al (2010) Pregnancy with epilepsy: obstetric and neonatal outcome of a controlled study. Seizure 19:112–119

Meador KJ, Baker G, Cohen MJ, Gaily E, Westerveld M (2007) Cognitive/behavioral teratogenetic effects of antiepileptic drugs. Epilepsy Behav 11:292–302

Meador K, Pennell PB, Harden CL et al (2008a) Pregnancy registries in epilepsy: a consensus statement on health outcomes. Neurology 71:1109–1117

Meador K, Reynolds MW, Crean S, Fahrbach K, Probst C (2008b) Pregnancy outcomes in women with epilepsy: a systematic review and analysis of published pregnancy registers and cohorts. Epilepsy Res 81:1–13

Meadow SR (1970) Congenital abnormalities and anticonvulsant drugs. Proc R Soc Med 63:48–49

Meyer JG (1973) The teratological effect of anticonvulsants and the effect of pregnancy and birth. Eur J Neurol 10:179–190

Morrow J, Russell A, Guthrie E et al (2006) Malformation risk of antiepileptic drugs in pregnancy: a prospective study from the UK Epilepsy and Pregnancy Register. J Neurol Neurosurg Psychiatry 77:193–198

Morrow JI, Hunt SJ, Russell AJ et al (2009) Folic acid use and major congenital malformations in offspring of women with epilepsy: a prospective study from the UK Epilepsy and Pregnancy Register. J Neurol Neurosurg Psychiatry 80:506–511

Nakane Y, Okuma T, Takahashi R et al (1980) Multi-institutional study on the teratogenicity and fetal toxicity of antiepileptic drugs: a report of a collaborative study group in Japan. Epilepsia 21:663–680

Olafsson E, Hallgrimsson JT, Hauser WA, Ludvigsson P, Gudnundsson G (1998) Pregnancies of women with epilepsy: a population-based study in Iceland. Epilepsia 39:887–892

Perucca E (2005) Birth defects after prenatal exposure to antiepileptic drugs. Lancet Neurol 4:781–786

Rischbieth RH (1979) Troxidone (trimethadione) embryopathy: case report with review of the literature. Clin Exp Neurol 16:251–256

Rothenberg SP, da Costa MP, Sequeira JM, Cracco J, Roberts JL, Weedon J, Quadros EV (2004) Autoantibodies against folate receptors in women with a pregnancy complicated by a neural-tube defect. N Engl J Med 350:134–142

Samrén EB, van Duijn CM, Koch S et al (1997) Maternal use of antiepileptic drugs and the risk of major congenital malformations: a joint European prospective study of human teratogenesis associated with maternal epilepsy. Epilepsia 38:981–990

Shapiro S, Hartz SC, Siskind V et al (1976) Anticonvulsants and parental epilepsy in the development of birth defects. Lancet 1:272–275

Shorvon SD, Reynolds EH (1977) Unnecessary polypharmacy for epilepsy. Br Med J 1:1635–1637

South J (1972) Teratogenic effects of anticonvulsants. Lancet 2:1154

Speidel BD, Mcadow SR (1972) Maternal epilepsy and abnormalities of the fetus and newborn. Lancet 2:839–843

Tamura T, Goldenberg RL, Chapman VR, Johnston KE, Ramey SL, Nelson KG (2005) Folate status of mothers during pregnancy and mental and psychomotor development. Pediatrics 116:703–798

Tomson T, Battino D (2012) Teratogenic effects of antiepileptic drugs. Lancet Neurol 11:803–813

Tomson T, Battino D, Bonizzoni E et al (2011) Dose-dependent risk of malformation with antiepileptic drugs: an analysis of data from the EURAP epilepsy and pregnancy registry. Lancet Neurol 10:609–617

Vajda FJE, O'Brien T, Hitchcock A, Graham J, Lander C, Eadie M (2007) The Australian antiepileptic drug in pregnancy register: aspects of data collection and analysis. J Clin Neurosci 14:936–942

Vajda FJE, O'Brien T, Hitchcock A, Graham J, Lander C, Eadie M (2008) The internal control group in a register of antiepileptic drug use in pregnancy. J Clin Neurosci 15:29–35

Vajda F, Hitchcock A, Graham J, O'Brien T, Lander C, Eadie M (2010) The teratogenic risk of antiepileptic drug polytherapy. Epilepsia 51:805–810

Vajda FJE, O'Brien TJ, Graham J, Lander CM, Eadie MJ (2013a) Dose-dependency of fetal malformations associated with valproate. Neurology 81:999–1003

Vajda FJE, O'Brien TJ, Lander CM, Graham J, Roten A, Eadie MJ (2013b) Tetratogenesis in repeated pregnancies in antiepileptic drug-treated women. Epilepsia 54:181–186

Vajda FJE, O'Brien TJ, Graham J, Lander CM, Eadie MJ (2014) The Australian register of antiepileptic drugs in pregnancy: changes over time in the epileptic population. J Clin Neurosci 21:1478–1482

Veiby G, Daltveit AK, Engelsen BA, Gilhus NE (2014) Fetal growth restriction and birth defects with newer and older antiepileptic drugs during pregnancy. J Neurol 261:579–588

Watson JD, Spellacy WN (1971) Neonatal effects of maternal treatment with the anticonvulsant drug diphenylhydantoin. Obstet Gynecol 37:881–885

Werler MA, Ahrens KA, Bosca JLF et al (2011) Use of antiepileptic medications in pregnancy in relation to risk of birth defects. Ann Epidemiol 21:842–850

Wide K, Winlladh B, Källén B (2004) Major malformations in infants exposed to antiepileptic drugs in utero, with emphasis on carbamazepine and valproic acid: a nation-wide, population-based register study. Acta Pediatr 93:174–176

Wyszynski DF, Nambisan M, Surve T, Alsdorf RM, Smith CR, Holmes LB, Antiepileptic Drug Pregnancy Registry (2005) Increased rate of major malformations in offspring exposed to valproate during pregnancy. Neurology 64:961–965

Yerby M (2003) Management issues for women with epilepsy: neural tube defects and folic acid supplementation. Neurology 61(Suppl 2):S23–S26

Chapter 9
Particular Antiepileptic Drugs and Foetal Malformations

Abstract This chapter attempts to discuss the published information concerning the risks of structural malformations occurring in foetuses exposed to those individual antiepileptic drugs that have been widely enough used in women with epilepsy for relevant data to be available. There appears to be persuasive evidence that valproate is a dose-related teratogen, with certain malformations such as neural tube defects seeming to be particularly associated with high maternal dosage of the drug. Evidence also points towards topiramate being a dose-related teratogen. On the basis of the available data the possibility that the remaining currently used drugs are teratogens cannot be excluded, but there appears to be enough evidence to indicate that any teratogenic hazard arising from exposure to them is quite small.

As will be apparent from the contents of the previous chapter, in the earlier years of the study of associations between intrauterine antiepileptic drug exposure and foetal malformations, there was a tendency for authors to write as if the malformations represented an unwanted class effect of the drugs. With the growth of knowledge as time passed, and as additional effective antiepileptic drugs became available, it became increasingly recognised that the degree of malformation hazard varied considerably between the individual agents. The present chapter attempts to discuss the information that is available concerning the individual antiepileptic drugs that have enjoyed some use in pregnancy in recent years.

Wlodarczyk et al. (2012) have provided a reasonably contemporary and thorough review of the literature concerning individual antiepileptic drugs and foetal malformations. Their paper includes a number of useful tabulations of previously published data. No attempt is made in the present chapter to reproduce all of the Wlodarczyk et al. material, which is a valuable source of information.

Phenobarbitone and Its Congeners

Phenobarbitone was among the antiepileptic drugs that featured in the early reports of a possible association between these agents and foetal malformations, but the drug was not singled out in these reports for a culprit role. However, after finding

M.J. Eadie, F.J.E. Vajda, *Antiepileptic Drugs and Pregnancy: A Guide for Prescribers*, DOI 10.1007/978-3-319-21434-4_9

congenital abnormalities in four of the offspring of 61 mothers who had been treated with phenobarbitone to try to prevent threatened abortions, Wheatley (1963) raised the possibility that the drug might be a teratogen. A few years later, Nelson and Forfar (1971) studied the possible association between various drugs and foetal malformations and noted that significantly more mothers than would have been expected had been taking phenobarbitone. In the earlier literature, there were other data concerning the outcomes of pregnancies exposed to phenobarbitone in women with epilepsy, but there was little explicit analysis of the phenobarbitone-related foetal hazard in its own right. Staples (1972) concluded that, up to his time of writing, there was no definite evidence incriminating the drug as a teratogen. Shapiro et al. (1976) also took the view that the drug did not cause dysmorphogenesis.

In their analysis of an international database of foetal malformations, Arpino et al. (2000) detected an association between exposure to phenobarbitone during pregnancy and the presence of oral clefts. Then Holmes et al. (2004) found a 6.5 % malformation rate in 77 offspring of mothers exposed to phenobarbitone therapy during pregnancy. This was more than four times the risk in an antiepileptic drug-unexposed control population. In a later analysis of an expanded population from the same source, Hernandez-Diaz et al. (2012) reported a 5.6 % increase in the malformation risk in 199 pregnancies in which phenobarbitone was used in antiepileptic drug monotherapy, compared with the rate in 51 antiepileptic drug-unexposed pregnancies. This increased risk was statistically significant. However, there was no evidence of a correlation between the phenobarbitone dose and the malformation risk. Tomson et al. (2011), in an analysis of 217 phenobarbitone-exposed foetuses whose records were contained in the EURAP register, found a statistically significant higher malformation rate when the maternal phenobarbitone dose exceeded 150 mg a day, as compared with the rate when lower doses had been used. The meta-analysis of Meador et al. (2008), which accumulated 945 pregnancies, found a phenobarbitone-associated malformation rate of 4.9 %, but there were no control data to permit comparisons being made.

Although it is possible that the same data may have appeared in more than one of the above reports, there now seems to probably be sufficient evidence to suggest that phenobarbitone is a teratogen. This knowledge may not have a great impact in Western medicine where the drug is tending to disappear from use in the age group in which pregnancy is likely, but it may have significant implications for less affluent communities globally where the drug is still in extensive and reasonably satisfactory use in treating epilepsy. No specific pattern of malformation appears to be particularly associated with exposure to the drug.

Phenytoin

There were two pregnancies which resulted in foetal malformations among 55 pregnancies exposed to phenytoin in monotherapy or polytherapy in the series of Janz and Fuchs (1964), and nine in 162 similarly exposed pregnancies in the report of

Speidel and Meadow (1972). Then Monson et al. (1973) specifically addressed the question of phenytoin exposure in pregnancy and the occurrence of foetal malformations. They found a 6.1 % malformation rate associated with exposure to the drug in 98 children, as compared with a 2.5 % rate in the pregnancies of over 50,000 non-epileptic women. Dravet et al. (1992) employed logistic regression analysis to find a 2.98 times increased malformation rate (95 % C.I. = 1.48, 6.05) in first trimester phenytoin-exposed foetuses, compared with a control group of 117,183 pregnancies.

Since those early reports, there has been relatively little further statistically significant evidence that phenytoin possesses any significant capacity for producing teratogenesis. When Wlodarczyk et al. (2012) reviewed the existing literature, they found nine relevant studies in which the drug had been used in monotherapy during pregnancy. In eight of these studies, the relative risk or odds ratio in favour of the drug being a teratogen exceeded 1.0, but in none to a statistically significant extent. In the most recent analysis of the Australian Pregnancy Register data, there was a foetal malformation rate of 2.4 % in 41 pregnancies exposed to phenytoin monotherapy, a relative risk of 1.49 (95 % C.I. = 0.30, 7.42) compared with the foetal malformation risk in women with epilepsy who did not take antiepileptic drugs in at least the early part of pregnancy. Logistic regression analysis of malformation risk on phenytoin dose in the Australian data showed a far from statistically significant trend for the risk to decrease rather than increase with increasing drug dose. From a statistical viewpoint, overall there seems to be little convincing recent evidence that phenytoin is an important human teratogen, though the possibility that it may be responsible for occasional foetal malformations cannot be excluded.

Despite this, over the years a substantial number of authors have written about a 'foetal hydantoin syndrome'. The idea seems to have been first proposed in print by Hanson and Smith (1975) after authors such as Loughnan et al. (1973), Hill et al. (1974), Danks et al. (1974) and Barr et al. (1974) had observed an increased frequency of digital hypoplasia and certain mid-face alterations in babies who had been exposed to the drug during pregnancy. As originally described, the syndrome involved relatively poor intrauterine growth and development, mild mental retardation, a facial appearance which was considered characteristic, skeletal abnormalities and, in particular, digital hypoplasia. Phelan et al. (1982) considered that the full syndrome could be recognised in some 11 % of phenytoin-exposed infants and incomplete forms in another 31 %, while Andermann et al. (1982) found hypoplasia of the phalanges in 22 % of phenytoin-exposed foetuses. Nearly all of these comparatively minor abnormalities became less noticeable as the affected infants grew older. Various subsequent authors, often on the basis of single instances, attempted to add additional features to the syndrome, and one or two began to expand the concept to that of a foetal anticonvulsant syndrome. A certain amount of animal laboratory investigation attempted to explain its mechanism, while clinical argument went on regarding whether it was a genuine entity, whether it could be diagnosed reliably in the absence of knowledge of the details of antiepileptic drug exposure in pregnancy and whether its features permitted its being distinguished from the subsequently described foetal carbamazepine and foetal valproate syndromes. Kini et al. (2006) reported that experienced dysmorphologists had failed to distinguish consistently between antiepileptic drug exposed and unexposed infants in photographs of the infants' facial features. As time has passed, interest in the matter seems to have dwindled, and the antiepileptic drug teratogenesis literature has tended to become more focussed on major and more clinically and cosmetically important malformations.

Ethosuximide

Ethosuximide is sometimes mentioned in the antiepileptic drug teratogenicity literature, but there is little indication that the drug is a significant cause of foetal malformations. The amount of information available is understandably small because nearly all the literature emanates from Western countries. In these countries, absence seizure disorders, the usual indication for the use of ethosuximide, are not often still active by the time women become pregnant, even though the disorders were active earlier in their lives. As well, because of a perhaps not adequately founded belief that using ethosuximide in monotherapy may facilitate the occurrence of convulsive seizures, the drug has often been co-prescribed with another antiepileptic drug such as phenytoin, carbamazepine or valproate. In these instances, any foetal malformations that developed, if they were not coincidental, might have been due to the co-administered drug.

Carbamazepine

There is considerably more information concerning the possible association between carbamazepine and foetal malformations than the amount that is available for the individual drugs discussed immediately above. This is probably so because carbamazepine has been in widespread use for some 40 years and is still commonly employed in Western countries in treating epilepsy in pregnant women. At a relatively early stage, the drug acquired a reputation for relative safety from the foetal point of view. This may have happened because no congenital abnormalities occurred in the pregnancies exposed to carbamazepine alone or together with other antiepileptic drugs, in the series described by Starreveld-Zimmerman et al. (1973). In that series there were 22 malformations among 247 live births to mothers who had taken other antiepileptic drugs during pregnancy.

Over the following years, various reports appeared concerning the likelihood of carbamazepine-associated teratogenesis. For instance, Kallen et al. (1989) and Kallen (1994) studied the data in the Swedish registry of malformed neonates and noted that a nonstatistically significant increase in the occurrence of spina bifida was associated with carbamazepine exposure. Lindhout and Omtzigt (1992) accepted that this particular association was a genuine one, while Little et al. (1993) reported the occurrence of a neural tube defect in a foetus that, at the age of 3 or 4 weeks of gestation, had been exposed to the high concentration of carbamazepine resulting from a single overdose of about 4800 mg, taken in a suicide attempt. Samrén et al. (1997) compared the outcome of 192 antiepileptic drug-exposed pregnancies in women with epilepsy with that in 158 untreated pregnancies. In relation to pregnancies involving carbamazepine intake, there was an increased hazard of foetal malformations (relative risk, 4.9; 95 % C.I. = 1.3, 18.0). Diav-Citrin et al. (2001) also described a statistically significantly increased hazard of foetal malformation associated with exposure to the drug during pregnancy as compared with matched and so-called 'general' controls (relative risk, 2.4; 95 % C.I. = 1.1, 4.56). Matalon et al. (2002), based on a meta-analysis of 1255 pregnancies, arrived at the view that carbamazepine increased the occurrence of foetal malformation rate (6.7 %) above its background value (2.34 %). Kaaja et al. (2003), in a logistic regression analysis of 740 antiepileptic drug-exposed pregnancies in women with epilepsy, found an odds ratio for carbamazepine-associated malformations of 2.5 (95 % C.I. = 1.0, 6.0) compared with the rate in 239 pregnancies not exposed to these drugs.

Thirteen of the relevant more major papers in the subsequent literature were summarised in the study of Wlodarczyk et al. (2012). These workers noted that the published major congenital malformation rates for carbamazepine monotherapy ranged between 2.2 and 6.3 %. Relative risk or odds ratio values were available for nine of the series analysed and were 1.0 or higher in eight of the nine, though statistically significant higher in only two. In the three largest series, those of Morrow et al. (2006) with 900 pregnancies, Hernandez-Diaz et al. (2007) with 873 pregnancies and Artama et al. (2005) with 805 pregnancies, the malformation rates were respectively, 2.2, 2.5 and 4.0 %.

There are a few relatively recent publications that were not included in the Wlodarczyk et al. (2012) analysis. Jentink et al. (2010) extracted from the literature a total of 2680 pregnancies in women with epilepsy exposed to carbamazepine monotherapy. There was a major congenital malformation rate of 3.3 % (95 % C.I. = 2.7, 4.2 %), with an increased spina bifida rate (odds ratio 2.6; 95 % C.I. = 1.2, 5.3) relative to that in antiepileptic drug-unexposed pregnancies. No definite association was found between carbamazepine and any other particular foetal malformation. Tomson et al. (2011), in 1402 carbamazepine-associated pregnancies drawn from the EURAP registry, found a malformation rate of 3.4 % (95 % C.I. = 1.11, 7.71 %) and produced evidence that the malformation rate was dose dependent. Holmes et al. (2011), in North American Registry data assessing major congenital malformations detected up to 3 months after the end of pregnancy, found a 2.9 % foetal malformation risk from carbamazepine exposure during pregnancy in women with epilepsy.

It seems likely that the meta-analyses and some of the literature review papers have included the same pregnancies that were previously included in other publications. Nevertheless the data seem sufficient to suggest that carbamazepine may have some capacity to be responsible for foetal malformations and probably to cause spina bifida. However, the degree of hazard appears to not greatly exceed that which applies for pregnancies in the untreated female epileptic and normal populations.

In the most recent Australian Pregnancy Register data, there were 346 pregnancies exposed to carbamazepine monotherapy, with a 5.5 % foetal malformation risk. The risk compared with that for pregnancies in women with epilepsy unexposed to antiepileptic drugs was not statistically significant (relative risk 1.68; 95 % C.I. = 0.64, 4.42). Logistic regression analysis of malformation risk on carbamazepine dose (Fig. 8.1) showed a nonstatistically significant tendency for the risk to increase with increasing dosage (P=0.405).

The existence of a foetal carbamazepine syndrome has been described. It comprised facial dysmorphism, congenital heart defects, skeletal abnormalities, renal agenesis, ambiguous genitalia and anal atresia (Akar et al. 2012). Some of these features had been described earlier by Jones et al. (1989), notably the facial appearances and fingernail hypoplasia, together with the overall developmental delay. Ornoy and Cohen (1996) identified such a carbamazepine syndrome in six of 47 neonates exposed to the drug. Some of the arguments as to whether such appearances constitute a recognisable syndrome specific to the drug have been mentioned in relation to phenytoin (above).

Valproate

Roughly a decade after it came into clinical use in Europe, suspicion began to arise that valproate might be a human teratogen. Robert and Guibaud (1982) noted an excessive number of instances of spina bifida among 71 malformations reported in the offspring of epileptic mothers in the Rhône Valley in France and found that there was an association between this particular malformation and exposure to valproate during pregnancy (Robert and Rosa 1983). Bjerkedal et al. (1982), Lindhout and Meinardi (1984) and Lindhout and Schmidt (1986) then reported further instances of the association, while Jager-Roman et al. (1986) described the presence of major malformations in 4 of 14 foetuses (28.6 %) exposed to valproate in monotherapy. Bailey et al. (1983) mentioned that the manufacturers of valproate had at that time held data on the outcome of 33 pregnancies which had been exposed to valproate and that there were four foetal malformations, including two meningomyelocoeles, in the material. Curran (1987) reported five instances of neural tube defects in foetuses exposed to valproate in utero. Thus within the span of a few years, there were grounds for strong suspicion that exposure to valproate during pregnancy carried a heightened risk of neural tube defects occurring in the foetus.

By this time Di Liberti et al. (1984) had proposed the existence of a characteristic identifiable syndrome (the foetal valproate syndrome) which they had recognised in all seven infants whom they had examined and who had been exposed to valproate during pregnancy. As described, the syndrome comprised changes in the epicanthic folds, a flat nasal bridge, a small upturned nose, a long upper lip with a relatively shallow philtrum, a thin upper vermillion border and downturned angles of the mouth. In two of their seven foetuses, hypospadias and delay in psychomotor development were present.

Over the subsequent years, this initial report was followed by numerous further accounts of the occurrence of this particular syndrome, some of the accounts attempting to add further features to the clinical picture. By 2001 Kozma (2001) had collected 69 instances from the literature and added two further examples. This writer at that time described the features of the syndrome as involving a consistent facial phenotype characterized by a small broad nose, small ears, flat philtrum, long upper lip with shallow philtrum and micrognathia or retrognathia. It was associated with multiple systemic and orthopaedic abnormalities (in 62 %), central nervous system dysfunction and altered physical growth. Minor skin defects were present in 30 %, cardiovascular abnormalities in 26 %, genital abnormalities in 22 % and lung abnormalities in 16 %. Brain, eye, kidney and hearing defects were less frequent, while neural tube defects occurred in 3 %. There was a substantial death rate during infancy in those affected (12 %), while another 23 % exhibited developmental defects or mental retardation.

This constellation of abnormalities did not limit the spectrum of abnormal developmental manifestations which later authors attempted to include in the syndrome, for instance, speech delay, joint laxity, glue ears and autistic features (Moore et al. 2000), the rare so-called Baller–Gerold syndrome that features malformation of the skull, face, forearm and hand bones (Lype et al. 2008) and septo-optic dysplasia (McMahon and Braddock 2001). Jacobsen et al. (2014) reported an increased risk of dental agenesis associated with valproate exposure in utero.

In the meanwhile, reports of larger-scale studies of the consequences of intrauterine valproate exposure had begun to appear (e.g. Koch et al. 1992; Kaaja et al. 2003; Artama et al. 2005; Wyszynski et al. 2005). These were among the 10 publications that Wlodarczyk et al. (2012) considered in their paper, in which they reported that the major congenital malformation rates associated with valproate exposure had ranged from 5.7 to 16.8 %. In the seven studies for which odds ratios or relative risks had been calculated, the values ranged between 2.52 and 5.94, in all instances being statistically significant at the $P<0.05$ level. Miki et al. (2014) subsequently published a meta-analysis of 58 cohort studies relevant to valproate-associated teratogenesis in humans, including some of those discussed immediately above.

In an analysis of the Australian Pregnancy Register data accumulated by late 2012, foetal malformations had occurred in 13.8 % of 253 pregnancies in which valproate had been used in monotherapy, a relative risk of 4.23 (95 % C.I. = 1.69, 10.57) compared with that for malformations in women with epilepsy who did not take antiepileptic drugs during at least the earlier months of pregnancy.

There thus seems quite strong evidence that valproate is a significant human teratogen. Further, a number of studies have shown that the malformation rate associated with the drug is dose dependent. Omtzigt et al. (1992) had noted that the occurrence of spina bifida was associated with statistically significantly higher valproate doses (mean 1640 ± 136 compared with 941 ± 48 mg per day). Canger et al. (1999) reached a similar conclusion. Samrén et al. (1999) reported that the malformation rate associated with valproate doses above 1000 mg per day was significantly higher than the rate for lower doses. Kaneko et al. (1999) plotted malformation rate against valproate dose and showed the malformation risk increased with drug dose. Vajda et al. (2004) and Vajda and Eadie (2005) observed in the data of the Australian Pregnancy Register that the valproate-associated malformation rate was substantially higher at daily drug doses in excess of 1400 mg a day during pregnancy and initially suggested that this value might distinguish between comparatively safe and unacceptably hazardous dosages from the foetal standpoint. Shortly afterwards, Vajda et al. (2006) reduced the cut-off dose to 1100 mg per day. Diav-Citrin et al. (2008) nominated a dose of 1000 mg a day as separating a 21.9 % malformation risk from a 2.5 % one. Later analyses of expanded data from the Australian Register, employing logistic regression, have shown that in practice there probably is no really safe valproate dosage from the standpoint of avoiding foetal malformation (Eadie 2008 and Figs. 8.1, 8.2 and 8.3).

The existence of this dose dependence in malformation rate associated with valproate has been confirmed in further studies (Bromfield et al. 2008; Tomson et al. 2011) and seems to be to be fairly generally accepted in the recent literature. The combination of the greater tendency of valproate to be associated with foetal malformations and the dose relatedness of the risk may explain much of the rather wide range of published values for the overall hazard of foetal malformation associated with intrauterine antiepileptic drug exposure in general. The more pregnancies exposed to valproate in a series of antiepileptic drug-treated pregnancies, the higher the malformation rate in that series will appear to be. Even in two series with equal proportions of valproate-exposed pregnancies, the overall malformation rate will be higher in the series with the greater mean valproate dose. As mentioned earlier (Chap. 8), the combination of the two factors also seems to explain the rather frequently described earlier finding that use of antiepileptic drugs in polytherapy was associated with higher malformation rates than use of the drugs in monotherapy.

Vajda et al. (2013b) have noted another phenomenon in relation to valproate dosage. At doses above 2000 mg a day, exposure to the drug tends to be statistically significantly associated with the occurrence of spina bifida and hypospadias and at lower doses with other malformations (Fig. 9.1). This suggests that the type of malformation associated with exposure to an antiepileptic drug may depend on the drug dose involved. This finding obviously needs confirmation, though that may be difficult to obtain because the already existing data about the dose dependence of the malformation risk associated with the drug has led to valproate being used in lower dosages, if it must be used in pregnant women. This use of lower dosages of valproate has been associated with a parallel decline in foetal malformation rates in the Australian data (Vajda et al. 2013b; Fig. 9.2).

Lamotrigine

Lamotrigine was first marketed in 1991, though its introduction into the United States was further delayed. The drug is increasingly being employed in the management of pregnant women with epilepsy and currently enjoys a reputation for being among the safest of the antiepileptic drugs from the teratogenicity point of view.

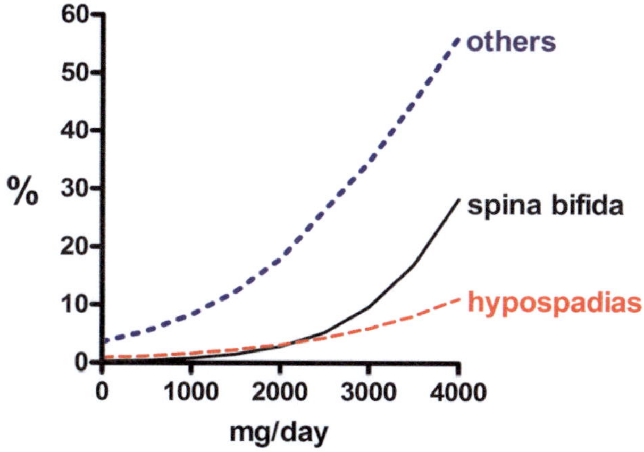

Fig. 9.1 Logistic regressions for risk of spina bifida (*continuous line*), hypospadias (*lower broken line*) and for all malformations except spina bifida and hypospadias (*upper dotted line*) on valproate dose. All regressions are statistically significant

Sabers et al. (2004) reported a 2.0 % malformation rate associated with foetal exposure to the drug. Morrow et al. (2006) analysed the data of the United Kingdom Register and found a major congenital malformation rate of 3.2 % (95 % C.I. = 2.1, 4.9 %) in 647 pregnancies in which the drug had been used in monotherapy. The malformation rate for lamotrigine was nonstatistically significantly higher than the 2.2 % rate for carbamazepine, the major comparator used (odds ratio 1.71; 95 % C.I. = 0.88, 3.32). Morrow et al. also noted that the frequency of malformations appeared to increase progressively through the lamotrigine dosage bands of (i) up to 100 mg per day, (ii) 100–200 mg per day and (iii) over 200 mg per day. The mean lamotrigine dose associated with malformations, 352.4 mg per day, was higher than the mean dose in pregnancies where there was no malformation (250.6 mg per day, $P<0.0001$). At much the same time, Vajda et al. (2006) described 65 pregnancies in which lamotrigine was used as the only epileptic drug and in which no foetal malformations had occurred, and Meador et al. (2006), by means of a literature review, traced 98 pregnancies involving lamotrigine monotherapy in which there was a serious outcome, including major congenital malformations, in only 1 %.

Cunnington et al. (2007) reported that there had been a major congenital malformation rate of 2.7 % (95 % C.I. = 1.8, 4.2 %) for 802 pregnancies in the records of the firm marketing the drug (this population probably included some or all of the pregnancies in the studies mentioned immediately above). Regression analysis found no relationship between the risk of malformations and the drug dose. In the North American Registry data, Holmes et al. (2008) calculated that there was a 2.3 % major congenital malformation rate for the drug. Compared with 206,224 antiepileptic drug-unexposed infants in whom there was a cleft palate or cleft lip rate of 0.07 %, they found a 10.4-fold increase in the incidence of cleft palates or lips in the pregnancies exposed to lamotrigine in monotherapy. Then Mawer et al. (2010) described a 5.4 % major congenital malformation rate in 227 pregnancies in

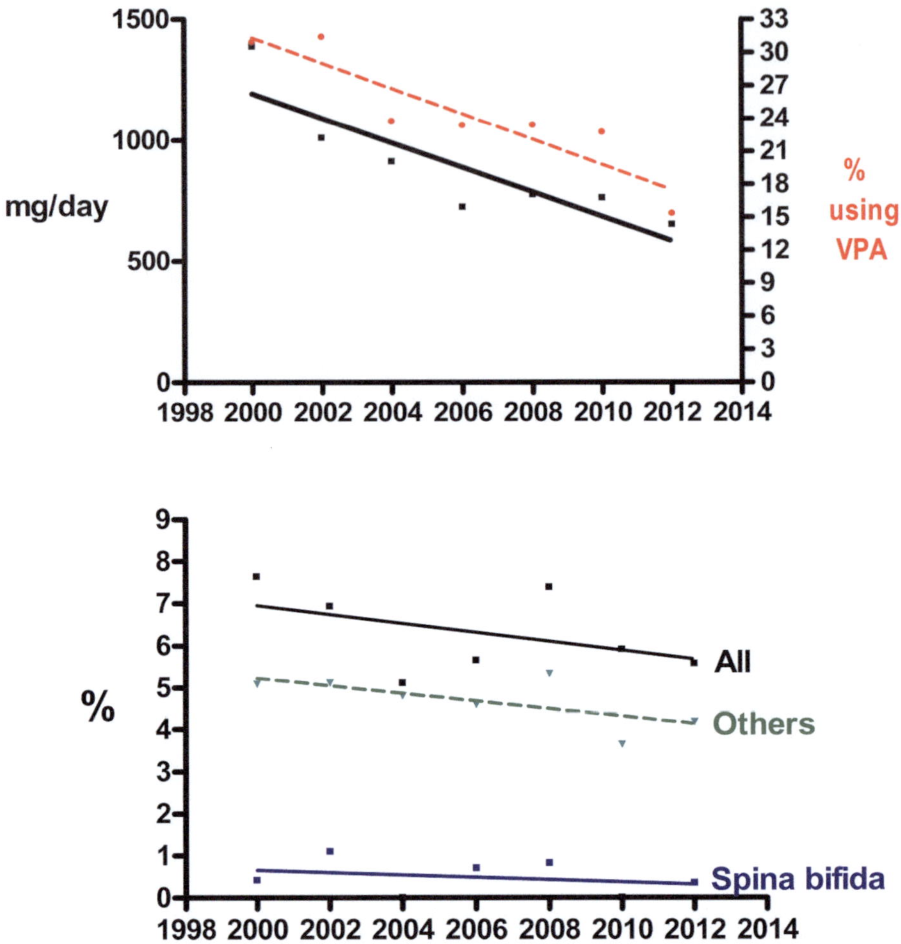

Fig. 9.2 *Top panel*: linear regressions on date for (i) mean valproate dose (*continuous line* – dose values shown on left 'y' axis) prescribed during consecutive 2-year periods between 1999 and 2014 and for (ii) the proportion of all pregnancies in the Australian Register that were prescribed valproate (percentage values shown on right 'y' axis; regression, *broken line*). *Lower panel*: linear regressions on dates for percentages of valproate exposed pregnancies in which (i) all types of malformation (*upper continuous line*) (ii) spina bifida only (*lower continuous line*) and (iii) all foetal malformations apart from spina bifida (*dashed line*) occurred. The slopes of all the linear regressions in both panels, except that for all other malformations, are statistically significant

lamotrigine-treated women with epilepsy, as compared with a 2.1 % rate in 315 matched control pregnancies ($P=0.23$). Vajda et al. (2010) found a 4.9 % malformation rate in 243 pregnancies exposed to lamotrigine monotherapy, as compared with a 3.4 % malformation rate in 118 pregnancies in women with epilepsy that was untreated during the critical period of organogenesis (odds ratio 1.48; 95 % C.I. = 0.46, 4.69). Unlike the situation for valproate, logistic regression for malformation risk plotted against increasing drug dose had a downward slope in the Vajda et al.

data. Molgaard-Nielsen and Hviid (2011) linked a Danish database of 837,795 live births between 1996 and 2008 with a database for national dispensed antiepileptic drugs. Major congenital malformations had occurred in 3.7 % of 1019 lamotrigine-exposed pregnancies, an adjusted prevalence odds ratio of 1.18 (95 % C.I. = 0.83, 1.68) compared with that which applied for the general population. In the same year Tomson et al. (2011), based on the EURAP data, quoted a major foetal malformation rate of 2.0 % for lamotrigine monotherapy in doses below 300 mg a day, based on the set of 1280 pregnancies in which the drug had been used in monotherapy. These authors stated that the malformation rate associated with lamotrigine was dose dependent. Holmes and Hernandez-Diaz (2012) described a 2 % foetal malformation rate in 1562 pregnancies exposed to lamotrigine in monotherapy (relative risk versus controls 1.8; 95 % C.I. = 0.7, 4.6).

Then Campbell et al. (2014) provided updated data from the United Kingdom Pregnancy Register at a stage when it contained 2198 pregnancies in which lamotrigine had been used as the sole antiepileptic drug. In these pregnancies there was a major congenital malformation rate of 2.3 % (95 % C.I. = 1.8, 3.1 %), and unlike the earlier analysis of this register's contents, the trend for the risk of malformation to increase with increasing drug dose was not statistically significant. Veiby et al. (2014), based on 833 Norwegian pregnancies in which lamotrigine was used in monotherapy, calculated a 3.4 % malformation rate with an odds ratio of 1.26 (95 % C.I. = 0.87, 1.84) compared with a control group of 771,412 antiepileptic drug-unexposed children. Vajda et al. (2014) studied data from the Australian Pregnancy Register at the end of 2013. There was a major congenital malformation rate of 4.6 % in the 307 lamotrigine monotherapy-exposed pregnancies, with a relative risk of malformation of 1.40 (0.51, 3.80) compared with 154 untreated pregnancies in women with epilepsy. Logistic regression analysis showed that the resulting regression line had a slight and nonstatistically significant downward slope for malformation risk on increasing drug dose (Fig. 8.2).

Thus there is a reasonable amount of relatively recent data concerning the foetal malformation hazard associated with use of lamotrigine in the pregnancies of women with epilepsy, though some of the material has probably been included more than once in the analysed data sets. Consistently, the malformation rates have been a little higher than those for the comparator populations that different groups of workers have chosen. However, none of the rates has been statistically significantly higher. Some studies have suggested that the foetal hazards from the drug may be dose related, though the evidence for this never achieved the $P<0.05$ level of statistical significance. Studies employing logistic regression have not suggested that such a dosage dependency exists. Interestingly, in the Australian data where regression analysis provided no evidence for a dose-dependent risk, when the malformation rate was correlated with the three lamotrigine dosage bands that Morrow et al. (2006) used, the malformation rate appeared to increase with dosage. However, if the highest dosage band was subdivided into two, the rate was lower for the new highest dosage range than for the immediately lower one. It seems reasonable to conclude that, if lamotrigine is a teratogen, its teratogenic potential is comparatively small.

Topiramate

Topiramate became available for therapeutic use in the mid-1990s and appears to have achieved a moderate penetration into the epilepsy market internationally. In its lower strengths, it has become quite extensively employed in migraine prevention.

Some information about foetal malformations associated with exposure to the drug in pregnancy has become available in recent years. In the study of Morrow et al. (2006), based on the United Kingdom Register, there were two foetal malformations in 28 pregnancies where topiramate was used in monotherapy (rate 7.1 %, uncorrected odds ratio relative to carbamazepine 2.7; 95 % C.I. = 0.58, 3.58). Hunt et al. (2008), in a further study based on the United Kingdom Register, described a 4.8 % malformation rate (95 % C.I. = 1.7, 13.3 %) in 70 live births to mothers who used the drug in monotherapy. They noted an incidence of oral clefts in the topiramate pregnancies that was 11 times that of the community background rate. Ornoy et al. (2008) found a 3.5 % major congenital malformation rate in 29 topiramate monotherapy-exposed pregnancies. Holmes et al. (2008) described a major congenital malformation rate of 4.1 % in 197 topiramate-exposed foetuses drawn from the records of the North American Registry. In an expanded data set comprising 359 pregnancies exposed to topiramate in monotherapy from the same registry, Holmes and Hernandez-Diaz (2012) calculated that there was a 4.2 % malformation rate that could be compared with the malformation rate in 442 unexposed control infants (relative risk 3.8; 95 % C.I. = 1.4, 10.6). Holmes and Hernandez-Diaz (2012) also noted a 1.4 % rate of facial clefts in their material, higher than the expected population rate for that abnormality, while Mines et al. (2014) observed a 0.36 % oral cleft rate in 1945 neonates exposed to topiramate in the first trimester of pregnancy, as compared with a 0.07 % rate in 13,614 offspring not exposed to the drug in utero.

In the Danish Registry data, Molgaard-Nielsen and Hviid (2011) found a malformation rate of 4.68 % for 108 infants exposed to topiramate in pregnancy (adjusted odds ratio 1.44; 95 % C.I. 0.58, 3.58), as compared with the rate in the unexposed infant population. Veiby et al. (2014) in 2600 children from Norway exposed to antiepileptic drugs during pregnancy found a higher, but not statistically significant, risk of malformations associated with intrauterine exposure to topiramate monotherapy (in 4.2 % of 48 infants; odds ratio 1.66; 95 % C.I. = 0.40, 6.85). Marguilis et al. (2012) obtained evidence of an association between first trimester exposure to topiramate and oral clefts in the foetus and a statistically significant risk of microcephaly. Vajda et al. (2014) traced 42 instances of topiramate use in monotherapy during pregnancy in the Australian Pregnancy Register. In these pregnancies there was a foetal malformation rate of 2.4 % (relative risk 0.73; 95 % C.I. = 0.09, 6.07) compared with the rate in 147 pregnancies in women with epilepsy in which no antiepileptic drug was taken in at least the first trimester of pregnancy. In addition, there were a further 85 pregnancies in the Register in which the drug had been used in combination with another antiepileptic agent. In these 85 pregnancies, the malformation rate was 14.1 % (relative risk compared with 147 untreated pregnancies in women with epilepsy from the Register 4.32; 95 % C.I. = 1.57, 11.05). The presence of valproate in a few of the topiramate polytherapy drug combinations did not seem capable of accounting for this higher malformation rate. Multivariate linear regression analysis with serial stripping of nonsignificant parameters was applied to the combined monotherapy and polytherapy data for all the pregnancies in the Register. There was a statistically significant ($P=0.013$) upward slope for the relationship between malformation risk and increasing topiramate dose (Vajda et al. 2013a). Further, when the relation between individual antiepileptic drug dosages and particular malformations was examined, there were statistically significant associations between topiramate dosage and both brain malformations and hypospadias, though not facial clefts (Fig. 9.3).

As mentioned in Chap. 8, the latest, as yet unpublished, analysis of the data of the Australian Pregnancy Register has provided further evidence that topiramate, at least when used together with any one of several other antiepileptic drugs, is a significant teratogen though, when used as the sole antiepileptic drug in pregnant women, the foetal malformation rate was not statistically significantly greater than that in pregnancies of women with epilepsy that was not treated with antiepileptic drugs.

There now seems to be sufficient evidence available to suggest that topiramate use in antiepileptic drug combinations in pregnancy, and perhaps when used alone, may be responsible for the occurrence of foetal malformations and that the malformation risk increases with increasing topiramate dosage. This dose dependence may be important because of the widespread contemporary use of topiramate in migraine prevention, where the drug dose is generally appreciably lower than that used in treating epilepsy. As further data accumulate, the degree of foetal hazard associated with topiramate, and perhaps the specificity of the risk for particular

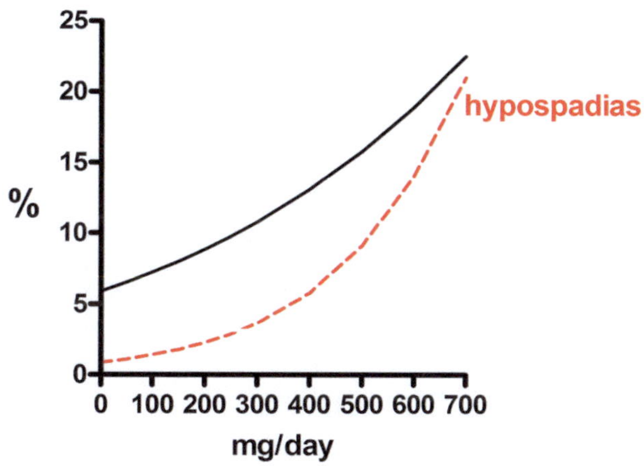

Fig. 9.3 Logistic regressions for risk of all foetal malformations (*continuous line*) and hypospadias (*broken line*) plotted against maternal topiramate dose

organ systems, may become better defined. However, there already probably is enough information to suggest the need for considerable caution in prescribing the drug in monotherapy for women capable of pregnancy, while its use combined with other antiepileptic drugs would be better avoided.

Levetiracetam

Levetiracetam, which came into therapeutic use a little later than the two drugs considered immediately above, seems to have achieved greater popularity among prescribers. It appears to be finding a place as one of the major antiepileptic drugs in contemporary clinical use. Until quite recently, the literature contained only a few reports of small numbers of pregnancies exposed the drug, with the opinion being expressed that it did not seem to constitute a particular hazard for the foetus. Then Molgaard-Nielsen and Hviid (2011) reported a series of 58 pregnancies exposed to the drug in monotherapy. There were no foetal malformations in the group. Hernandez-Diaz et al. (2012) noted a 2.4 % malformation rate in 84 pregnancies from the North American Registry which had been exposed to levetiracetam in monotherapy. There was a relative risk of 2.2 (95 % C.I. = 0.8, 6.4) compared with the malformation rate in pregnancies not exposed to the drug. In 304 pregnancies recorded in the United Kingdom Register and treated with the drug, Mahwinney et al. (2013) described a 0.70 % malformation rate (95 % C.I. = 0.19, 2.51 %). Subsequently, Veiby et al. (2014) found a foetal malformation rate of 1.7 % in 118 pregnancies in women with epilepsy managed with levetiracetam monotherapy, with an adjusted odds ratio of 0.63 (95 % C.I. = 0.16, 2.55) compared with 777,412 pregnancies in women not taking antiepileptic drugs. Chaudhry et al. (2014), in their review of the literature, found record of 1213 pregnancies that had been exposed to levetiracetam monotherapy. There were 27 major congenital malformations in these pregnancies, a 2.2 % malformation rate (95 % C.I. = 1.53, 3.22), whereas a 1–3 % malformation rate would have been expected in the general population. These authors noticed that the malformation rate was higher when levetiracetam was used as part of antiepileptic drug polytherapy.

In an analysis of the records of the Australian Pregnancy Register, Vajda et al. (2014b) found a 2.4 % foetal malformation rate in 84 pregnancies in which levetiracetam monotherapy had been employed. The risk relative to that in women with untreated epilepsy was 0.75 (95 % C.I. = 0.15, 3.76). Multivariate logistic regression for malformation risk on dosage of all of the antiepileptic drugs used in the Register population (Fig. 8.2) found that there was a nonstatistically significant trend for the risk to increase with increasing levetiracetam dose ($P=0.76$).

Sufficient information is now available to suggest that levetiracetam, used in monotherapy, probably exposes the foetus in utero to little or no additional hazard of being born malformed.

Gabapentin

Gabapentin was introduced in therapeutics fairly soon after lamotrigine but, outside North America, does not seem to have been employed extensively in treating epilepsy. Relatively little published information exists concerning its hazards for the foetus.

Montouris (2003) analysed data for 44 live births from 51 pregnancies collected in the register of gabapentin-treated pregnancies maintained by the pharmaceutical firm that marketed the drug. She stated that use of gabapentin in pregnancy did not increase the risk of foetal malformations. However, gabapentin had been used in monotherapy in only 11 of these pregnancies. No malformations had occurred in this subset, but there were two major malformations and one minor one in the 33 pregnancies that involved gabapentin use in polytherapy. The data really do not permit reliable conclusions.

Molgaard-Nielsen and Hviid (2011) cited a 1.7 % foetal malformation rate for 59 gabapentin-exposed pregnancies, compared with a 2.4 % malformation rate in Danish infants not exposed to the drug during pregnancy. Holmes and Hernandez-Diaz (2012), in their own series of 145 pregnancies, found a 0.7 % foetal malformation rate but indicated that they could not extract adequate numerical data from the literature to warrant a more definite opinion about the foetal safety of the drug. Fujii et al. (2013) compared the outcome of 223 gabapentin-treated pregnancies (only 34 % in women with epilepsy) with 223 pregnancies in which the drug had not been used, the comparator pregnancies not necessarily being those of women with epilepsy. The foetal malformation rates were similar in both groups. As of the end of 2013, the Australian Pregnancy Register contained only 14 pregnancies in which the drug has been used in monotherapy. There were no foetal abnormalities.

Thus, in the limited available data, there appears little to indicate that gabapentin treatment in pregnancy constitutes a foetal hazard. On the other hand, the amount of data available is probably insufficient to warrant any assertion that the drug is safe from the foetal standpoint.

Oxcarbazepine

Oxcarbazepine became available in some countries as long ago as 1990 but does not seem to have achieved any considerable market penetration outside Europe. Some information relative to the drug's hazards for the development of normal foetal morphology is available.

Kaaja et al. (2003) noted a statistically significant association between oxcarbazepine intake and foetal malformation, but in a study involving only 9 pregnancies. Meischenguiser et al. (2004) reported on the outcome of 55 pregnancies in which the drug had been used (in polytherapy in 20). Only one foetal malformation occurred, and that was in the polytherapy subset. Sabers et al. (2004) noted a foetal malformation rate of 5 % (95 % C.I. = 0.7, 18.2 %) in 37 pregnancies in which the drug had been used in mono- or polytherapy. Artama et al. (2005) recorded a solitary instance of foetal malformation in 99 pregnancies exposed to oxcarbazepine monotherapy. Montouris (2005), from the records of the pharmaceutical company marketing the drug, obtained data from 248 pregnancies exposed to oxcarbazepine in monotherapy and found a 2.4 % malformation rate when a 2.0–4.0 % rate would have been expected to be present in the general population. It seems likely that some of the pregnancies considered in this paper would have already been reported in some of the publications discussed immediately above. Molgaard-Nielsen and Hviid (2011) studied 393 pregnancies exposed the drug in monotherapy and found a malformation rate of 2.8 %, with an adjusted odds ratio of 0.86 (95 % C.I. = 0.46, 1.59) when compared with the malformation rate in their large population of Danish normal pregnancies. Hernandez-Diaz et al. (2012) described a foetal malformation rate of 2.2 % in 182 pregnancies in which oxcarbazepine had been used in monotherapy, with a relative risk of 2.0 (95 % C.I. = 0.5, 7.4) in comparison with a population of drug-unexposed pregnancies. The drug has been too little used in the pregnancies recorded in the Australian Register to justify drawing conclusions.

The amount of information currently available is hardly sufficient to permit secure conclusions about the drug's teratogenicity, though there is as yet nothing to suggest that it is particularly dangerous from the foetal malformation point of view.

Benzodiazepines

A number of 1,4-benzodiazepines, e.g. diazepam, nitrazepam, clonazepam, lorazepam and also one 1,5-benzodiazepine (clobazam), have at times been used to treat epilepsy and are still taken by some pregnant women with the disorder. It has not been possible to trace publications dealing with the foetal safety of these drugs in such women, though there seems little reason to suspect that it would differ from their safety when taken by pregnant women in general, in whom the drugs may be used as tranquillisers and for other purposes. Except for diazepam, which has sometimes been considered as a separate entity, the literature has tended to regard the possible consequences of intrauterine exposure to these drugs on foetal body structure in terms of a class effect. Safra and Oakey (1975) published data which suggested that the intake of diazepam during pregnancy might correlate with the occurrence of palate and lip clefts, though these authors accepted that the finding might simply be due to chance. Rosenberg et al. (1983) studied 445 infants who were born with cleft lip with or without cleft palate and another 166 with cleft palate only after being exposed to benzodiazepines in the first four months of pregnancy and compared them with 2498 controls who had other malformations. The relative risks for the two groups of clefts were 1.0 and 0.8 respectively and, after adjustment for potential confounding factors, became 0.8 for each group. Despite this, suspicion lingers in the literature that there may be a relationship between such oral clefts and intrauterine exposure to benzodiazepines.

McElhatton (1994) detected no increase over the expected background malformation rate in the rate of occurrence of foetal malformations associated with benzodiazepine intake in pregnancy. Dolovich et al. (1998) carried out a meta-analysis of the data that were available in the literature from infants who had been exposed to benzodiazepines in the first trimester of pregnancy. They found no association between the drugs and the presence of major congenital malformations (odds ratio 0.90; 95 % C.I. = 0.61, 1.35) and also none between the drugs and oral clefts (odds ratio 1.19; 95 % C.I. = 0.34, 4.15). However, they remarked that pooled case–control studies have tended to find a raised incidence of oral clefts in association with benzodiazepine administration in pregnancy. Bonnot et al. (2003) obtained statistically significant evidence for an association between lorazepam intake and anal atresia. Lin et al. (2004) recorded the birth of one malformed infant in 33 pregnancies exposed to clonazepam monotherapy in the first trimester. Kjaer et al. (2007) found an odds ratio of 1.2 (95 % C.I. = 1.0, 1.4) for foetal malformations in infants exposed to lorazepam in pregnancy when compared with a large collection of over 35,000 births. Enato et al. (2011) calculated a benzodiazepine-associated foetal malformation odds ratio of 1.07 (95 % C.I. = 0.91, 1.25) when compared with the outcome of studies involving over 1 million normal pregnancies.

At the time of writing, the Australian Register of Antiepileptic Drugs in Pregnancy contained records of 24 pregnancies in which clonazepam had been used in monotherapy. None of these pregnancies resulted in a foetal malformation. There was a total of 104 pregnancies where the drug had been used alone or with other antiepileptic agents. In this group there was a foetal malformation rate of 4.8 %. Logistic regression of malformation risk on drug dose for the full Register data set showed a regression line for clonazepam which had a slight and not statistically significant downward slope ($P=0.53$) as the drug dose increased.

Benzodiazepines have been in extensive use for over a half a century and statistical data such as those cited above exist. There has been little clinical reason to suspect that the drugs may be significant teratogens. It is therefore probably reasonable to conclude that their use in treating epilepsy in pregnancy is unlikely to involve a significantly increased risk of foetal malformations occurring.

Zonisamide

The only information traced is that Kondo et al. (1996) described a 7.7 % foetal malformation rate in 26 pregnancies in which intrauterine exposure to zonisamide was involved. However, both of the affected infants had been exposed to the drug in antiepileptic drug combinations.

Other Antiepileptic Drugs

A number of other marketed antiepileptic drugs are sometimes used in pregnancy. Several have been available for some years, e.g. sulthiame, felbamate, stiripentol and tiagabine, but have been employed too infrequently in pregnancy for useful data concerning their foetal safety to be available in the public domain. Others, e.g. lacosamide, eslicarbazepine, pregabalin and perampanel, have become generally available too recently for there to have been enough time or extensive enough use in pregnancy for sufficient information about their hazards for the foetus to yet be available.

Antiepileptic Drugs in Combination

As mentioned earlier in this and the previous chapters, there have been rather numerous statements in the literature to the effect that foetal malformation rates are higher when antiepileptic drugs are used in combination in pregnant women as compared with when they are used in monotherapy. However, there now seems to be reasonably good evidence that, so long as valproate or topiramate is not a member of the drug combinations, the malformation risk is not greater than that which applies for each drug used alone. As yet, there does not appear to have been any careful study of the possibility that combining two antiepileptic drugs, apart from valproate and topiramate, increases the risk of foetal malformation over that which applies for each drug used alone. The existing data suggest that any teratogenic potential of the commonly used antiepileptic drugs apart from valproate and topiramate is relatively small so that it would probably require a very large collection of data on pregnant women with epilepsy before this possibility of additive risk could be assessed adequately. In the present state of knowledge, the prudent course may be to accept that there could be a slightly higher risk.

References

Akar M, Dilli D, Yilmaz Y, Erdeve O, Oyuz S, Uras N, Dilmen U (2012) A case of fetal carbamazepine syndrome with right hemihypoplasia of the entire body. Genet Couns 23:19–24

Andermann E, Dansky L, Andermann F, Loughnan PM, Gibbons J (1982) Minor congenital malformations and dermatoglyphic alterations in the offspring of epileptic women: a clinical investigation of the teratogenic effect of anticonvulsant medication. In: Janz D, Bossi L, Dam M, Helge H, Richens A, Schmidt D (eds) Epilepsy, pregnancy and the child. Raven, New York, pp 235–249

Arpino C, Bresarini S, Robert W et al (2000) Teratogenic effects of antiepileptic drugs: use of an international database on malformation and drug exposure (MADRE). Epilepsia 41:1436–1443

Artama M, Auvinen A, Raudaskoski T, Isojarvi I, Isojarvi J (2005) Antiepileptic drug use of women with epilepsy and congenital malformations in the offspring. Neurology 64:1874–1878

Bailey CJ, Pool RW, Poskitt EME, Harris F (1983) Valproic abnormality and fetal abnormality. Br Med J 286:190

Barr MJ, Pozanski AK, Schmickel RD (1974) Digital hypoplasia and anticonvulsants during gestation; a teratogenic syndrome? J Pediatr 84:254–257

Bjerkedal T, Czeizel A, Goujard J et al (1982) Valproic acid and spina bifida. Lancet 2:1096

Bonnot O, Vollset SE, Godet PF, d'Amato T, Dalery J, Robert E (2003) In utero exposure to benzodiazepine: is there a risk for anal atresia with lorazepam? Encéphale 29:553–559

Bromfield EB, Dworetzky BA, Wyszynski DF, Smith CR, Baldwin EJ, Holmes LB (2008) Valproate teratogenicity and epilepsy syndromes. Epilepsia 49:2122–2124

Campbell E, Kennedy F, Russell A et al (2014) Malformation risks of antiepileptic drug monotherapies in pregnancy: updated results from the UK and Ireland Epilepsy and Pregnancy Registers. J Neurol Neurosurg Psychiatry 85:1029–1034

Canger R, Battino D, Canevini MP et al (1999) Malformations in offspring of women with epilepsy: a prospective study. Epilepsia 40:1231–1236

Chaudhry SA, Jong G, Koren G (2014) The fetal safety of levetiracetam. Reprod Toxicol 46C:40–45

Cunnington M, Ferber S, Quartey G, International Lamotrigine Pregnancy Registry Scientific Advisory Committee (2007) Effect of dose on the frequency of major birth defects following fetal exposure to lamotrigine monotherapy in an international observational study. Epilepsia 48:1207–1210

Curran MAW (1987) The management of epilepsy in women of child-bearing age and the Australian experience of valproate in pregnancy. Clin Exp Neurol 23:145–148

Danks DM, Barry JE, Sheffield LJ (1974) Digital hypoplasia and anticonvulsants during pregnancy. J Pediatr 85:877

Di Liberti JH, Farndon RA, Dennis NR, Curry CJR (1984) The fetal valproate syndrome. Am J Med Genet 19:473–481

Diav-Citrin O, Shectman S, Arnon J, Ornoy A (2001) Is carbamazepine teratogenic? A prospective controlled study of 210 pregnancies. Neurology 57:321–324

Diav-Cirtin O, Shechhman S, Bar-Oz, Cantrell D, Amon J, Ornoy A (2008) Pregtnancy outcome after in utero exposure to valproate - evidence of dose relationship in teratogenic effect. CNS Drugs 22: 325–335

Dolovich LR, Addis A, Vaillancourt JM, Power JD, Koren G, Einarson TR (1998) Benzodiazepine use in pregnancy and major malformations or oral cleft: meta-analysis of cohort and case–control studies. Br Med J 317:839–843

Dravet C, Julian C, Legras C et al (1992) Epilepsy, antiepileptic drugs, and malformations in children of women with epilepsy: a French prospective cohort study. Neurology 42(Suppl 5):75–82

Eadie MJ (2008) Antiepileptic drugs as human teratogens. Expert Opin Drug Saf 7:195–201

Enato E, Moretti M, Koren G (2011) The fetal safety of benzodiazepines: an updated meta-analysis. J Obstet Gynaecol Can 33:46–48

Fujii H, Goel A, Bernard N et al (2013) Pregnancy outcomes following gabapentin use. Results of a prospective comparative study. Neurology 80:1565–1570

Hanson JW, Smith DW (1975) The fetal hydantoin syndrome. J Pediatr 87:285–290

Hernandez-Diaz S, Smith CR, Wyzszynski D (2007) Risk of major malformations among infants exposed to carbamazepine during pregnancy. Proc 47th Teratol Soc Meet Birth Defects Res (Part A) 79:357 (Cited by Wlodarczyl 2012, *loc cit*)

Hernandez-Diaz S, Smith CR, Shen A et al (2012) Comparative study of antiepileptic drugs during pregnancy. Neurology 78:1692–1699

Hill RM, Verniaud WM, Horning MD, McCulley LB, Morgan NF (1974) Infants exposed in utero to antiepileptic drugs. Am J Dis Child 127:645–653

Holmes LB, Hernandez-Diaz S (2012) Newer anticonvulsants: lamotrigine, topiramate and gabapentin. Birth Defects Res (Part A) 94:599–606

Holmes LB, Wyszynski DF, Lieberman E, for the AED Pregnancy Registry (2004) The AED (antiepileptic drug) pregnancy registry. A 6-year experience. Arch Neurol 61:673–678
Holmes LB, Baldwin EJ, Smith CR, Habecker E, Glassman L, Wong SL, Wyuszynski DF (2008) Increased frequency of isolated cleft palate in infants exposed to lamotrigine during pregnancy. Neurology 70:2152–2158
Holmes LB, Mittendorf R, Shen A, Smith CR, Hernandez-Diaz S (2011) Fetal effects of anticonvulsant polytherapies. Arch Neurol 68:1275–1281
Hunt S, Russell A, Smithson WH et al (2008) Topiramate in pregnancy. Preliminary experience from the UK Epilepsy and Pregnancy Register. Neurology 71:272–276
Jacobsen PE, Henriksen TB, Haubek D, Østergaard JR (2014) Prenatal exposure to antiepileptic drugs and dental agenesis. PLoS One 9, e84420
Jager-Roman E, Deichl A, Jakob S (1986) Fetal growth, major malformations, and minor anomalies in infants born to women receiving valproic acid. J Pediatr 108:997–1004
Janz D, Fuchs U (1964) Are anti-epileptic drugs harmful when given during pregnancy? Ger Med Mont 9:20–22
Jentink J, Dolk H, Loane MA, Wellesley D, Game E, de Jong-van den Berg L, EUROCAT Antiepileptic Study Group (2010) Intrauterine exposure to carbamazepine and specific congenital malformations: systematic review and case–control study. Br Med J 341:c6581
Jones KL, Lacro RV, Johnson KA, Adams J (1989) Pattern of malformations in children of women treated with carbamazepine during pregnancy. N Engl J Med 320:1661–1666
Kaaja E, Kaaja R, Hiilesmaa V (2003) Major malformations in offspring of women with epilepsy. Neurology 60:575–579
Kallen AJ (1994) Maternal carbamazepine and infant spina bifida. Reprod Toxicol 8:203–205
Kallen B, Robert E, Mastroiacovo P, Martinez-Frias ML, Castilla EE, Cocchi G (1989) Anticonvulsant drugs and malformations is there a drug specificity? Eur J Epidemiol 5:31–36
Kaneko S, Battino D, Andermann E et al (1999) Congenital malformations due to antiepileptic drugs. Epilepsy Res 33:145–158
Kini U, Adab N, Vinten J, Fryer A, Clayton-Smith J, Liverpool and Manchester Neurodevelopmental Study Group (2006) Dysmorphic features: an important clue to the diagnosis and severity of fetal anticonvulsant syndromes. Arch Dis Child Neonatal Ed 91:F90–F95
Kjaer D, Horvath-Puhó E, Christensen J, Vestergaard M, Czeizel AE, Sørensen HT, Olsen J (2007) Use of phenytoin, phenobarbital, or diazepam during pregnancy and the risk of congenital abnormalities: a case-time-control study. Pharmacoepidemiol Drug Saf 16:181–188
Koch S, Losche G, Jager-Romän C, Jakob S, Rating D, Deichl A, Helge H (1992) Major and minor birth malformations and antiepileptic drugs. Neurology 42(4 Suppl 5):83–88
Kondo T, Kaneko S, Amano Y, Egawa I (1996) Preliminary report of teratogenic effect of zonisamide in the offspring of treated women with epilepsy. Epilepsia 37:1242–1244
Kozma C (2001) Valproic acid embryopathy: report of two siblings with further expansion of the phenotypic abnormalities and a review of the literature. Am J Med Genet (Part A) 98:168–175
Lin AE, Peller AJ, Westgate M-N, Houda K, Franz A, Holmes LB (2004) Clonazepam use in pregnancy and the risk of malformation. Birth Defects Res (Part A) 70:534–536
Lindhout D, Meinardi H (1984) Spina bifida and in utero exposure to valproate. Lancet 2:396
Lindhout D, Omtzigt JG (1992) Pregnancy and the risk of teratogenicity. Epilepsia 33(Suppl 4):S41–S48
Lindhout D, Schmidt D (1986) In-utero exposure to valproate and neural-tube defects. Lancet 2:1392–1393
Little BB, Santos-Ramos R, Newell JF, Mayberry MC (1993) Megadose carbamazepine during the period of neural tube closure. Obstet Gynecol 82:705–708
Loughnan PM, Gold H, Vance JC (1973) Phenytoin teratogenicity in man. Lancet 1:70–72
Lype M, Henry P, Aravind C, Arun K (2008) Baller-Gerold syndrome: further evidence for association with prenatal exposure to valproate. Ann Indian Acad Neurol 11:52–55
Mahwinney E, Craig J, Morrow J et al (2013) Levetiracetam in pregnancy. Results from the UK and Ireland epilepsy and pregnancy registers. Neurology 80:401–405

Marguilis AV, Mitchell AA, Gilboa SM et al (2012) Use of topiramate in pregnancy and risk of oral clefts. Am J Obstet Gynecol 207:405 e1–e7

Matalon S, Schectman S, Goldzweig G, Ornoy A (2002) The teratogenic effect of carbamazepine: a meta-analysis of 1255 exposures. Reprod Toxicol 16:9–17

Mawer G, Briggs M, Baker GA et al (2010) Pregnancy with epilepsy: obstetric and neonatal outcome of a controlled study. Seizure 19:112–119

McElhatton PR (1994) The effect of benzodiazepine use during pregnancy and lactation. Reprod Toxicol 8:461–475

McMahon CL, Braddock SR (2001) Septo-optic dysplasia as a manifestation of valproic acid embryopathy. Teratology 64:83–86

Meador KJ, Baker JA, Finnell RH et al (2006) In utero fetal drug exposure. Fetal death and malformations. Neurology 67:407–412

Meador K, Reynolds MW, Crean S, Fahrbach K, Probst C (2008) Pregnancy outcomes in women with epilepsy: a systematic review and analysis of published pregnancy registers and cohorts. Epilepsy Res 81:1–13

Meischenguiser R, D'Giano CH, Ferraro SM (2004) Oxcarbazepine in pregnancy: clinical experience in Argentina. Epilepsy Behav 5:163–167

Miki T, Reo T, Tohru K, Joseph B, Gideon K, Elizabeth U, Shinya I (2014) Risks of congenital malformations in offspring exposed to valproic acid in utero: Emergence of the signals over the last 30 years. J Popul Ther Clin Pharmacol 21:2 (e277)

Mines D, Tennis P, Curkendall SM et al (2014) Topiramate use in pregnancy and the birth prevalence of oral clefts. Pharmacoepidemiol Drug Saf 23:1017–1025

Molgaard-Nielsen D, Hviid A (2011) Newer-generation antiepileptic drugs and the risk of major birth defects. J Am Med Assoc 305:1996–2002

Monson RR, Rosenberg L, Hartz SC, Shapiro S, Heinonen OP, Stone D (1973) Diphenylhydantoin and selected congenital malformations. N Engl J Med 289:1049–1052

Montouris G (2003) Gabapentin exposure in human pregnancy: results from the Gabapentin Pregnancy Registry. Epilepsy Behav 4:310–317

Montouris G (2005) Safety of the newer antiepileptic drug oxcarbazepine during pregnancy. Curr Med Res Opin 21:693–701

Moore SJ, Turpenny P, Quinn A, Glover S, Lloyd DJ, Montgomery T, Dean JC (2000) A clinical study of 57 children with fetal anticonvulsant syndromes. J Med Genet 37:489–497

Morrow J, Russell A, Guthrie E et al (2006) Malformation risk of antiepileptic drugs in pregnancy: a prospective study from the UK Epilepsy and Pregnancy Register. J Neurol Neurosurg Psychiatry 77:193–198

Nelson MM, Forfar IO (1971) Association between drugs administered during pregnancy and congenital abnormalities in the fetus. Br Med J 1:523–527

Omtzigt JG, Los FJ, Grobbee DE et al (1992) The risk of spina bifida aperta after first trimester exposure to valproate in a prenatal cohort. Neurology 42(Suppl 5):119–125

Ornoy A, Cohen E (1996) Outcome of children born to epileptic mothers treated with carbamazepine during pregnancy. Arch Dis Child 75:517–520

Ornoy A, Zvi N, Arnon J, Waajnberg R, Schectman S, Diav-Citrin O (2008) The outcome of pregnancy following topiramate treatment: a study of 52 pregnancies. Reprod Toxicol 25:388–389

Phelan MC, Pellock JM, Nance WE (1982) Discordant expression of the fetal hydantoin syndrome in heteropaternal dizygotic twins. N Engl J Med 307:99–101

Robert E, Guibaud P (1982) Maternal valproic acid and congenital neural tube defects. Lancet 2:937

Robert E, Rosa F (1983) Valproate and birth defects. Lancet 2:1142

Rosenberg L, Mitchall AA, Parsells JL, Pashayan H, Louik C, Shapiro S (1983) Lack of relation of oral clefts to diazepam use during pregnancy. N Engl J Med 309:1282–1285

Sabers A, Dam M, a-Rogvi-Hansen B et al (2004) Epilepsy and pregnancy: lamotrigine as main drug used. Acta Neurol Scand 109:9–13

Safra MJ, Oakey GPJ (1975) Association between cleft lip with or without cleft palate and prenatal exposure to diazepam. Lancet 2:478–480

Samrén EB, van Duijn CM, Koch S et al (1997) Maternal use of antiepileptic drugs and the risk of major congenital malformations: a joint European prospective study of human teratogenesis associated with maternal epilepsy. Epilepsia 38:981–990

Samrén EB, van Duijn CM, Lieve Christiaens GCM, Hofman A, Lindhout D (1999) Antiepileptic drug regimens and major congenital abnormalities in the offspring. Ann Neurol 46:739–746

Shapiro S, Hartz SC, Siskind V et al (1976) Anticonvulsants and parental epilepsy in the development of birth defects. Lancet 1:272–275

Speidel BD, Meadow SR (1972) Maternal epilepsy and abnormalities of the fetus and newborn. Lancet 2:839–843

Staples RE (1972) Teratology. In: Penry JK, Schmidt RP, Woodbury DM (eds) Antiepileptic drugs. Raven, New York, pp 55–62

Starreveld-Zimmerman AAE, Van Der Kolk WJ, Meinardi H, Elshove J (1973) Are anticonvulsants teratogenic? Lancet 2:48–49

Tomson T, Battino D, Bonizzoni E et al (2011) Dose-dependent risk of malformation with antiepileptic drugs: an analysis of data from the EURAP epilepsy and pregnancy registry. Lancet Neurol 10:609–617

Vajda FJE, Eadie MJ (2005) Maternal valproate dosage and foetal malformations. Acta Neurol Scand 112:137–143

Vajda FJ, O'Brien TJ, Hitchcock A, Graham J, Cook M, Lander C, Eadie MJ (2004) Critical relationship between sodium valproate dose and human teratogenicity: results of the Australian register of anti-epileptic drugs in pregnancy. J Clin Neurosci 11:854–858

Vajda F, Hitchcock A, Graham J, Solinas C, O'Brien TJ, Lander CM, Eadie MJ (2006) Foetal malformations and seizure control: 52 months data of the Register, Australian Pregnancy. Eur J Neurol 13:645–654

Vajda FJE, Graham J, Hitchock AA, O'Brien TJ, Lander CM, Eadie MJ (2010) Is lamotrigine a significant human teratogen? Observations from the Australian Pregnancy Register. Seizure 19:555–561

Vajda FJE, O'Brien TJ, Graham J, Lander CM, Eadie MJ (2013a) Associations between particular types of fetal malformation and antiepileptic drug exposure. Acta Neurol Scand 128:228–234

Vajda FJE, O'Brien TJ, Graham J, Lander CM, Eadie MJ (2013b) Dose-dependency of fetal malformations associated with valproate. Neurology 81:999–1003

Vajda FJE, O'Brien TJ, Lander CM, Graham J, Eadie MJ (2014) The teratogenicity of the newer antiepileptic drugs – an update. Ácta Neurol Scand 130: 234–238

Veiby G, Daltveit AK, Engelsen BA, Gilhus NE (2014) Fetal growth restriction and birth defects with newer and older antiepileptic drugs during pregnancy. J Neurol 261:579–588

Wheatley D (1963) Drugs in pregnancy survey. Practitioner 191:775–780

Wlodarczyk BJ, Palacios AM, George TM, Finnell TH (2012) Antiepileptic drugs and pregnancy outcomes. Am J Med Genet A 158A:2071–2090

Wyszynski DF, Nambisan M, Surve T, Alsdorf RM, Smith CR, Holmes LB, Antiepileptic Drug Pregnancy Registry (2005) Increased rate of major malformations in offspring exposed to valproate during pregnancy. Neurology 64:961–965

Chapter 10
Antiepileptic Drugs, Cognition and Neurodevelopment

Abstract Antiepileptic drug exposure in utero may have adverse effects on the developing brain, as has been shown in experimental animals. Exposure in the first trimester of human pregnancy may be associated with the occurrence of physical malformations in the foetus but, in addition, foetal valproate exposure poses a significant risk for the cognitive development of the infant, an effect that is dose dependent. Carbamazepine and lamotrigine exposures appear to hold a lesser risk for cognitive development, while the risks associated with exposure to the other antiepileptic drugs are uncertain. Further, evidence has become available that intrauterine valproate exposure may be associated with the development of autism-spectrum disorder in childhood. Not enough data exists to clarify the situation in this regard for the other antiepileptic drugs.

The highly important possibility that antiepileptic drug exposure during pregnancy may be associated with the presence of adverse consequences for cognition and neurobehavioral development in the infant and child has been rather intensively investigated in recent years. The situation in this regard has been progressively clarified in a series of publications from the collaborative NEAD (Neurodevelopmental Effects of Antiepileptic Drugs) studies carried out by Meador and colleagues, who have been collecting data and presenting interim analyses of a well-designed, comprehensive prospective investigation.

The actual recognition of cognitive and developmental adverse effects of antiepileptic drugs presents a more considerable challenge than observations and analysis of data related to physical malformations in the foetus and infant. The relevant data concerning intellectual functioning need to be obtained from prospective quantitative observational studies carried out in an area where human experimentation is unethical and the examinations and follow-up that are required have many limitations. Babies are not easy subjects for intellectual testing. Numerous potential confounders exist that make the assessment task very complex. Such confounders include parental factors such as educational level, socioeconomic status, drug taking (including tobacco and alcohol), concurrent illnesses and disorders that occur during pregnancy, family history, inherited illnesses, mental disorders, nutrition, folate intake, as well as environmental factors other than the above, and in addition

M.J. Eadie, F.J.E. Vajda, *Antiepileptic Drugs and Pregnancy: A Guide for Prescribers*, DOI 10.1007/978-3-319-21434-4_10

among other factors the maternal epilepsy syndrome that is being treated and the effects of multiple or uncontrolled seizures during pregnancy.

Although many anecdotal reports had existed about impaired neurodevelopmental outcomes in the offspring of women with antiepileptic drug-treated epilepsies, it was not until relatively recently that prospectively recruited collections of in utero antiepileptic drug-exposed infants have been systematically explored and the findings about intellectual impairment followed up in a cohort of antiepileptic drug-exposed infants at progressively increasing ages during childhood (Meador et al. 2013).

Adverse Effects of Antiepileptic Drugs on the Developing Brain

Foetuses exposed to antiepileptic drugs during the first trimester of pregnancy, the primary period of organogenesis, have an elevated risk of congenital physical malformations, including defects that can affect the brain. The most obvious and serious of these are neural tube defects. The neural tube closes by the end of the third week after conception. This is the most vulnerable period for the development of neural tube malformations induced by antiepileptic drugs. It is also a time that often proves to be too early for the prospective mother to realise that she is pregnant. In the past, it was recommended that, after the first few weeks of pregnancy had passed, during which there was intense concern for the adverse effects of antiepileptic drugs on the brain, attention should shift to focus on seizure control throughout the remainder of pregnancy. This recommendation will now need to be revised, because it appears that the drug-related cognitive and developmental issues affecting the baby may originate throughout the whole length of pregnancy. Human brain development is a long, highly complex process that involves neurogenesis, synaptogenesis, apoptosis, synaptic pruning, glial development and myelination. It probably extends not only throughout gestation but also continues postnatally, through infancy, childhood, the teenage years and possibly beyond. The cellular processes involved in brain development are multiple, occurring in a parallel but interrelated manner, occurring in different brain regions and in different cellular types at different times. Antiepileptic drugs have been shown in experimental animals to have effects on all of these processes. The results of an insult to brain structure and function will depend on the processes which are most active in the time window when the insult occurs. The duration of the insult from antiepileptic drugs may extend throughout the entire duration of gestation. Kaindl et al. (2006) and Ikonomidou et al. (2007) have reported findings which lead to a better understanding of the potential adverse neurobiological effects that antiepileptic drugs can produce in the developing brains of experimental animals.

Obtaining objective clinical evidence of intrauterine brain damage in humans is easiest for the anatomical abnormalities that develop early in pregnancy. These produce structural malformations such as abnormal limbs or bones, or spina bifida, which are readily visible objective endpoints that are recognisable at birth. It is more difficult to identify abnormalities that develop later in pregnancy. Such disturbances of cognition, personality, behaviour and motor development may be due to multiple possible causes (Blom et al. 2006) and tend not to become obvious until well after birth.

Mechanisms of Behavioural Teratogenesis

Earlier animal experimental studies provided evidence of the adverse effects of postnatal phenobarbitone treatment on brain development in infant rats, resulting in reduced brain weights (Schain and Watanabe 1975), reduction in neuronal numbers in the hippocampus (Bergman et al. 1982) and cerebellum (Fishman et al. 1983), neurocognitive deficits (Rogel-Fuchs et al. 1992) and behavioural abnormalities that comprised increased aggression and overactivity (Diaz and Schain 1978). Phenobarbitone treatment in young animals with post-kainic acid-induced status epilepticus resulted in fewer seizures, as compared with saline-treated rats (Mikati et al. 1994), but also resulted in a worse neurocognitive performance (Bolanos et al. 1998).

Valproic acid is a histone deacetylase inhibitor, and it is possible that differential teratogenesis exists in B6 and D2 strain mice because of strain differences in histone acetylation. B6 mice foetuses are more susceptible than D2 foetuses to digit and vertebral malformations, but D2 mice are more susceptible to rib malformations. Downing et al. (2010) observed strain differences in acetylation of histones H3 and H4 in both the embryo and placenta following in utero valproate exposure. However, additional studies are needed to determine the roles of these changes in mediating teratogenesis, though the findings suggest that genetic factors, both maternal and foetal, may play a part in causing valproate-associated foetal malformations. Clonazepam, diazepam, phenobarbitone, phenytoin and valproate, as well as vigabatrin, have been observed to produce widespread neuronal apoptosis in neonatal rat brains (Bittigau et al. 2002, 2003; Asimiadou et al. 2005; Meador et al. 2007; Stefovska et al. 2008; Ikonomidou and Turski 2010). This effect is dose dependent and may occur at blood concentrations that would be therapeutically relevant in humans. Two antiepileptic drugs, each given at below apoptosis threshold dosages, can still trigger the full apoptotic response. Antiepileptics which do not produce apoptosis in monotherapy, including carbamazepine, lamotrigine and topiramate (Glier et al. 2004; Manthey et al. 2005; Kim et al. 2007), can enhance apoptosis induced by another agent (Katz et al. 2007). This suggests that antiepileptic drug polytherapy could increase the risk of neurodevelopmental problems in antiepileptic drug-exposed foetuses. Levetiracetam is the only antiepileptic drug among those tested thus far that does not produce apoptosis in monotherapy or enhance apoptosis produced by other antiepileptic drugs (Manthey et al. 2005). This information provides another indication that the availability of levetiracetam may offer a major advance in foetal safety in pregnancy (Shallcross et al. 2011; Vajda et al. 2014).

Human Cognitive Development

The impact on the cognitive and behavioural development of the offspring produced by foetal exposure to maternal antiepileptic drugs has emerged in recent times as an area of major concern in relation to the use of these drugs in pregnant women with epilepsy (Palac and Meador 2011). Pregnancy registers have contributed prospective data on women with epilepsy and their offspring in regard to many factors, including the intelligence of the offspring, though the different registers have employed different timings for their postpartum data collections (Vajda et al. 2007). Each of the individual registers has other weaknesses (see Chap. 8 and Meador et al. 2008). Nevertheless, enough information is now available from the registers to warrant making women with epilepsy who are planning a pregnancy aware of the possible neurobehavioral consequences of foetal antiepileptic drug exposure. In humans, foetal exposure, particularly to valproate or to antiepileptic drug polytherapy, may be associated with an increased risk of cognitive impairment and diminished verbal abilities in the offspring (Nadebaum et al. 2011a; Meador et al. 2013).

Cognitive Effects of Maternal Epilepsy per se

In a prospective study (Gaily et al. 2004), and in a blinded retrospective study (Holmes et al. 2000), no IQ differences were found between children of women with epilepsy that was not treated with antiepileptic drugs and healthy control children (Gedzelman and Meador 2012). Two prospective population-based studies (Gaily et al. 1988, 2004) found that there was no IQ impairment in children exposed in utero to self-limiting generalised tonic–clonic seizures (i.e. no status epilepticus was involved). However, a retrospective study (Adab et al. 2004) showed that the verbal IQ was significantly reduced in children who had been exposed to more than four generalised tonic–clonic maternal seizures during pregnancy. Based on case reports, prolonged seizures and status epilepticus are considered to provide a serious threat to both mother and foetus (Hiilesmaa 1996).

Other Factors Possibly Affecting Cognitive and Behavioural Development in Humans

Heritability accounts for 30–50 % of phenotypic variance in human IQ. The correlation coefficient between the IQs of monozygotic twins reared together is 0.85 and for those reared apart 0.67 (Sattler 1992). The correlation coefficient between parental and child IQ is 0.42 (Kaufman 1990). Maternal education and socioeconomic status correlate less closely with the child's IQ (correlation coefficient = 0.298). The paternal IQ co-varies with the maternal IQ. Children's IQs may also be affected by complications of pregnancy or severe childhood illnesses. Obstetrical complications and malnutrition do not generally appear to have an overall substantial effect on IQs, though individual children may be severely affected. Drug abuse in pregnancy influences foetal development, socioeconomic status is correlated with behavioural adaptation and social variables are known to predispose to biomedical risks. Other possible factors to be considered include gender, ethnic origin, geography, maternal age and parity. Approximately half of the patients with low IQs carry more than one risk factor (Meador et al. 2001). Although the majority of children born to women with epilepsy are normal, the somatic and functional development of these children, as a group, is reduced (Delgado-Escueta and Janz 1992).

Reported Antiepileptic Drug-Associated Effects on Human Cognitive Development

Antiepileptic drugs may decrease cell membrane excitability, increase postsynaptic inhibition or alter synchronisation of neural networks to decrease the excessive neuronal excitability that is associated with seizure development. Common side effects of decreasing neuronal excitability include slowed motor and psychomotor speed, poorer attention spans and mild memory impairment (Meador 2005). Treatment decisions made in childhood may have lifelong implications for cognitive ability (Loring and Meador 2001; Meador 2005).

Prenatal exposure to phenobarbitone, phenytoin, primidone and carbamazepine has been associated with reduced head circumferences (Hanson et al. 1976; Majewski et al. 1981; Gaily et al. 1990) and reduced psychomotor development of infants (Deblay et al. 1982). However, other studies did not support the correlation with phenytoin exposure (Smith et al 1986, 1994; Dodrill and Wilensky 1992; Pulliainen and Jokelainen 1994, 1995). Unfortunately, neurocognitive tests in young children appear to have a relatively poor reliability so that a long follow-up period may be required to obtain a valid assessment of this parameter. Selection biases may have been present in some studies concerning the matter, and multiple confounders such as those listed above may have been operative. The interpretation of the numerous studies on the differential effects of antiepileptic drugs on neurodevelopment remained controversial, until the publication of the multicentre, prospective series of NEAD studies.

Farwell et al. (1990) had studied 217 children (at 8 and 36 months) randomly assigned to 2 years treatment with phenobarbitone (4–5 mg/kg/day) or placebo. After 2 years (on treatment), the mean corrected IQ was 7.03 lower in the phenobarbitone-treated children. Six months after the drug had been discontinued, the mean IQ remained 5.2 points lower in the group that had been assigned to phenobarbitone. In the follow-up study, 139 children were re-tested 3–5 years later: the phenobarbitone-treated group performed significantly lower than the placebo group on WRAT-R, a reading achievement standard score.

Longer-term outcomes of children born to women with epilepsy were reported by Adab et al. (2004) from the UK. These workers performed a retrospective study of the prevalence of cognitive delay and possible associated dysmorphic features in children exposed to antiepileptic drugs in utero. The participants were aged between 6 months and 16 years. Structured interviews, hospital records, clinical examinations and psychometric tests (Wechsler) were used to assess the extents of drug exposure and the IQs. Of 249 children, 41 had been exposed to sodium valproate, 52 to carbamazepine, 21 to phenytoin and 49 to antiepileptic drug polytherapy, while 80 were unexposed to antiepileptic drugs. The mean verbal IQ was significantly lower in the valproate group compared with the unexposed and the other monotherapy groups. Both valproate exposure and frequent tonic–clonic seizures in pregnancy were significantly associated with a lower verbal IQ despite adjusting for other confounding factors. This study identified valproate as posing potential risks for developmental delay and cognitive impairment and was the first to suggest that frequent tonic–clonic seizures in the pregnant woman had a similar effect. Like many others in this field, this study may be criticised for some methodological flaws, perhaps in particular, the potential for ascertainment bias. Nevertheless, the study heightened existing concerns regarding the risks of in utero exposure to valproate during pregnancy.

A Finnish study (Gaily et al. 2004) of the effects of foetal antiepileptic drug exposure on cognition involved the intakes of carbamazepine ($N=73$), phenytoin ($N=48$), lamotrigine ($N=84$) and valproate ($N=53$). At 4 years of age, the IQs of the children showed statistically significant differences in favour of the first three drugs compared with valproate. The mean IQ values were, for carbamazepine 98, for lamotrigine 101, for phenytoin 99 and for valproate 92.

Neurocognitive effects of exposure to carbamazepine in utero have been reported in three further smaller population-based studies that showed no significant associations between prenatal exposure to the drug and poorer cognitive outcomes (Scolnik et al. 1994; Wide et al. 2002; Eriksson et al. 2005). A number of small population and clinic-based studies have found associations between intrauterine phenobarbitone and phenytoin exposures and lower IQs than those in unexposed controls, but these agents have not been established as posing a risk independent of maternal IQ (Vanoverloop et al. 1992; Reinisch et al. 1995). Although animal studies, referred to earlier, had shown that foetal exposure to antiepileptic drugs, at doses lower than the thresholds that are required to produce physical congenital malformations, can be associated with cognitive and behavioural abnormalities, the cognitive effects of human foetal exposure to antiepileptic drugs were not convincingly demonstrated until the NEAD data became available.

The NEAD Study

The NEAD study was a prospective, observational, investigation carried out in the United States and Britain. For the study, between 1999 and 2004, Meador and colleagues enrolled pregnant women with epilepsy who were taking a single antiepileptic agent (carbamazepine, lamotrigine, phenytoin or valproate). The primary analysis was planned to involve a comparison of neurodevelopmental outcomes 6 years after exposure to the different antiepileptic drugs in utero. However, a planned interim analysis of cognitive outcomes at 3 years of age showed that children who had been exposed to valproate in utero had significantly lower IQ scores than those who had been exposed to the other antiepileptic drugs. The degree of neurodevelopmental impairment was valproate dose dependent (Meador et al. 2009). This interim report had compared 258 children exposed to antiepileptic drug monotherapy in utero (73 exposed to carbamazepine, 84 to lamotrigine, 48 to phenytoin and 53 to valproate). IQ adjustments were made to compensate for effects of maternal IQ, maternal age, antiepileptic drug dose, gestational age at birth and maternal use of folate before conception. The mean adjusted IQ was 101 for children exposed to lamotrigine, 99 for those exposed to phenytoin, 98 for those exposed to carbamazepine but 92 for those exposed to valproate. The children's IQs were significantly related to maternal IQs in those exposed to carbamazepine, lamotrigine and phenytoin, but not in those exposed to valproate.

These findings, together with the obvious concern about high-dose intrauterine valproate exposure being related to the development of physical foetal malformations (see Chaps. 8 and 9), would support a recommendation that valproate should not be used as a first-choice antiepileptic drug in women of childbearing potential. These Meador et al. (2009) findings also indicate that foetal exposure to carbamazepine and lamotrigine is relatively safe in respect to adversely altering cognition in children exposed to them in utero. This is a very significant and welcome finding from the standpoint of counselling women about risks of antiepileptic drug therapy in pregnancy.

Results from the NEAD cohort at 6 years of age were published in 2013, as planned (Meador et al. 2013). At this stage, 305 mothers and 311 children were included in the primary analysis. The children's IQs at this age were lower after exposure to valproate (mean 97; 95 % C.I. = 94–101), than after exposure to the other three drugs (lamotrigine mean IQ 108, 95 % C.I. = 105–111; carbamazepine mean IQ 105, 95 % C.I. = 102–108; phenytoin mean IQ 108, 95 % C.I. = 104–112). The children exposed to valproate did poorly in verbal and memory measures, as well as in measures of nonverbal and executive functions and in a dose-related manner that was statistically significant. Verbal abilities were more affected than nonverbal ones and there was evidence of benefit being derived from peri-conception folate administration. The latter findings were consistent with some, but not all, other published studies. The authors mentioned that a limitation of this landmark study may have resulted from the loss of a number of participants to follow-up. Nevertheless, the IQ values at 6 years correlated strongly with those in the earlier report, at 3 years, described above.

Other Recent Investigations

Cummings et al. (2011) carried out a blinded cohort study which employed control subjects. The study involved 186 children aged 8 years or less (of whom 142 had been exposed to antiepileptic drugs in utero). The children were prospectively ascertained through the UK Epilepsy and Pregnancy Register. It was found that those exposed to sodium valproate in utero were more likely to have evidence of neurodevelopmental delay than the controls. In the control population ($N=42$), two children (4.8 %) showed delay (one significant, one mild). In the valproate group ($N=58$), 23 children (39.6 %) showed delay, in five significant, in 18 mild. Ten children (20.4 %) exposed to carbamazepine in utero ($N=49$) also demonstrated some degree of neurodevelopmental delay, of significant degree in two and mild in eight. However, those children exposed to lamotrigine in utero appeared to have similar neurodevelopmental outcomes to the control subjects, only one of the 35 (2.9 %) exhibiting delay.

Findings from the Australian Pregnancy Register also suggest that an association exists between exposure to valproate in pregnancy and lower IQs in the offspring, the IQ decrease being dose dependent. This finding, and that of the Meador et al. (2013) study described above, raise the possibility that lower valproate doses may be relatively safer from the neurodevelopmental point of view (Nadebaum et al. 2011a). However, it is recognised that there is considerable individual variability in the IQs among children exposed to similar valproate doses. The Australian study assessed the offspring of pregnancies in women with epilepsy who had participated in the Register and attempted to test the children when they were between 2 and 7 years of age. Children in the younger age groups are regarded as difficult test subjects, whose assessment may require the development of special methods. Children born to women with epilepsy that were exposed in utero to levetiracetam ($N=51$) were assessed for early cognitive development and compared with children exposed in utero to valproate ($N=44$) and also with a group of 97 children not exposed to antiepileptic drugs. The children were recruited prospectively and were assessed using the Griffiths Mental Development Scale (1996) when they were aged less than 24 months. The children exposed to levetiracetam obtained higher mean developmental scores than children exposed to valproate ($P<0.001$). Those exposed to levetiracetam did not differ from control children in regard to the overall developmental quotient ($P=0.62$). There thus was evidence that children under the age of 24 months exposed to levetiracetam in utero are not at an increased risk of delayed early cognitive development. The importance of this study lies in the possible future increased employment of levetiracetam in pregnant women who do not respond to or cannot tolerate lamotrigine and who are reluctant to take valproate or in whom that drug is contraindicated. In the future, levetiracetam may come to be considered an alternative medication to valproate in treating focal and also generalised epilepsy syndromes in women capable of pregnancy.

Another recent study (Shallcross et al. 2011) compared neurodevelopment in children exposed in utero to levetiracetam ($N=55$), to valproate ($N=44$) or to no antiepileptic drugs ($N=97$). It demonstrated high rates of neurodevelopmental delay in the valproate-exposed group, but no significant difference between the levetiracetam and the untreated control groups. The levetiracetam findings are again very reassuring in view of the possible expanded use of the drug in pregnancy referred to above.

Evidence of adverse cognitive effects from intrauterine exposure to tiagabine and gabapentin is not available, but oxcarbazepine appears not to affect cognitive function in healthy infants (Molgaard-Nielsen and Hviid 2011).

Overall, there is growing evidence of an association between in utero exposure to antiepileptic drugs (at least when they are used to treat epilepsy) and neurodevelopmental delay or behavioural change in the child. There are multiple lines of evidence indicating that these changes are more common with in utero exposure to valproate. Opinions among clinicians have differed as to how conclusive the current data are. A review (Nicolai et al. 2008) had concluded that, although the available studies raised concerns, particularly in relation to valproate, a valid risk estimate for antiepileptic drug use during pregnancy on neurodevelopment was not possible so that no definite conclusions could be drawn. However, the evidence accumulated since the time of that review appears to be increasingly compelling in incriminating valproate.

Large, well-controlled prospective studies with longer term follow-up will probably be needed to answer the important questions about specific cognitive risks posed by the traditional antiepileptic drugs and the newer ones that will probably come into increasing use. However, in the meanwhile, the ethical question is likely to arise as to whether, in view of the amount of evidence already available, it is justifiable to continue to expose human foetuses to substances that may impair neurodevelopment when at least one apparently safer and effective alternative already exists in the form of levetiracetam.

Language Impairment

Nadebaum et al. (2011b) reported on language function in women with epilepsy treated with antiepileptic drugs and in their children. Language skills were assessed using Clinical Evaluation of Language Fundamentals (CELF) scores. Histories were obtained from prospectively collected records. The mean CELF-4 Core Language scores of children exposed in utero to valproate in monotherapy or polytherapy were significantly below the standardised test mean. Language scores of children exposed to carbamazepine or lamotrigine in monotherapy, or to antiepileptic drug polytherapy that did not include valproate, were not significantly different from normal. First-trimester valproate dosage was negatively correlated with language scores and also significantly predicted language scores after controlling for other group differences. Foetal exposure to valproate thus appeared to be associated with an increased risk of language impairment in childhood.

Verbal Intellectual Impairment

A recent study using the Wechsler Intelligence Scale for children (Nadebaum et al. 2011b) evaluated the cognitive impact of prenatal exposure to valproate monotherapy and to antiepileptic drug polytherapy that did not include valproate, in two groups each comprising 57 school-aged children. Information on the maternal epilepsy, on the pregnancy involved and on the child's medical history was obtained prospectively. Both groups had elevated frequencies (15.8–40.0 %) of extremely low (0.70) or borderline (0.70–0.79) full-scale IQs. Verbal comprehension and working memory scores in both groups fell significantly below the standardised test mean, while Perceptual Reasoning and Processing Speed scores were relatively intact. Multivariate analysis of covariance revealed significant main effects of valproate on Verbal Comprehension and Working Memory and of polytherapy on Verbal Comprehension and Processing Speed, suggesting that valproate has a dose-related negative impact on verbal intellectual abilities and may also affect working memory.

In the most recent United Kingdom study, the risk to children's IQs associated with frequently prescribed antiepileptic drugs was investigated by Baker et al. (2015). Children born to women with epilepsy ($N=243$) and to women without epilepsy ($N=287$) were recruited during pregnancy and then followed prospectively. It was possible to assess, blindly, 408 of the children at 6 years of age. The adjusted mean IQ was 9.7 points lower for children exposed to high-dose valproate (above 800 mg daily), with a similar significant effect of the drug observed for the verbal, nonverbal and spatial subscales. Children exposed in utero to high-dose valproate had an eightfold increased need of educational intervention relative to the control children. Valproate at doses below 800 mg daily was not associated with a reduced IQ but was still associated with impaired verbal abilities and a sixfold increase in the occurrence of educational intervention. In utero exposure to carbamazepine or lamotrigine did not have a significant effect on IQ, but carbamazepine exposure was associated with reduced verbal abilities. School-aged children exposed to valproate at maternal doses above 800 mg daily continued to experience significantly poorer cognitive development than control children or children exposed to lamotrigine and carbamazepine. These findings corroborate the outcomes of the NEAD study. The Baker et al. (2015) study again raises the question of whether there is a safe dose of valproate, at least from the cognitive viewpoint. It also suggests that carbamazepine probably has significant effects on the intellectual status of offspring exposed to it in utero. Tomson and Klein (2015) considered that this latter issue is not yet settled, as there does not appear to be a dose-related effect in regard to carbamazepine, and individual criteria of intellectual function did not appear to be significantly impaired, especially spatial and nonverbal subclasses.

Cortical Thickness and Antiepileptic Drug Exposure

Wood et al. (2014) reported a possible correlation between valproate dose-related cognitive changes and cerebral anatomical changes recognised on magnetic resonance imaging. This study of 16 children exposed to valproate prenatally, as compared with controls, has provided preliminary insights into a putative neural structural basis that may underlie the intellectual difficulties experienced by some valproate-exposed children. A close relationship was found between the thickness of the left hemisphere cerebral cortex and verbal skills in the children and also an association between the thickness and the maternal valproate dosage. There was a significant difference between the two groups of subjects, with the normal asymmetry of the inferior frontal gyri being absent in the valproate-exposed children.

Autism

Earlier research based on retrospective pregnancy records raised the possibility that there was an elevated autism risk related to antiepileptic drug exposure during pregnancy. Rasalam et al. (2005) reported that 26 (10 %) of 260 children exposed to antiepileptic drugs in utero were found to have social or behavioural difficulties. Twelve fulfilled the DSM-IV criteria for autism-spectrum disorder. Nine had been exposed to valproate (five in monotherapy) and five to carbamazepine (two in monotherapy). Unfortunately, there were no control subjects included in the study and there was a high potential for bias. Several other studies based on small case series had also found associations between autism and in utero antiepileptic drug exposure, almost always exposure to valproate (Christianson et al. 1994; Moore et al. 2000; Williams et al. 2001). In a more recent Liverpool study, seven of 249 children (2.8 %) exposed to antiepileptic drugs in utero were diagnosed with autism-spectrum disorders, compared with 3 of 336 (0.9 %) antiepileptic drug-unexposed controls (Bromley et al. 2008). Of the seven children with autism, four (6.3 %) were among the 64 who had been exposed to valproate in monotherapy. The antiepileptic drug exposure was characterised in affected children by the presence of pervasive impairments in several areas of neurodevelopment, such as reciprocal social interaction skills and communication skills, and by the presence of stereotyped behaviour, interests and activities. The Cochrane report (Bromley et al. 2008) stated that evidence existed that postnatal antiepileptic drug exposure can also damage the brain. However this is an area that is very difficult to study clinically, because confounders make the finding difficult to interpret.

A more recent study was aimed at systematic evaluation of autism-spectrum disorder traits in a sample of prospectively recruited children exposed to antiepileptic drugs. The study population was recruited via the Australian Pregnancy Register after exclusion of children with major malformations or epilepsy (Wood et al. 2015). Assessments were conducted blind to drug exposure status, the evaluation of autism-spectrum traits being performed by trained clinical research staff using the Conners Autism Rating Scale (CARS). Data on 103 exposed children aged 6–8 years revealed that the scores of 11 children (10.7 %) exceeded the CARS threshold. Of the 11, two were among the 26 exposed to valproate monotherapy (7.7 %), two were in the 32 exposed to carbamazepine monotherapy (6.3 %) and seven were in the 15 exposed to antiepileptic drug polytherapy that included valproate (46.7 %). No child exposed to antiepileptic drug polytherapy that did not include valproate ($N=19$) had scores that exceeded the CARS threshold. There was a significant relationship between first trimester valproate dose and CARS scores ($r=0.56$, $P<0.05$). This investigation appears to be the first prospective study that has systematically screened for autism after foetal antiepileptic drug exposure. It demonstrated a higher rate of autism traits, particularly in relation to valproate polytherapy, than the rates that had previously been noted in the general population. However, the finding may reflect the higher valproate doses prescribed in the polytherapy subgroup.

Overall, the available evidence suggests that foetal valproate exposure poses a significant risk for cognitive development in the child and that this risk is dose related. Carbamazepine and lamotrigine exposures appear to constitute a lower risk for cognitive development, while the risks associated with the other antiepileptic drugs are uncertain. There also is concern that intrauterine valproate exposure may be associated with the development of autism-spectrum disorder in childhood, but not enough data exist to clarify the situation in this regard as it involves the other antiepileptic drugs.

References

Adab N, Kini U, Vinten J et al (2004) The longer term outcome of children born to mothers with epilepsy. J Neurol Neurosurg Psychiatry 75:1575–1583

Asimiadou S, Bittigau P, Felderhoff-Mueser U et al (2005) Protection with estradiol in developmental models of apoptotic neurodegeneration. Ann Neurol 58:266–276

Baker GA, Bromley RL, Brigg SM et al (2015) IQ at 6 years after in utero exposure to antiepileptic drugs. A controlled cohort study. Neurology 84:382–390

Bergman A, Feigenbaum JJ, Yanai J (1982) Neuronal losses in mice following both prenatal and neonatal exposure to phenobarbital. Acta Anat 114:185–192

Bittigau P, Sifringer M, Genz K et al (2002) Aeds and apoptotic neurodegeneration in the developing brain. Proc Natl Acad Sci U S A 99:15089–15094

Bittigau P, Sifringer M, Ikonomidou C (2003) Antiepileptic drugs and apoptosis. Ann NY Acad Sci 993:103–114

Blom HJ, Shaw GM, den Heijer MS, Finnell RH (2006) Neural tube defects and folate; case far from closed. Nat Rev Neurosci 7:724–731

Bolanos AR, Sarkisian M, Yang Y et al (1998) Comparison of valproate and phenobarbital treatment after status epilepticus in rats. Neurology 51:41–48

Bromley RL, Mawer G, Clayton-Smith J, Baker GA, Liverpool and Manchester Neurodevelopment Group (2008) Autism spectrum disorders following in utero exposure to antiepileptic drugs. Neurology 71:1923–1924

Christianson AL, Chesler N, Kromberg JG (1994) Fetal valproate syndrome: clinical and neurodevelopmental features in two sibling pairs. Dev Med Child Neurol 36:361–369

Cummings C, Stewart M, Stevenson M, Morrow J, Nelson J (2011) Neurodevelopment of children exposed to lamotrigine, sodium valproate and carbamazepine. Arch Dis Child 96:643–647

Deblay MF, Vert P. André M (1982) Children of epileptic mothers. Nouv Presse Med 11: 173–176

Delgado-Escueta AV, Janz D (1992) Consensus guidelines: preconception counselling, management, and care of the pregnant woman with epilepsy. Neurology 42(4 Suppl 5):149–160

Diaz J, Schain RJ (1978) Phenobarbital: effects of long-term administration on behavior and brain of artificially reared rats. Science 199:90–91

Dodrill CB, Wilensky AJ (1992) Neuropsychological abilities before and after 5 years of stable antiepileptic drug therapy. Epilepsia 33:327–334

Downing C, Biers J, Larson C et al (2010) Genetic and maternal effects on valproic acid teratogeness in C57BL/6J and DBA/2J mice. Toxicol Sci 116:632–639

Eriksson K, Viinikainen K, Mönkkönen A, Aikiä M, Nieminen P, Heinonen S, Kälviäinen R (2005) Children exposed to valproate in utero – population based evaluation of risks and confounding factors for long-term neurocognitive development. Epilepsy Res 65:189–200

Farwell JR, Lee YJ, Hirtz DG, Sulzbacher SI, Ellenberg JH, Nelson KB (1990) Phenobarbital for febrile seizures – effects on intelligence and on seizure recurrence. N Engl J Med 322:364–369. Erratum in: N Engl J Med (1992); 326:144

Fishman RH, Ornoy A, Yanai J (1983) Ultrastructural evidence of long-lasting cerebellar degeneration after early exposure to phenobarbital in mice. Exp Neurol 79:212–222

Gaily E, Kantola-Sorsa F, Granstrom MI (1988) Intelligence of children of epileptic mothers. J Pediatr 113:677–684

Gaily EK, Granström ML, Hiilesmaa VK, Bardy AH (1990) Head circumference in children of epileptic mothers: contributions of drug exposure and genetic background. Epilepsy Res 5:217–222

Gaily E, Kantola-Sorsa F, Hiilesmaa V et al (2004) Normal intelligence in children with prenatal exposure to carbamazepine. Neurology 62:28–32

Gedzelman E, Meador KJ (2012) Aeds in women with epilepsy during pregnancy. Ther Adv Drug Saf 3:71–87

Glier C, Dzietko M, Bittigau P, Jarosz B, Korobowicz E, Ikonomidou C (2004) Therapeutic doses of topiramate are not toxic to the developing rat brain. Exp Neurol 187:403–409

Hanson JW, Myrianthopoulos NC, Harvey MA, Smith DW (1976) Risk to the offspring of women treated with hydantoin anticonvulsants, with emphasis on fetal hydantoin syndrome. J Pediatr 89:662–668

Hiilesmaa V (1996) Effects of maternal seizures on the fetus. In: Tomson T, Gram L, Sillanpaa M, Johanessen S (eds) Epilepsy and pregnancy. Wrightson Biomedical Publishing, Peterfield, pp 135–141

Holmes LB, Rosenberger PB, Harvey EA, Khoshbin S, Ryan L (2000) Intelligence and physical features of children of women with epilepsy. Teratology 61:196–202

Ikonomidou C, Turski L (2010) Aeds and brain development. Epilepsy Res 88:11–22

Ikonomidou C, Scheer I, Wilhelm T et al (2007) Brain morphology alterations in the basal ganglia and the hypothalamus following prenatal exposure to antiepileptic drugs. Eur J Paediatr Neurol 11:297–301

Kaindl AM, Asimiadou S, Manthey D, Hagen MV, Turski L, Ikonomidou C (2006) Aeds and the developing brain. Cell Mol Life Sci 63:399–413

Katz I, Kim J, Gale K, Kondratyev A (2007) Effects of lamotrigine alone and in combination with MK-801, phenobarbital, of phenytoin on cell death in the neonatal rat brain. J Pharmacol Exp Ther 322:494–500

Kaufman AS (1990) Assessing adolescent and adult intelligence. Allyn & Bacon, Boston

Kim J, Kondratyev A, Gale K (2007) Antiepileptic drug-induced neuronal cell death in the immature brain: effects of carbamazepine, topiramate, and levetiracetam as monotherapy *versus* polytherapy. J Pharmacol Exp Ther 323:165–173

Loring DW, Meador KJ (2001) Cognitive and behavioral effects of epilepsy treatment. Epilepsia 42(Suppl 8):24–32

Majewski F, Steger M, Richter B, Gill J, Rabe F (1981) The teratogenicity of hydantoins and barbiturates in humans, with considerations on the etiology of malformations and cerebral disturbances in the children of epileptic parents. Int J Biol Res Pregnancy 2:37–45

Manthey D, Asimiadou S, Stefovska V et al (2005) Sulthiame but not levetiracetam exerts neurotoxic effect in the developing rat brain. Exp Neurol 193:497–503

Meador KJ (2005) Cognitive effects of epilepsy and of antiepileptic medications. In: Wyllie E (ed) The treatment of epilepsy. Principles and practices, 4th edn. Lippincott Williams & Wilkins, Philadelphia, pp 1185–1195

Meador KJ, Gilliam FG, Kanner AM, Pellock JM (2001) Cognitive and behavioral effects of antiepileptic drugs. Epilepsy Behav 2:SS1–SS17

Meador KJ, Baker G, Cohen MJ, Gaily E, Westerveld M (2007) Cognitive/behavioral teratogenetic effects of antiepileptic drugs. Epilepsy Behav 11:292–302

Meador K, Reynolds MW, Crean S, Fahrbach K, Probst C (2008) Pregnancy outcomes in women with epilepsy: a systematic review and analysis of published pregnancy registers and cohorts. Epilepsy Res 81:1–13

Meador KJ, Baker GA, Browning N et al (2009) Cognitive function at 3 years of age after fetal exposure to antiepileptic drugs. N Engl J Med 360:1597–1605

Meador KJ, Baker GA, Browning N et al (2013) Fetal antiepileptic drug exposure and cognitive outcomes at age 6 years (NEAD study): a prospective observational study. Lancet Neurol 12:244–252

Mikati MA, Holmes GL, Chronopoulos A et al (1994) Phenobarbital modifies seizure-related brain injury in the developing brain. Ann Neurol 36:425–433

Molgaard-Nielsen D, Hviid A (2011) Newer-generation antiepileptic drugs and the risk of major birth defects. JAMA 305:1996–2002

Moore SJ, Turnpenny P, Quinn A, Glover S, Lloyd DJ, Montgomery T, Dean JC (2000) A clinical study of 57 children with fetal anticonvulsant syndromes. J Med Genet 37:489–497

Nadebaum C, Anderson V, Vajda F, Reutens D, Barton S, Wood A (2011a) The Australian brain and cognition and antiepileptic drugs study: IQ in school-aged children exposed to sodium valproate and polytherapy. J Int Neuropsychol Soc 17:133–142

Nadebaum C, Anderson VA, Vajda F, Reutens DC, Barton S, Wood AG (2011b) Language skills of school-aged children prenatally exposed to antiepileptic drugs. Neurology 76:719–726

Nicolai J, Vles JSH, Aldenkamp AP (2008) Neurodevelopmental delay in children exposed to antiepileptic drugs *in utero*: a critical review directed at structural study basis. J Neurol Sci 271:1–14

Palac S, Meador KJ (2011) Aeds and neurodevelopment: an update. Curr Neurol Neurosci Rep 11:423–427

Pulliainen V, Jokelainen M (1994) Effects of phenytoin and carbamazepine on cognitive functions in newly diagnosed epileptic patients. Acta Neurol Scand 89:81–86

Pulliainen V, Jokelainen M (1995) Comparing the cognitive effects of phenytoin and carbamazepine in long-term monotherapy: a two-year follow-up. Epilepsia 36:1195–1202

Rasalam AD, Hailey H, Williams JH, Moore SJ, Turnpenny PD, Lloyd DJ, Dean JC (2005) Characteristics of fetal anticonvulsant syndrome associated autistic disorder. Dev Med Child Neurol 47:551–555

Reinisch JM, Sanders SA, Mortensen EL, Rubin DB (1995) In utero exposure to phenobarbital and intelligence deficits in adult men. JAMA 274:1518–1525

Rogel-Fuchs Y, Newman ME, Trombka D, Zahalka EA, Yanai J (1992) Hippocampal cholinergic alterations and related behavioral deficits after early exposure to phenobarbital. Brain Res Bull 29:1–6

Sattler JM (1992) Assessment of children's intelligence and special abilities. Allyn & Bacon, Boston

Schain RJ, Watanabe K (1975) Effect of chronic phenobarbital administration upon brain growth of the infant rat. Exp Neurol 47:509–515

Scolnik D, Nulman I, Rovet J et al (1994) Neurodevelopment of children exposed in utero to phenytoin and carbamazepine monotherapy. JAMA 271:767–770. Erratum in JAMA (1994); 271:1745

Shallcross R, Bromley RL, Irwin B et al (2011) Child development following in utero exposure: levetiracetam vs sodium valproate. Neurology 76:383–389

Smith DB, Craft BR, Collins J et al (1986) Behavioral characteristics of epilepsy patients compared with normal controls. Epilepsia 27:760–768

Smith KR Jr, Goulding PM, Wilderman D et al (1994) Neurobehavioral effects of phenytoin and carbamazepine in patients recovering from brain trauma: a comparative study. Arch Neurol 51:653–660

Stefovska VG, Uckermann O, Czuczwar M et al (2008) Sedative and anticonvulsant drugs suppress postnatal neurogenesis. Ann Neurol 64:434–445

Tomson T, Klein P (2015) Fine-tuning risk assessment with antiepileptic drug use in pregnancy. Neurology 84:339–340

Vajda FJE, O'Brien T, Hitchcock A, Graham J, Lander C, Eadie M (2007) The Australian antiepileptic drug in pregnancy register: aspects of data collection and analysis. J Clin Neurosci 14:936–942

Vajda FJE, O'Brien TJ, Lander CM, Graham J, Eadie MJ (2014) The teratogenicity of the newer antiepileptic drugs – an update. Acta Neurol Scand 130:234–238

Vanoverloop D, Schnell RR, Harvey EA, Holmes LB (1992) The effects of prenatal exposure to phenytoin and other anticonvulsants on intellectual function at 4 to 8 years of age. Neurotoxicol Teratol 14:329–335

Wide K, Henning E, Tomson T, Winbladh B (2002) Psychomotor development in preschool children exposed to antiepileptic drugs in utero. Acta Paediatr 91:409–414

Williams G, King J, Cunningham M, Stephan M, Kerr B, Hersh JH (2001) Fetal valproate syndrome and autism: additional evidence of an association. Dev Med Child Neurol 43:202–206

Wood AG, Chen J, Barton S et al (2014) Altered cortical thickness following prenatal sodium valproate exposure. Ann Clin Transl Neurol 1:497–501

Wood AG, Nadebaum C, Anderson VA, Reutens DC, Barton S, O'Brien TJ, Vajda FJE (2015) Prospective assessment of autism traits in children exposed to antiepileptic drugs during pregnancy. Epilepsia 56:1047–1055

Part III
Antiepileptic Drug Use and Pregnancy

Chapter 11
Antiepileptic Drug Therapy: Management Issues and Pregnancy

Abstract This chapter draws on material discussed in earlier chapters in an attempt to provide a scientifically based discussion of the management of antiepileptic drug therapy in women with epilepsy who are planning pregnancy, while pregnant and in the postpartum period. The aim of the management is to maintain optimal control of epileptic seizures at all times while also minimising the risks to the foetus from developing structural malformations while still in utero and from encountering neurodevelopmental problems during infancy and childhood. The information regarding the management of antiepileptic drug therapy in pregnant women with epilepsy should also, for the most part, be applicable to the use of these drugs in pregnant women for indications other than epilepsy.

Managing epilepsy in women presents potentially more complex problems than managing the same disorder in men. This is so particularly because of issues related to pregnancy, a situation where appropriate management must take into account the welfares of both the woman concerned and that of her baby. Although epileptic seizure disorders may become manifest for the first time during the course of pregnancy, the great majority of women with epilepsy who enter pregnancy do so with the therapeutic management of their seizure disorders already instituted.

The following account attempts to consider the use of antiepileptic drugs in the woman who already possesses, or is likely to possess in the reasonably near future, reproductive capacity. It deals with her situation (i) before pregnancy, (ii) during pregnancy and (iii) in the postpartum period.

Before Pregnancy

Prior to pregnancy, it is desirable to have organised the antiepileptic drug treatment of the woman with epilepsy so that it provides the greatest advantage it can for her and for any baby that she may subsequently carry in her uterus. As well, the potential mother needs to have been provided with an understanding of the issues that are likely to arise in relation to her antiepileptic drug therapy during her pregnancy, and afterwards, and of how these issues may be managed.

M.J. Eadie, F.J.E. Vajda, *Antiepileptic Drugs and Pregnancy: A Guide for Prescribers*, DOI 10.1007/978-3-319-21434-4_11

The burdens that may result from having suffered epileptic seizure include the uncertainties arising from the possibility of further seizures occurring, the possibly of seizures causing physical injury, the small increased risk of sudden unexplained death occurring, the restrictions imposed on various aspects of daily living including vehicle driving and participation in sporting and certain recreational activities, the limitation of alcohol intake and the possibility that prescribed antiepileptic medications may cause adverse effects. Discrimination in relation to employment and employment prospects may still be encountered today by those with epilepsy. This situation exists despite the best efforts made by the medical profession, by recognised epilepsy associations whose memberships include scientists and paramedical personnel and by patient advocacy groups to remedy this situation, mainly through better educating the general community. A further major burden appears to arise from the fears of women with epilepsy that the children to whom they give birth may inherit their disorder and also may be born with physical malformations or with lower than average intellects.

The Initiation of Antiepileptic Drug Therapy

After adequate discussion of these issues with the woman concerned, if it is agreed that antiepileptic drug treatment is expected to hold overall advantages for her and her prospective offspring in any pregnancy that occurs, the matter of the most appropriate antiepileptic drug therapy in her situation has to be considered, even if she is already taking an antiepileptic drug, or drugs. If future pregnancy was not an issue, the decision about the choice of drug would be based mainly on the type of epileptic seizure disorder that was present and required treatment. However, in women who could become pregnant during the anticipated durations of their antiepileptic drug intake, the welfare of any foetuses that are conceived must also be considered in choosing the most appropriate drug. It will nearly always be easier to organise this choice of agent at the outset of treatment or early in its course than to attempt it later, often when pregnancy either is imminent, or already exists.

From the foetal harm point of view, it appears desirable that the antiepileptic drug that is chosen is not valproate and also probably not topiramate, if that is at all possible. The degree of teratogenicity associated with the other antiepileptic drugs in contemporary use is relatively small, perhaps virtually negligible, and there is no consistent evidence that it is dose related, unlike the situations in relation to valproate and topiramate.

The Initial Choice of an Antiepileptic Drug

Information on the selection of so-called first-line drugs for treating the two main categories of epilepsy syndromes, genetic generalised and focal (partial) epilepsies, is widely available but needs to be adapted to individual patients' situations. The use of the more recently introduced second-generation antiepileptic drugs, with their improved tolerability profiles and comparable efficacies, increases the chances of achieving successful therapy, but it also poses a challenge for making the most appropriate choice of agent for the woman who may become pregnant (Pennell 2005; Perucca 2005). These newer drugs have not yet been thoroughly evaluated for their human teratogenicity over sufficiently long periods. As well, not all second-generation antiepileptic drugs are available worldwide. Regional and traditional prescribing differences, cost factors and lack of availability of specialist care may further complicate decisions as to choice of appropriate agent for a given woman (Tomson et al. 2007a).

Women with Genetic/Idiopathic Generalised Epilepsies

Valproate: Valproate, often marketed as its sodium salt, is generally accepted as being the most effective agent for preventing the seizures of the genetic generalised epilepsies. Unfortunately, valproate is also the antiepileptic drug with the greatest potential for being associated with foetal malformations (Chaps. 8 and 9) and also with cognitive and other neurodevelopmental problems in the offspring of pregnancy (Chap. 10). There is therefore reason to consider the relative expected efficacies of all the available appropriate drugs and also the disadvantages their use entails from the foetal standpoint, before deciding to prescribe valproate in preference to alternative agents in women with epilepsy who may become pregnant while they continue to need seizure-suppressing drug therapy.

Lamotrigine: The relative safety of lamotrigine from the standpoint of teratogenesis clearly favours this drug over valproate, but unfortunately lamotrigine is overall less effective in achieving seizure control in pregnant women as compared not only with valproate but also with another relatively new antiepileptic drug, viz. levetiracetam (Vajda et al. 2014). Early reviews of lamotrigine and its clinical application in epilepsy suggested that the drug would probably provide an excellent treatment option for patients with generalised epilepsies in pregnancy, a view that for a time subsequently became generally accepted (Choi and Morrell 2003). However, the increasingly reported problem of plasma lamotrigine levels falling relative to drug dose in each trimester (Pennell et al. 2008), the need for the drug's slow introduction and its lesser seizure-preventing efficacy have tended to make its use less attractive (Vajda et al. 2006a). As well, Morrow et al. (2006) reported that in utero lamotrigine exposure could be associated with the occurrence of dose-related foetal malformations, and other studies have suggested that the drug is not free of responsibility for producing foetal malformations, though the degree of hazard is low, compared with that which applies for valproate (see Chap. 9).

Ethosuximide: Ethosuximide, an older drug for which there is virtually no evidence of teratogenicity (see Chap. 9), may be used to treat absence seizures in preference to valproate, if absences are the only type of seizure that is present (Glauser et al. 2013). In a controlled clinical trial, randomly allocated ethosuximide ($N=156$), valproic acid ($N=148$) and lamotrigine ($N=149$) were compared in treating childhood absence epilepsy. Drug doses were incrementally increased until seizure freedom was obtained, or the maximal allowable or highest tolerable dose was reached, or a criterion indicating treatment failure was met. Freedom-from-failure rates for ethosuximide and valproic acid were similar (53 and 58 %, respectively), both being higher than the rate for lamotrigine (29 %). There were no significant differences among the three drugs with regard to discontinuation of intake because of adverse events. Attentional dysfunction was more common with valproic acid than with ethosuximide (in 49 % of the children compared with 33 %). The findings of this study suggests that, in women of childbearing potential who have genetic generalised epilepsies that are manifested only as absence seizures, itself an uncommon situation, ethosuximide may provide more appropriate monotherapy than lamotrigine in relation to seizure control efficacy and be safer than valproate in relation to avoiding teratogenesis. However, there is not enough evidence to know the situation regarding ethosuximide and neurodevelopmental impairment.

Other possibilities: Levetiracetam, zonisamide and topiramate appear to be less effective than valproate in treating genetic generalised epilepsies, though on the basis of currently available evidence in terms of teratogenicity the first two appear to be more acceptable. However, the evidence regarding relative teratogenic hazards is not as extensive as might be desirable. Topiramate probably is less well tolerated than levetiracetam and zonisamide, and the evidence that it is a dose-related teratogen further deters its use.

Valproate and the European Medicines Authority: In 2014 the European Medicines Authority issued a statement which in its effect has restricted physicians' choice of antiepileptic medications within the European Union. The statement declared that it is inadvisable to prescribe valproate for women of childbearing age who suffer from epilepsy and also for such women at earlier stages in their lives, because of the documented teratogenicity of the drug. The wording employed was 'This medicine should not be used in women of child-bearing potential unless clearly necessary' and should only be used in situations 'where other treatments are ineffective or not tolerated'. References were cited in the declaration that supported this statement, but comments by the European Pregnancy Registry (EURAP) and a statement from the International League Against Epilepsy, which represents all countries worldwide in terms of epilepsy management, were not included (Meador et al. 2008, 2009, 2013; Bromley et al. 2008; Cummings et al. 2011; Thomas 2011; Christensen et al. 2013; Cohen et al. 2013).

This action by the European Medicines Authority is appropriate up to a point, but the statement may have different implications in Europe than in other parts of the world. From a regulator's perspective such a statement is understandable, but it fails to give appropriate weight to the harm that may result from failure to employ the most effective available therapy for a major type of epilepsy. To limit prescription of the drug to situations where all other potential useful therapy has first been found wanting may endanger women's lives and the lives of their foetuses if, for instance, otherwise avoidable status epilepticus were to occur.

Women with Focal (Partial) Epilepsies

Overall, focal epilepsies are more difficult to treat effectively than genetic generalised ones, but a wider choice of reasonably satisfactory antiepileptic drugs is available for their management. The choice between these drugs in women with epilepsy is based on a comparison of the risk–benefit ratio that would be expected to apply in each given individual. Initially, antiepileptic drug monotherapy is almost always tried, and if this fails combinations of antiepileptic drugs, preferably drugs with different mechanisms of action, are employed. In the future, the choice of drug may be made more efficiently if more robust documentation of efficacy of newer antiepileptic drugs can be obtained from epilepsy syndrome-oriented trials than was possible from, as in the past, trials based on seizure types.

There is little persuasive evidence that any one of the rather substantial number of antiepileptic drugs that are effective in managing focal epilepsies is appreciably more effective than its fellows. However, there is rather widespread acceptance that the older agents such as phenobarbitone and phenytoin probably have more adverse effects and are often more difficult to use, than the newer agents. Carbamazepine, despite being available for half a century, still enjoys substantial use but valproate's adverse effects on the foetus limit its use for focal epilepsies because there are a number of at least equally effective alternatives. Inevitably, in more affluent countries, the more recently introduced antiepileptic drugs are becoming the preferred agents for managing focal epilepsies, though globally phenobarbitone probably remains the most widely used antiepileptic agent (Kwan and Brodie 2004).

Lamotrigine is of particular interest in relation to women with focal epilepsies. It was originally introduced into therapeutics in 1994 for the treatment of this type of epilepsy, but its indications were later extended to include genetic generalised epilepsies (see above). Some adverse effects attributable to the drug may be serious, including rashes and immunological disturbances ranging as far as a full-blown Stevens–Johnson syndrome, which may be fatal. Slowly incremented dosages of the drug may reduce its unwanted effects. A desirable feature is that lamotrigine administration may produce a mood elevation. There is no generally accepted therapeutic range of plasma concentrations of the drug, and an individual therapeutic window needs to be established for each patient who takes the drug (Vajda et al. 1999; Perucca 2001).

Levetiracetam, marketed in 2005, has a pharmacokinetic profile which approximates to the ideal characteristics for an antiepileptic drug. It is involved in few known drug interactions and has a considerable margin of safety (Patsalos 2000; Mula et al. 2003) and probably possesses greater antiepileptic efficacy than the other new antiepileptic drugs (Tomson et al. 2007b; Weintraub et al. 2007). In clinical practice, its use may be associated with dose-related cognitive slowing and emotional disturbances, which are less than ideal for women with epilepsy, who may already be emotionally stressed.

Topiramate is approved in a number of countries for the treatment of both focal and genetic generalised epilepsies, though the growing evidence of its teratogenicity does not yet seem to have been perhaps sufficiently been taken into account.

Oxcarbazepine has been used safely in Scandinavia for over two decades. In focal seizures it has an efficacy comparable to that of valproate and phenytoin, in both adults and in children. It is generally better tolerated than carbamazepine, but its use is associated with a higher incidence of laboratory abnormalities, especially hyponatraemia. Insufficient data are available in regards to its effectiveness, acceptability and foetal safety in pregnancy. Gabapentin is generally perceived to be less effective than the other alternatives for focal epilepsies but appears remarkably safe at usual dosages. Little information is available regarding its efficacy in pregnancy. Zonisamide appears to have no significant associated teratogenicity as yet reported. Lacosamide has not been extensively used in pregnancy and little information is available concerning its teratogenicity. As mentioned above, all the drugs named in this paragraph are coming to be used increasingly in focal epilepsy in pregnant women, being prescribed according to individual needs and preferences (Boon et al. 2012). However, they have not yet found their definitive places in the management of focal seizure disorder in pregnant women.

The Further Management of Antiepileptic Drug Therapy Before Pregnancy

It is hoped that, once the woman with epilepsy is established on appropriate antiepileptic drug therapy, there will be sufficient time before pregnancy occurs to ascertain that the aim of her treatment has been achieved. Ideally, she should have been kept free of all clinical manifestations of her epilepsy and have experienced no adverse effects from her drug therapy. She should also be in a situation where her treatment offers her the least risk of worsened seizure control in any pregnancy that she undertakes and also in a situation in which any foetus that she carries will not suffer physical or intellectual maldevelopment because of her antiepileptic drug intake.

Seizure control during pregnancy has been shown to be better when no seizures have occurred in a woman's pre-pregnancy 9 months or year (Chap. 7). Control over shorter periods before pregnancy is still associated with advantages from the standpoint of seizure freedom during pregnancy, while the data of Fig. 7.1 suggest that no considerable additional dividends may accrue from having periods of pre-pregnancy seizure control that exceed 1–2 years. It is often stated in the literature that, if valproate is to be used, it should be employed in the lowest possible dose, though in practice achieving this endpoint may require months of dosage adjustments. This advice may be prudent but, if the possible alternatives to its use have already proved unsatisfactory in a woman, she may have an epilepsy that is rather difficult to control. In this case, relatively high valproate doses may be required to obtain seizure control. After that control is achieved, the effort to find the lowest effective dose of the drug may involve trialling dose reductions that in the end compromise earlier hard-won seizure suppression and, if pregnancy occurs, may still leave her foetus with a significant risk of being born malformed. In a way, the situation may be easier to manage if the woman's epilepsy has been impossible to control for some time despite the best therapeutic endeavours. From the social disadvantage standpoint, paradoxically, such a woman has less to lose than the woman whose controlled seizures have been permitted to recur while seeking the lowest effective valproate dose. If valproate must be used in a woman with an intractable seizure disorder, it may be realistic to keep its dosage low enough to avoid worsening of seizure control during pregnancy rather than attempting to obtain complete seizure control, even though this policy may expose the woman to the hazards of injury or rarely death, in relation to seizures, in the hope of minimising foetal harm.

To obtain seizure control prior to pregnancy, if the first antiepileptic drug that was prescribed has failed, ideally various other potentially appropriate antiepileptic drugs would be tried in monotherapy before drug combinations were employed. In practice, rather than abruptly ceasing the first drug and immediately commencing intake of a second one, a progressive transition between the two agents is often arranged. If a completely satisfactory clinical situation is attained during the transition, the patient may be left taking a combination of agents. There has been considerable mention in the literature that the use of antiepileptic drug combinations, i.e. polytherapy, is associated with increased risks of foetal malformations occurring (Nakane et al. 1980; Kaneko et al. 1992; Lindhout and Omtzigt 1992; Samrén et al. 1997; Morrow et al. 2006). However, as discussed in Chap. 8, several relatively recent studies have demonstrated that the heightened malformation risk is determined by the presence of valproate in the combinations and not simply by the presence of any two or more antiepileptic drugs (Artama et al. 2005; Vajda et al. 2010b; Mawer et al. 2010; Holmes et al. 2011). As mentioned in Chaps. 8 and 9, there is now evidence that topiramate may play a similar role to valproate in antiepileptic drug combinations. Further, the possibility of pharmacokinetic interactions occurring between members of other antiepileptic drug combination may make a scientific approach to their handling more difficult to apply in practice. The magnitudes of such interactions may change as drug disposition parameters alter during the course of pregnancy and afterwards (see Chap. 3).

In an ideal situation, once antiepileptic drug therapy has been adjusted before pregnancy to achieve the best achievable compromise between seizure control and preservation of the welfare of any prospective foetus, knowledge of the steady-state plasma concentration of antiepileptic drugs associated with this satisfactory situation becomes a valuable, perhaps almost essential, guidepost for managing the treatment situation during the course of pregnancy.

Pre-pregnancy Advice

Qualitative research suggests that many women with epilepsy remain uninformed about the risks and other issues associated with epilepsy and pregnancy. They may, as a result, make uninformed and sometimes inappropriate decisions. Evidence suggests that many women with epilepsy want to receive more information – particularly about the risks that exposure to antiepileptic drugs may hold for their offspring – and that they wish to receive it well in advance of beginning to take an antiepileptic drug or to plan pregnancy. Women aged below 35 years, in particular, seem to seek the most information (McGrath et al. 2014). There also may be other matters which have not occurred to them at the stage when they ask for information, but which they should know about. Leaving aside aspects that are predominantly matters of obstetric concern and practice, this information relevant to antiepileptic drug therapy in pregnancy can be provided below in the form of answers to questions that women with epilepsy who are considering pregnancy may well ask.

Will I have a malformed baby?

Here the first point to be made is that any pregnant woman has some risk of giving birth to a baby with a malformation. The risk is of the order of 2 or 3 per 100, and the malformations can range in severity between the cosmetically almost trivial and the catastrophic, though many of the latter can be detected during pregnancy and appropriate action considered at that stage. The woman with epilepsy needs to realise that the essential matter that she should appreciate is the extent to which her antiepileptic drug use increases her risk of giving birth to a malformed baby above the general population background risk of this happening.

In the present state of knowledge, it is possible to state that, with the exception of valproate and topiramate, the increase risk associated with the longer established antiepileptic drugs that remain in common use is probably a real one but so small that it cannot be demonstrated unambiguously in the available statistics. For practical purposes, it would be almost negligible for the individual woman. Unfortunately, it cannot be stated definitely that any of the newer antiepileptic drugs is associated with less risk of birth defects than the older agents (excluding valproate and topiramate). There simply is not enough information available regarding some of the recently introduced drugs such as lacosamide and perampanel to permit any firm advice. This is a situation that is likely to continue for some time. Further, it needs to be pointed out that there is now evidence that some of the risk of a malformed baby being born to a woman with an antiepileptic drug-treated seizure disorder is related to genetic factors (see Chap. 8). It is therefore important to ascertain whether the woman concerned has a family history or past history of births of malformed babies. Such a history could significantly increase the woman's hazard of having a malformed baby and may suggest the need for genetic counselling.

If the woman with epilepsy is taking valproate or topiramate, she should be made aware that her risk of a malformed baby due to exposure to the drug is increased and that the risk increases with increasing drug dosages, with higher doses of valproate than are now customarily used being associated in particular with the occurrence of neural tube defects (Vajda et al. 2013). There is no standard pattern of malformation associated with either of these two drugs. Some of the malformations are relatively minor, and they and others may be surgically remediable. In addition to the hazard of giving birth to a malformed baby, the woman taking valproate need to be told that relatively recent investigations have shown that babies born to mothers taking valproate, even if not physically malformed at birth, are more likely to prove less intelligent than their peers and are also more likely to develop behavioural disturbances and autism spectrum manifestations. It is not yet possible to indicate the degree of risk of these latter situations occurring. For topiramate exposure in pregnancy, the dose-related malformations appear to be mainly facial clefts and hypospadias, both at least to an extent remediable surgically. The prospective mother certainly should be made aware of this matter. There does not appear to be sufficient evidence available to permit any definite statement regarding the possibility of neurodevelopmental problems associated with intrauterine exposure to this drug.

Overall, if the woman with epilepsy that is treated with antiepileptic drugs is not taking valproate or perhaps topiramate or one of the very recently available drugs for which the relevant information is not yet available and has no previous or family history of potentially inheritable foetal malformations, the answer to the question posed above should not be likely to deter her from becoming pregnant.

Will the drugs increase my risk of miscarriage or other pregnancy problem?

In so far as consequences of taking antiepileptic drugs are concerned, as distinct from the effects of seizures occurring, there does not appear to be clear-cut evidence of an increased hazard.

What will happen if I do not take antiepileptic drugs when pregnant?

This question arises out of the widespread community awareness that any therapeutic drug intake during pregnancy is undesirable from the foetal standpoint and from the more specific knowledge that foetal malformation and other hazards may be associated with intrauterine antiepileptic drug exposure.

It seems entirely reasonable to expect that the increased foetal malformation risk associated with antiepileptic drug exposure in utero would be avoided if a woman were to cease her antiepileptic drug intake before the time of conception and continued not to take these drugs during at least the first trimester of pregnancy, the critical stage for organogenesis. Doing this would in practice involve ceasing the drugs before conception occurs, as taking such action once it is realised that pregnancy exists may be too late to achieve the desired outcome. Unfortunately, as far as can be ascertained, there is little published evidence that such cessation of therapy does reduce the malformation risk to the level of the community background one, but on the other hand, there is no evidence that it does not. In so far as foetal neurodevelopmental problems are concerned, an issue that at present mainly concerns valproate, it seems likely that intake of the drug would have to be avoided throughout the entire duration of pregnancy and possibly also while breastfeeding.

The possible benefits for the baby in this scenario have to be balanced against possible disadvantages for the mother, and some of the maternal disadvantages may possibly extend to the baby. There is the likelihood of seizure control worsening, perhaps with status epilepticus occurring and perhaps damaging the mother or foetus or interrupting the pregnancy. Loss of seizure control in more advanced and complicated societies may impose various limitations on the mother, particularly in relation to vehicle driving. This restriction may reduce her capacity to care for other members of her family, as well as the baby whose welfare she has tried to protect by avoiding antiepileptic drug intake.

The possibility might be considered that a more teratogenic drug could be replaced with a less teratogenic but perhaps also less effective antiepileptic one for the duration of the pregnancy or for part of it. In the woman with apparently fully controlled epilepsy before pregnancy, unless the substitution was carried out long enough before conception to be sure that seizure control was maintained, the various limitations imposed by potentially uncontrolled epilepsy would again apply, as well as the further problems that might arise from any return of seizures. If the woman's epilepsy was already incompletely controlled before pregnancy, the same social disadvantages would already apply, but difficulties could arise from increased frequency or severity of seizures. As well, the substituting drug might produce adverse effects in the woman now taking it.

A decision to interrupt, or modify, antiepileptic drug therapy in preparation for pregnancy needs to be made on the basis of a clear and realistic understanding of the issues likely to be involved. The experience of the Australian Pregnancy Register suggests that some women with epilepsy do take this decision, being prepared to deliberately sacrifice their own welfare for the potential benefit of their foetuses. Thus Vajda et al. (2015) recorded that in the Register, 148 of the women with epilepsy had entered pregnancy when not taking antiepileptic drugs. The intake of these drugs had been ceased in the few months prior to pregnancy in 41.9 % of these women, usually with the explicit aim of avoiding foetal exposure to the effects of these agents. In this subset of the original 148 untreated pregnancies, seizures had been experienced in 48.4 % during the pregnancy, and by term antiepileptic drug intake had been resumed in 56.4 %.

Will I be able to breastfeed?

So long as no other potential contraindication exists, the short answer here would nearly always be 'yes', in so far as the effects of maternal antiepileptic drug intake was the issue. This answer is based on certain information, as follows.

Human milk is not simply a food. It is a complex, sophisticated and highly integrated human infant support system. The ability of lactation to provide this support results from its provision of both non-nutritive and food components. In addition, many, if not most, women regard breastfeeding as an integral and important part of the experience of motherhood (Pack 2006). The concerns of women who are taking antiepileptic drugs in regard to breastfeeding relate mainly to the possibility that drugs taken by the mother will pass into the child and cause immediate adverse effects such as impaired alertness and a decrease ability to thrive (Vajda et al. 2010a).

Earlier chapters of this book contain information regarding the simultaneous dispositions of individual antiepileptic drugs in breast milk, in other maternal body fluids and in the blood plasma of the breastfed infant. The drug concentration ratios between these various fluids show rather considerable ranges of variation. However, with few exceptions, the drug concentrations in the infants' blood plasmas do not exceed their more or less simultaneous concentration values in maternal plasma.

This suggests that, if the mother is not adversely affected by the drug taken, the baby, particularly if it has already been exposed to the drug throughout pregnancy, is also unlikely to be affected, though it certainly does not guarantee that this will be the case. Nonetheless, the American Academy of Neurology (2009) found it necessary to state that the clinical consequences for the newborn of ingesting antiepileptic drugs via breast milk remained sorely underexplored, a situation that produces anxiety in women with epilepsy who are considering pregnancy or are pregnant (Harden et al. 2009). Since that time, the situation in this regard has been further clarified.

The findings of a recent large-scale population-based study of babies who were exposed in utero to any of the three commonly used antiepileptic drugs valproate, lamotrigine and carbamazepine (the Norwegian Mother and Child Cohort study) have become available (Veiby et al. 2013a, b). This study reported the cognitive outcomes of breastfed babies at early time points, beginning at 6 months of age, and also shed light on the question of the possible adverse effects of breastfeeding for periods of 6–12 months in women with antiepileptic drug-treated epilepsy. The women were enrolled early in pregnancy, at 13–17 weeks. Validated techniques were used to assess cognitive outcomes that comprised motor skills, language, social skills and behaviour of babies, at 6 months (N=78,744), at 18 months (N=61,351) and at 36 months (N=44,147). Control data were obtained from the babies of women without epilepsy, and there also were internal comparator groups of babies of untreated women with epilepsy and the babies of fathers with epilepsy. Fine motor skills were assessed at all the time points studied. In utero exposure to the drugs was associated with impaired fine motor and social skills detectable as early as 6 months after birth, particularly in cases where the mothers were receiving antiepileptic drug polytherapy. This finding is in keeping with a previous study in which similar results were documented in children at 3 years of age (Meador et al. 2012). The three drugs studied seemed to show comparable effects on cognition. This is surprising, as in earlier studies valproate had been shown to be associated with the least favourable outcomes in this regard (Pennell 2005). At 36 months of age, the offspring who had shown cognitive impairment at earlier time points continued to show impairment, regardless of what their breastfeeding status had been. The results suggest that, in general, breastfeeding is safe in women treated with valproate, lamotrigine or carbamazepine and whose babies had already been exposed to these agents while in utero. Babies of untreated women with epilepsy and babies of fathers with epilepsy had no cognitive impairment when compared with babies who had non-epileptic parents. Continuous breastfeeding was associated with less cognitive impairment at 6 and 18 months than no breastfeeding or breastfeeding for less than 6 months.

A report of a prospective observational multicentre study of long-term antiepileptic drug use, examining cognitive functions in children at the age of 6 years in relation to previous breastfeeding, has also become available. Meador et al. (2010) had previously found that breastfeeding in mothers taking antiepileptic drugs appeared to have no adverse effects on the offspring's IQs at the age of 3 years. However, the IQ at the age of 6 years provides a better predictor of school performance and adult abilities. The Meador et al. (2014) breastfeeding study enrolled participants in Britain and the United States, 42.9 % of the children involved being breastfed. The primary endpoint was the differential ability IQ. Secondary endpoints included verbal and non-verbal memory and executive functions. The IQs at 6 years of age were found to be related to the drug that had been taken during breastfeeding, the adjusted IQ for offspring exposed to valproate being 7–13 points lower than those for the other drugs studied. The IQs were negatively correlated with the drug doses and positively correlated with maternal IQs (the higher the maternal IQ, the higher the child's). Folate supplementation and breastfeeding were both correlated with higher maternal IQs. Verbal memory scores were higher for breastfed children. No adverse effects were observed related to breast milk intake. The rigorous methodology and controlled nature of this study adds significantly to the perception that, in women taking antiepileptic drugs apart from valproate, breastfeeding is safe and beneficial from the infant's cognitive viewpoint.

There is a further, perhaps more pragmatic, argument in favour of women who have taken antiepileptic drug therapy during pregnancy undertaking breastfeeding. If they do not, in effect the baby undergoes abruptly withdrawal from antiepileptic drug exposure at the time of birth, producing the hazard of drug withdrawal effects such as irritability and, possibly, seizures. If the baby is breastfed and weaned progressively at a later appropriate time, the gradual cessation of intake of a substance with general sedative properties is less likely to cause problems.

Overall, the available evidence appears rather strongly in favour of breastfeeding in the situation discussed.

Will my epilepsy get worse during the pregnancy or afterwards?

The literature indicates the long-standing existence of some controversy as to whether epilepsy worsens, remains unaltered or improves during pregnancy (Knight and Rhind 1975; Schmidt 1982; Gjerde et al. 1988; Schaffler 1990; Vidović and Della Marina 1994; Costa et al. 2005). As discussed in Chap. 7, the interpretation of the situation is confounded by the effects of pregnancy on antiepileptic drug disposition (Chap. 3) and also by whether action has been taken to counter the consequences of this altered drug disposition. These potential confounding factors have often not been considered in the published reports.

A relatively recent study based on the Australian Pregnancy Register found that pregnancy had little overall influence on the control of epileptic seizure disorders in which no attempt had been made to influence the patterns of antiepileptic drug prescribing (Vajda et al. 2008). Seizures during pregnancy occurred in 49.7 % of 841 antiepileptic drug-treated pregnancies in the women with epilepsy. Epilepsies that were active in the year before pregnancy tended to be associated with an increased risk of intrapartum and postpartum seizures, while the risk of seizures during pregnancy was 50–70% lower if the pre-pregnancy year had been seizure-free. A recent large observational study involving 3,806 pregnancies in 3,451 women with epilepsy from the EURAP database reported that 66.6 % of the pregnancies treated with carbamazepine, lamotrigine, phenobarbitone or valproate, all in monotherapy, were seizure-free throughout (Battino et al. 2013). Women with genetic generalised epilepsies were more likely to continue to be seizure-free throughout pregnancy

(73.6 %) than women with focal (localisation-related) epilepsies (59.5 %; $P<0.0001$). Seizure control worsened during 15.8 % of pregnancies. The antiepileptic drug dose had been increased during 26.0 % of the pregnancies and a second antiepileptic drug added to the initial drug in 2.6 %. Compared with pregnancies managed with the other drugs used in monotherapy, pregnancies treated with lamotrigine had been less likely to remain seizure-free (58.2 %; $P<0.0001$), with increased numbers of generalised tonic–clonic seizures being experienced in 21.1 % ($P<0.0001$). There was a greater chance of deterioration in seizure control from the first to the second or third trimesters in the lamotrigine-treated pregnancies (in 19.9 %; $P<0.01$). More (47.7 %; $P<0.0001$) had required an increased antiepileptic drug dosage.

Being aware of the substantial fall in the ratio of plasma concentration to dose of lamotrigine during pregnancy, the reported poorer seizure control in pregnancy treated with the drug and the arguments for monitoring plasma lamotrigine concentrations in pregnancy (Sabres et al. 2004; Vajda et al. 2006b), Sabers and Petrenaite (2009) adopted a proactive policy in adjusting the lamotrigine dosage during pregnancy to maintain the drug's plasma concentrations at their pre-pregnancy values. This course of action resulted in better seizure control being maintained during pregnancy. This experience can be extrapolated to suggest that epilepsy is unlikely to worsen during pregnancy if plasma concentrations of antiepileptic drugs are maintained at those levels that were present prior to pregnancy, so long as the epilepsy itself is not secondary to some pathological state that is not itself controlled.

There thus appears justification for claiming that pregnancy is unlikely to worsen during pregnancy if its treatment is managed optimally according to the current state of knowledge.

Will my having drug-treated epilepsy influence my obstetric management?

In its own right, antiepileptic drug treatment should not make a difference, unless its failure results in worsening seizures which may constitute an indication for action on the part of the obstetrician involved.

Will my baby have epilepsy?

The answer to this question is relevant to antiepileptic drug therapy only in so far as certain antiepileptic drugs may be the preferred agents for epilepsies which are potentially inheritable.

Additional Information

There are further items of information that would usually be provided to women with epilepsy who are contemplating pregnancy or are in early pregnancy.

Before pregnancy, or in early pregnancy, arrangements should exist for an obstetrician to undertake the main responsibility for the conduct of the woman's pregnancy, with supporting advice from a neurologist or other medical practitioner with expertise in the management of epilepsy. Delivery in a well-equipped obstetrical centre is advisable, as complications at term tend to be more common in women with epilepsy (Yerby 2003; Sabers 2009).

It is commonly recommended that folic acid 0.4 to 5 mg daily be taken for at least 6 weeks before a planned pregnancy, with the intake continuing into the first few months of pregnancy. This recommendation is based mainly on studies in pregnant normal female populations, without epilepsy, as discussed in more detail in Chap. 8. There is no evidence for its value in reducing the incidence of neural tube defects and other malformations in the offspring of women with antiepileptic drug-treated seizure disorders. However, it is generally thought that such use of folic acid is likely to be harmless, and the substance itself is inexpensive.

Information should be provided regarding the investigations that are likely to be performed in preparation for pregnancy and during pregnancy, both as a general check on the woman's health and to obtain early evidence of the presence of foetal abnormalities. These investigations include routing blood examinations and serum biochemical investigations. Ultrasonography is likely to be carried out on more than one occasion. The procedure can identify the majority of major physical defects in the foetus. In most instances, neural tube defects can be detected in utero by detailed ultrasonography and by measuring levels of alpha-fetoprotein in maternal serum or amniotic fluid. In particular, women being treated with valproate should be made aware of these diagnostic procedures that may be carried out in the early stages of gestation (Koren and Kennedy 1999). On first presentation in pregnancy, an ultrasonogram is likely to be obtained to define the gestational age more accurately than may be possible from the dates of the most recent missed menstrual period. Routine ultrasonography at 11–13 weeks is intended to identify the more severe foetal defects, such as anencephaly. Maternal serum alpha-fetoprotein testing and repeat anatomical ultrasonography at 16 weeks should be able to identify abnormalities such as orofacial clefts, heart defects and caudal neural tube defects. A late ultrasound in the third trimester may be performed to check foetal growth, the volume of fluid around the baby and the position of the placenta (Palomaki et al. 2013; Yerby et al. 2004; Bianchi et al. 2012; Garfield and Armstrong 2012). A larger than normal value in an ultrasound measurement of the foetus's nape of neck raises the possibility of Down syndrome.

A Prenatal Testing Fact sheet has been prepared by the NCHPEG (National Coalition for Health Professional Education in Genetics) and the National Society of Counsellors. The sheet advises professionals of an option for testing for trisomy 21 and other chromosomal abnormalities. It is based on detection of foetal DNA, which is normally cleared from the blood in a few hours. Quantitative differences in chromosome fragments can distinguish foetuses with certain chromosome abnormalities. The test is performed after 10 weeks of pregnancy. It is non-invasive, uses maternal blood and may detect trisomy 21, 18 and sometimes 13. The test is claimed to be highly sensitive and specific for detecting these abnormalities.

If plasma antiepileptic drug monitoring is to be carried out during pregnancy, a schedule for the measurements should be organised in advance. The optimal interval between measurements may be arguable, but the measurements may sometimes be carried out as frequently as monthly during pregnancy.

Near term, it is likely that vitamin K supplementation will be prescribed (Shorvon 2002).

During the Course of Pregnancy

Continuing Management into Pregnancy

Leaving aside all matters particular to obstetric interests, if a woman with epilepsy enters pregnancy with the various arrangements described above already organised, so long as her epilepsy is not due to active pathology, it is unlikely that there will be difficulty in managing her antiepileptic drug therapy in the coming months. However, the possible effects of the pregnancy-related alterations in antiepileptic drug disposition have to be kept in mind and, if indicated, appropriate action taken to prevent their possible consequences.

The clearances of all the commonly used antiepileptic drugs, with the probable but not certain exception of carbamazepine when used in monotherapy, may be expected to increase during pregnancy. Therefore antiepileptic drug dosage increases, particularly dosages of lamotrigine where the increment may be of the order of a doubling or trebling, may be anticipated. The increase in clearance often begins, and sometimes achieves most of its final magnitude, in the first trimester. It is therefore important, if antiepileptic drug therapy is to be used scientifically, and it is hoped, effectively, that monitoring plasma concentration of antiepileptic drugs should begin in the first few weeks of pregnancy and that pre-pregnancy plasma drug concentration values should be available. Dose adjustments should be made to maintain plasma drug concentrations at values close to those which existed at the time of optimal seizure control shortly before pregnancy. Such concentrations are therapeutic ones for the individual woman concerned and should provide a more appropriate yardstick for managing the drug therapy in that individual than the so-called 'therapeutic' or 'target' range values can. This range is a population parameter, and also one that usually has not been determined by any rigorous statistical approach. In adjusting antiepileptic drug dosages, it is necessary to keep in mind that steady-state plasma concentrations of some of these drugs, e.g. phenytoin and carbamazepine, do not increase in linear proportion to the size of a dosage increase. Only one dose increase often proves necessary during the course of a pregnancy, though sometimes a second increment is required. Increases are not often needed in the final trimester of pregnancy. Although it would be logical to carry out the plasma level monitoring at intervals determined by the time course of the behaviour of the drug concentrations, in practice it often proves easier to have the measurements done at pre-planned intervals which permit their reasonable contemporary results being available at the times of routine contact with the overseeing obstetrician.

In the third trimester of pregnancy, plasma protein concentrations tend to fall. For protein-bound antiepileptic drugs, this fall results in there being higher concentrations of protein-unbound (biologically available) drug present relative to the total plasma drug concentration, the parameter that is usually measured. Therefore, in the last trimester, those responsible for antiepileptic drug dosage adjustment tend in their minds to reduce the individual 'yardstick' whole plasma drug concentration before considering any further dosage increase. Of course, it is possible to handle this matter more scientifically by measuring drug concentrations in plasma water or, for some antiepileptic drugs (e.g. phenytoin, carbamazepine, lamotrigine), in the woman's saliva. However, clinicians usually do not find this necessary, perhaps because third trimester plasma drug concentration to dose ratios often tend to be comparatively stable, the changes having occurred earlier.

Of course, even with such an anticipatory preventive approach, seizure control may deteriorate during pregnancy. This occurrence necessitates assessment of the cause of the worsening and then taking appropriate remedial action, if possible. In this connection, knowledge of the plasma drug concentration to dose ratio is often helpful, since any marked departure from recent values may suggest a basis for the worsening, e.g. non-compliance with prescribed dosage.

Management When Presenting and Already Pregnant

In contrast to the above relatively organised and tidy situation, women with antiepileptic drug-treated epilepsy may present for the first time when already pregnant. In that case, the planned conduct described above will need modification, and a few aspects may not be feasible, e.g. pre-pregnancy folate supplementation.

If a woman presents early enough in pregnancy for there to be a reasonable prospect of reducing the hazard of foetal maldevelopment, an orderly substitution of a less teratogenic antiepileptic drug for valproate or topiramate may be possible, though there is likely to be a need for haste, and it is important that any too abrupt change of therapy does not itself harm the foetus, as might occur if, for instance, prolonged maternal status epilepticus were to occur as a withdrawal phenomenon.

In the more usual situation that there is no opportunity to influence antiepileptic drug therapy until after the first trimester of pregnancy, in the past the advice usually given would have been to adjust antiepileptic drug therapy only as necessary to maintain or improve seizure control. It would have been argued that, if a drug such as valproate was being taken, it would have already produced any teratogenic effect of which it was capable. However, the more recently available information on the relationship between intrauterine valproate exposure and neurodevelopmental issues in the foetus raises the question of whether, if feasible, valproate should be replaced with an alternative agent irrespective of the stage of pregnancy. If there were a potentially equipotent or more potent and safe alternative available, the appropriate course would probably be to replace the valproate. Unfortunately, in most such circumstances there will be no better alternative to valproate from the epilepsy control standpoint and it will already too late to avoid any teratogenic and perhaps any neurodevelopmental consequences. As yet, there do not seem to be publications in the literature that provide information on the outcomes of persisting with, or replacing, valproate in such circumstances.

If plasma concentration monitoring is to be employed, information may not be available regarding the drug's plasma concentration in the individual before pregnancy and its correlation with control of her seizures. If this is the case, it may be necessary to use the less desirable guidepost of the population therapeutic range of drug concentrations to guide the sizes of clinically indicated dosage alterations. Although values for these ranges are available in the literature (Patsalos et al. 2008), particularly for the newer drugs, the figures do not appear to be securely based on adequate correlations of drug concentration and clinical effectiveness in the various seizure disorder types in which the agents have been employed in monotherapy.

After Pregnancy

The issues relevant to breastfeeding have been dealt with above, in relation to a question frequently raised by women taking antiepileptic drugs and planning pregnancy.

From the antiepileptic drug aspect, the main issue in the postnatal weeks is the return of the pattern of drug disposition to its pre-pregnancy situation. This process nearly always appears to be underway within the first fortnight of giving birth and occasionally seems to be nearly completed within that time period though it can extend for as long as 3 months after giving birth. In the early postpartum weeks, there is a tendency for mothers and other family members to focus their main attention on the new baby. As a result, maternal lack of well-being and complaints of tiredness may be attributed to 'getting over the pregnancy and birth', or to the strain of coping with a new baby, or be considered a manifestation of postpartum depression. Instead, the problem may be antiepileptic drug overdosage due to failure to lower the dose soon enough as the pregnancy-induced increased clearance of the drug resolves. There is something to be said for measuring plasma concentrations of antiepileptic drugs weekly or fortnightly after childbirth, until the levels have returned to their clinically satisfactory individual pre-pregnancy ones and remain at these levels. In the interval antiepileptic drug doses should be adjusted in the light of the changing plasma drug concentrations.

Disorders Other than Epilepsy

All the foregoing material in this chapter has been concerned with the management of antiepileptic drug therapy in women with epilepsy before, during and immediately after pregnancy. However, as mentioned earlier in this book, in recent years there has been increasing use of antiepileptic drugs in treating a variety of disorders apart from epilepsy, mainly various psychiatric illnesses and also for migraine prophylaxis and the relief of neuropathic pain and several other uncommon conditions. Women taking the drugs for these latter indications may become pregnant. They then face issues analogous to those that confront women with epilepsy in the same circumstance, but as well as similarities, there may be certain differences in their situations, and these differences may vary with individual circumstances.

During pregnancy, the dispositions of any antiepileptic drug that is being taken may be expected to behave as it would in pregnant women with epilepsy, unless pharmacokinetic interactions occur between the antiepileptic drug and any other drug that is also being taken. Similarly, the foetal hazards from an antiepileptic drug that is taken would be expected to be similar to those that apply in women with epilepsy treated with the same antiepileptic drug. Where there may be differences in (i) the effects of pregnancy on the course of the disorder being treated; (ii) the expected efficacy of, and hazards from, any drug that might be substituted for a potentially teratogenic antiepileptic drug that was being taken; and (iii) the degree of hazard to the well-being of the woman concerned and possibly to her foetus, if alteration of antiepileptic drug therapy resulted in impaired control of the disorder being treated.

As an example of an instance where some of the above factors would be relevant, consider the situations of two otherwise similar women planning to become pregnant, one suffering from bipolar disorder and taking valproate as a mood stabiliser and the other taking the same drug in the same dose for migraine prophylaxis. If they continue to take valproate throughout pregnancy, both are likely to require similar degrees of dosage adjustment to maintain the plasma valproate concentrations that were satisfactory prior to pregnancy. Assuming neither has a family history of foetal malformations, each probably faces a similar risk of giving birth to a malformed foetus. If they both ceased taking valproate to reduce their hazards of teratogenesis, the woman with bipolar disorder has the choice of going untreated or of taking a drug of possible lesser efficacy and probably uncertain teratogenic potential and with the risk that worsening of her psychiatric illness may for instance result in her suicide. However, if the woman taking valproate to prevent migraine ceases the drug, she often may need to take little further action in relation to the pregnancy if she is prepared to put up with a few migraine attacks, as that disorder usually becomes less active or inactive in pregnancy, while death in migraine attacks is a great rarity. Decisions about her management in relation to pregnancy seem more easily made and more clear cut than in the hypothetical woman with bipolar disorder, but basically the management of antiepileptic drug therapy in disorders other than epilepsy, as in epilepsy, is a matter of trying to achieve the best reconciliation between the factors discussed above, as they are recognised to apply in each given individual. If this reconciliation involves a change in antiepileptic drug, it will generally be desirable to make the change gradually rather than abruptly, so long as there is no clinical urgency involved in the situation.

In the present book, it would scarcely be practicable to go into further detail in relation to these matters as they apply in the various psychiatric and other disorders in which antiepileptic drugs are currently used. The experience of the use of these drugs in treating epilepsy in pregnant women provides the precedent and model for their use in pregnancy for managing other disorders. This state of affairs is likely to continue to apply, at least until studies become available that establish the actual situation for each disorder so treated and thereby permit more detailed and more particular advice.

References

Artama M, Auvinen A, Raudaskoski T, Isojarvi I, Isojarvi J (2005) Antiepileptic drug use of women with epilepsy and congenital malformations in the offspring. Neurology 64:1874–1878

Battino D, Tomson T, Bonizzoni E et al (2013) Seizure control and treatment changes in pregnancy: observations from the EURAP epilepsy pregnancy registry. Epilepsia 54:1621–1627

Bianchi DW, Platt LD, Goldberg JD et al (2012) Genome-wide fetal aneuploidy detection by maternal plasma DNA sequencing. Obstet Gynecol 119:890–901

Boon P, Engelborghs S, Hauman H et al (2012) Recommendations for the treatment of epilepsy in adult patients in general practice in Belgium: an update. Acta Neurol Belg 112:119–131

Bromley RL, Mawer G, Clayton-Smith J, Baker GA, Liverpool and Manchester Neurodevelopment Group (2008) Autism spectrum disorders following in utero exposure to antiepileptic drugs. Neurology 71:1923–1924

Choi H, Morrell MJ (2003) Review of lamotrigine and its clinical applications in epilepsy. Exp Opin Pharmacother 4:243–251

Christensen J, Grønborg TK, Sørensen MJ, Schendel D, Parner ET, Pedersen LH, Vestergaard M (2013) Prenatal valproate exposure and risk of autism spectrum disorders and childhood autism. JAMA 309:1696–1703

Cohen MJ, Meador KJ, Browning N et al (2013) Fetal antiepileptic drug exposure: adaptive and emotional/behavioral functioning at age 6 years. Epilepsy Behav 29:308–315

Costa AL, Lopes-Cendes I, Guerreiro CA (2005) Seizure frequency during pregnancy and the puerperium. Int J Gynaecol Obstet 88:148–149

Cummings C, Stewart M, Stevenson M, Morrow J, Nelson J (2011) Neurodevelopment of children exposed to lamotrigine, sodium valproate and carbamazepine. Arch Dis Child 96:643–647

Garfield SS, Armstrong SO (2012) Clinical and cost consequences of incorporating a novel non-invasive prenatal test into the diagnostic pathway for fetal trisomies. J Manage Care Med 15:34–41

Gjerde IO, Strandjord RE, Ulstein M (1988) The course of epilepsy during pregnancy: a study of 78 cases. Acta Neurol Scand 78:198–205

Glauser T, Ben-Menachem E, Bourgeois B et al (2013) Updated ILAE evidence review of antiepileptic drug efficacy and effectiveness as initial monotherapy for epileptic seizures and syndromes. Epilepsia 54:551–563

Harden C, Hopp J, Ting TY et al (2009) Management issues for women with epilepsy – focus on pregnancy (an evidence-based review): 1. Obstetrical complications and change in seizure frequency. Epilepsia 50:1229–1236

Holmes LB, Mittendorf R, Shen A, Smith CR, Hernandez-Diaz S (2011) Fetal effects of anticonvulsant polytherapies. Arch Neurol 68:1275–1281

Kaneko S, Utami K, Kondo T et al (1992) Malformations in infants of mothers with epilepsy receiving antiepileptic drugs. Neurology 42(Suppl 5):68–74

Knight AH, Rhind EG (1975) Epilepsy and pregnancy: a study of 153 pregnancies in 59 patients. Epilepsia 16:99–110

Koren G, Kennedy D (1999) Safe use of valproic acid during pregnancy [Motherisk Update]. Can Fam Physician 45:1451–1453

Kwan P, Brodie MJ (2004) Phenobarbital for the treatment of epilepsy in the 21st century: a critical review. Epilepsia 45:1141–1149

Lindhout D, Omtzigt JG (1992) Pregnancy and the risk of teratogenicity. Epilepsia 33(Suppl 4):S41–S48

Mawer G, Briggs M, Baker GA et al (2010) Pregnancy with epilepsy: obstetric and neonatal outcome of a controlled study. Seizure 19:112–119

McGrath A, Sharpe L, Lah S, Parratt K (2014) Pregnancy-related knowledge and information needs of women with epilepsy: a systematic review. Epilepsy Behav 31:246–266

Meador K, Reynolds MW, Crean S, Fahrbach K, Probst C (2008) Pregnancy outcomes in women with epilepsy: a systematic review and analysis of published pregnancy registers and cohorts. Epilepsy Res 81:1–13

Meador KJ, Baker GA, Browning N et al (2009) Cognitive function at 3 years of age after fetal exposure to antiepileptic drugs. N Engl J Med 360:1597–1605

Meador KJ, Baker GA, Browning N et al (2010) Effects of breastfeeding in children of women taking antiepileptic drugs. Neurology 75:1954–1960

Meador KJ, Baker GA, Browning N et al (2012) Effects of fetal antiepileptic drug exposure: outcomes at age 4.5 years. Neurology 78:1207–1214

Meador KJ, Baker GA, Browning N et al (2013) Fetal antiepileptic drug exposure and cognitive outcomes at age 6 years study): a prospective observational study. Lancet Neurol 12:244–252

Meador KJ, Baker GA, Browning N et al (2014) Breastfeeding in children of women taking antiepileptic drugs: cognitive outcomes at age 6 years. JAMA Pediatr 168:729–736

Morrow J, Russell A, Guthrie E et al (2006) Malformation risk of antiepileptic drugs in pregnancy: a prospective study from the UK Epilepsy and Pregnancy Register. J Neurol Neurosurg Psychiatry 77:193–198

Mula M, Trimble MR, Yuen A et al (2003) Psychiatric adverse events during levetiracetam therapy. Neurology 61:704–706

Nakane Y, Okuma T, Takahashi R et al (1980) Multi-institutional study on the teratogenicity and fetal toxicity of antiepileptic drugs: a report of a collaborative study group in Japan. Epilepsia 21:663–680

Pack AM (2006) Therapy insight: clinical management of pregnant women with epilepsy. Nat Clin Pract Neurol 2:190–200

Palomaki GE, Knight GJ, Ashwood ER, Best RG, Haddow JE (2013) Screening for Down syndrome in the United States: results of surveys in 2011 and 2012. Arch Pathol Lab Med 137:921–926

Patsalos PN (2000) Pharmacokinetic profile of levetiracetam: toward ideal characteristics. Pharmacol Ther 85:77–85

Patsalos PN, Berry DJ, Bourgeois BF et al (2008) Antiepileptic drugs - best practice guidelines for therapeutic drug monitoring: a position paper by the subcommission on therapeutic drug monitoring, I.L.A.E. Commission on Therapeutic Strategies. Epilepsia 49:1239–1276

Pennell PB (2005) Using current evidence in selecting antiepileptic drugs for use during pregnancy. Epilepsy Curr 5(2):45–51

Pennell PB, Peng L, Newport DJ et al (2008) Lamotrigine in pregnancy: clearance, therapeutic drug monitoring, and seizure frequency. Neurology 70:2130–2136

Perucca E (2001) Clinical pharmacology and therapeutic use of the new antiepileptic drugs. Fundam Clin Pharmacol 15:405–417

Perucca E (2005) An introduction to antiepileptic drugs. Epilepsia 46(Suppl 4):31–37

Sabers A (2009) Influences on seizure activity in pregnant women with epilepsy. Epilepsy Behav 15:230

Sabers A, Petrenaite V (2009) Seizure frequency in pregnant women treated with lamotrigine monotherapy. Epilepsia 50:2163–2166

Sabers A, Dam M, a-Rogvi-Hansen B et al (2004) Epilepsy and pregnancy: lamotrigine as main drug used. Acta Neurol Scand 109:9–13

Samrén EB, van Duijn CM, Koch S et al (1997) Maternal use of antiepileptic drugs and the risk of major congenital malformations: a joint European prospective study of human teratogenesis associated with maternal epilepsy. Epilepsia 38:981–990

Schaffler L (1990) Epilepsy and pregnancy. Schweiz Med Wochenschr 120:1508–1516

Schmidt D (1982) The effect of pregnancy on the natural history of epilepsy: review of the literature. In: Janz D, Bossi L, Dam M, Helge H, Richens A, Schmidt D (eds) Epilepsy, pregnancy, and the child. Raven, New York, pp 3–14

Shorvon S (2002) Commentary. Antiepileptic drug therapy during pregnancy: the neurologist's perspective Antiepileptic medication in pregnancy. J Med Genet 39:248–250

Thomas SV (2011) Managing epilepsy in pregnancy. Neurol India 59:59–65

Tomson T, Battino D, French J et al (2007a) Antiepileptic drug exposure and major congenital malformations: the role of the pregnancy registries. Epilepsy Behav 11:277–282

Tomson T, Palm R, Kallen K et al (2007b) Pharmacokinetics of levetiracetam during pregnancy, delivery, in the neonatal period, and lactation. Nat Clin Pract Neurol 310:538–539

Vajda FJE, Angelis-Stoforidis P, Eadie MJ (1999) Utility of plasma lamotrigine concentration: Concept of the plasma therapeutic range for individual patients. J Neurol 246(Suppl 1):185

Vajda FJE, Lander CM, O'Brien TJ et al (2006a) Foetal malformations and seizure control: 52 months data reported from the Australian Register of Pregnancies. Eur J Neurol 13:645–654

Vajda F, Solinas C, Graham J, Hitchcock A, Eadie M (2006b) The case for lamotrigine monitoring in pregnancy. J Clin Neurosci 13:103–104

Vajda FJE, Hitchcock A, Graham J, O'Brien T, Lander C, Eadie M (2008) Seizure control in antiepileptic drug-treated pregnancy. Epilepsia 49:172–175

Vajda FJE, Dodd S, Horgan D (2010a) Lamotrigine in epilepsy, pregnancy and psychiatry – a drug for all seasons? J Clin Neurosci 20:13–16

Vajda F, Hitchcock A, Graham J, O'Brien T, Lander C, Eadie M (2010b) The teratogenic risk of antiepileptic drug polytherapy. Epilepsia 51:805–810

Vajda FJE, O'Brien TJ, Graham J, Lander CM, Eadie MJ (2013) Dose-dependency of fetal malformations associated with valproate. Neurology 81:999–1003

Vajda FJE, O'Brien T, Lander C, Graham J, Eadie M (2014) The efficacy of the newer antiepileptic drugs in controlling seizures in pregnancy. Epilepsia 55:1229–1234

Vajda FJ, O'Brien TJ, Graham J, Lander CM, Eadie MJ (2015) The outcomes of pregnancy in women with untreated epilepsy. Seizure 24:77–81

Veiby G, Daltveit AK, Schjølberg S et al (2013a) Exposure to antiepileptic drugs in utero and child development: a prospective population-based study. Epilepsia 54:1462–1472

Veiby G, Engelsen BA, Gilhus NE (2013b) Early child development and exposure to antiepileptic drugs prenatally and through breastfeeding: a prospective cohort study on children of women with epilepsy. JAMA Neurol 70:1367–1374

Vidović MI, Della Marina BM (1994) Trimestral changes of seizure frequency in pregnant epileptic women. Acta Med Croatica 48:85–87

Weintraub D, Buchsbaum R, Resor SR Jr, Hirsch LJ (2007) Psychiatric and behavioral side effects of the newer antiepileptic drugs in adults with epilepsy. Epilepsy Behav 10:105–110

Yerby M (2003) Management issues for women with epilepsy: neural tube defects and folic acid supplementation. Neurology 61(Suppl 2):S23–S26

Yerby MS, Kaplan P, Tran T (2004) Risks and management of pregnancy in women with epilepsy. Cleve Clin J Med 71(S25):825–837

Chapter 12
Antiepileptic Drugs and Pregnancy: The Future

Abstract The study of the interaction between antiepileptic drugs and the pregnant human female body that has gone on over the better part of half a century has provided evidence that the currently available drugs are inactivated more quickly during pregnancy and that they possess to various degrees responsibility for the occurrence of malformations in the body structures of foetuses exposed to them, and also, at least in the case of valproate, for impaired neurodevelopment in infancy and childhood. As the drugs in current use come to be replaced by newer agents, there will be a need to maintain, and hopefully expand, the current data-collecting mechanisms that have so far provided the information about the teratogenicity of the antiepileptic drugs. While application of knowledge that is already available has made possible both better epileptic seizure control in pregnancy, and a reduced incidence of foetal malformations, it is uncertain how widely this knowledge has been disseminated and, after dissemination, has been applied. The available knowledge also points to other matters that warrant investigation.

Over the course of some 30–40 years, medicine has accumulated a good deal of information concerning antiepileptic drugs and their use in pregnant women. From a practical standpoint, perhaps the most important items of knowledge that have emerged from this work are that (i) nearly all antiepileptic drugs are cleared from the maternal body more rapidly during pregnancy, whether or not this increased elimination is due to heightened metabolic activity or to greater renal excretion of un-metabolised drug and (ii) intrauterine exposure of the foetus to at least some of these drugs results in the hazard of physical malformation occurring in the foetus and, after birth, in the possibility of disordered neurodevelopment in the infant. At least in theory, the application of this knowledge should have ensured better control of antiepileptic drug-treated seizure disorders during pregnancy, and the avoidance to some extent of the hazards that an injudicious choice of antiepileptic drug therapy may impose on the physical, intellectual and behavioural development of the foetus and infant.

As mentioned at several places earlier in this book, there are reports that the attempted adjustment of antiepileptic drug dosages at appropriate stages during the course of pregnancy, particularly if guided by knowledge of circulating concentrations of antiepileptic drugs and pre-pregnancy reference drug concentration values,

M.J. Eadie, F.J.E. Vajda, *Antiepileptic Drugs and Pregnancy: A Guide for Prescribers*, DOI 10.1007/978-3-319-21434-4_12

appears to have had some success in preventing any worsening of epileptic seizure control in pregnant women. Through this means, some of the disadvantages that having active epilepsy is likely to produce for the prospective mother's pattern of living may be minimised, or avoided entirely. The recognition that certain antiepileptic drugs that are currently in common use during pregnancy in Western countries, notably valproate and topiramate, are particularly prone to be associated with the occurrence of foetal malformations, and for the hazard of such malformations to worsen as the dosages of these drugs increase, has altered prescribing practice in relation to valproate, at least among those sections of the Australian medical profession who have appreciated the drug's dangers for the foetus. As illustrated in Fig. 9.2, over the years during which the Australian Pregnancy Register has been collecting information, both the mean daily valproate dose in those women with epilepsy prescribed the drug and the proportion of pregnant women receiving the drug have tended to fall progressively, accompanied by a degree of downward trend in the numbers of malformed foetuses reported to the Register. Unfortunately, from this register's data, it is impossible to know whether there has been a similar change in prescribing behaviour among the Australian medical profession more generally, let alone among medical practitioners globally. It is also impossible to know whether those who are using the drug to treat disorders other than epilepsy, especially various psychiatric conditions, have been influenced by this knowledge concerning the foetal hazards arising from intrauterine valproate exposure. Valproate dosages used in psychiatry and in some other medical specialties sometimes appear to be high relative to those likely to be used in treating epilepsies. If so, there may be a particular danger of foetal malformations occurring if women treated with such dosages find themselves pregnant unexpectedly. They then face the possibility of abrupt withdrawal of potentially teratogenic medication, a process that may produce its own problems, without any certainty that this course of action is not being taken already too late to avoid foetal damage. The information concerning topiramate and its teratogenic potential is too recent to have yet had time to exert any widespread influence.

As well as these practical dividends, the accumulated information that has been obtained regarding the behaviour of antiepileptic drugs in human pregnancy has raised a number of interesting scientific questions whose answers, though they may not yield immediate practical dividends for women with epilepsy, may open future possibilities. For instance, although there is already a reasonable general understanding of the mechanisms responsible for the increased antiepileptic drug clearance that occurs during pregnancy, neither the detailed renal nor the metabolic mechanisms involved in the clearance increases have been anything like thoroughly explored.

There has been little attempt to study the possible relationships between circulating concentrations of antiepileptic drugs and the risks of developing specific patterns of foetal malformation. Such attempted correlations in the past certainly paid dividends in improving the control of epileptic seizures. However, in practice, there would probably be considerable difficulty in organising the drug concentration measurements so that they were carried out not only at the appropriate time in the first weeks of pregnancy but also at the appropriate stage of the dosage interval, because it is not known, for instance, when are the critical times for particular patterns of foetal damage to occur. Is it the time of peak circulating drug concentrations or the time of the trough steady-state ones, that would be more relevant? Further, it is not certain whether the teratogenic potential of a drug resides in the parent substance, or in a drug metabolite, or metabolites. Up to perhaps 50 women would have to be studied to obtain the relevant drug concentration data for correlation with a single incidence of a malformation. The logistics of such a study, carried out in a sufficient number of pregnancies, would probably prove both challenging and expensive.

In connection with foetal exposure to the antiepileptic drugs established as definite (valproate) or probable teratogens (topiramate), there is a need to explain the rather wide range of expression of their effects on the physical development of the foetus, unlike the much more structure-specific malformation pattern associated with a teratogen such as thalidomide. Conceivably, both antiepileptic drugs could simply facilitate teratogenesis non-specifically, but both have particular dosage-related associations with specific malformations (valproate and spina bifida, Fig. 9.1; topiramate and hypospadias, Fig. 9.3). Both valproate and topiramate have numerous known biotransformation products (Chaps. 4 and 5). Some of their metabolites are known to lack antiepileptic activity, and a similar absence of such activity is assumed for most of the others. But lack of antiepileptic activity may not necessarily equate with lack of teratogenic culpability. It has been shown that there is an association between maternal intake of valproate in doses over 2000 mg per day and the occurrence of neural tube defects in the foetus (Chap. 9). The predominant pathway of valproate metabolism, at least in the non-pregnant state, changes progressively as the drug dose increases. At lower doses, fatty acid beta oxidation preponderates, but as the dose becomes higher, the body's beta oxidative capacity seems to become saturated. Increasing proportions of the drug dose are then cleared through glucuronide conjugation and probably through minor metabolic pathways. Assuming that such dosage-related shifts in valproate's metabolic pathway predominance also occur in pregnancy, something that does not appear to have been established, is it possible that valproate glucuronide exposure is responsible for the occurrence of neural tube defects but is not responsible for some of the other patterns of foetal malformations associated with the drug? Or, is it that at higher valproate doses more of the drug is diverted along one of the several minor metabolic pathways described for the drug, e.g. omega or omega-1 oxidation, and that one or more of these metabolites can damage the development of the neuraxis? The Australian Pregnancy Register data are consistent with topiramate, when used as the sole antiepileptic drug, not being teratogenic, but being a significant teratogen when used together with any one of several other antiepileptic drugs. In view of this, is it possible that topiramate per se is not harmful to the developing foetus but that some metabolite or metabolites whose formation is increased in the presence of other antiepileptic drugs may damage the foetus in utero? These are interesting though speculative possibilities. One can have little idea where their exploration might ultimately lead. Nevertheless, in the present state of knowledge, they seem reasonable hypotheses that warrant investigation, providing that the appropriate studies are seen as logistically feasible and ethically justifiable.

For the more immediate future, there are a few somewhat pressing matters that seem worth considering.

It would be very helpful to know with certainty which of the currently available antiepileptic drugs are definitely human teratogens, which of the ones likely to become available in the foreseeable future will prove to be teratogens and which are safe from the foetal standpoint. The evidence that valproate is a teratogen is already persuasive, and the evidence is becoming increasingly strong that topiramate also is a teratogen. There are also some observations that would raise suspicion regarding phenobarbitone and carbamazepine and, to a lesser extent, lamotrigine, among the more common currently available drugs. The evidence incriminating these latter drugs in teratogenesis may not have consistently been statistically significant, but it does produce an uneasy sense that the availability of more extensive data might see some of them incriminated.

A significant part of the more extensive data so far available concerning teratogenesis related to antiepileptic drugs has come from national or community statistics, some of which have been collected retrospectively. These latter statistics are likely to have been amassed with variable degrees of enthusiasm and competence by different people. Statistics derived from pregnancy registers, while prospective, are unlikely to have captured the relevant information from anything like the majority of pregnant women with epilepsy in the communities from which the registers have obtained their information. Further, there may have been a tendency for women whose epilepsies in pregnancy have required expert advice or management to be recruited into the registers. Therefore, the register data may not necessarily be fully representative of the general situation of pregnant women with epilepsy. Accepting that registers, with their voluntary recruitment policies, are still likely to prove more reliable than governmental statistics usually collected for different purposes, it seems likely that it will nearly always continue to be impossible in practice to collect high-quality information from all the pregnancies in women with antiepileptic drug-treated epilepsy in the wider community. Comprehensive data will be unobtainable unless some form of compulsory registration of pregnancies in women with epilepsy is imposed. Such an imposition would raise issues of cost and individuals' rights to privacy, the latter in a situation where retention of privacy rights could hardly be shown to cause significant immediate harm to the wider community. Nevertheless, more extensive data, and also data for the antiepileptic drugs that are still to come into common use in pregnant women, will continue to be needed. The best solution in practice may lie in trying to obtain higher voluntary recruitment rates for women with treated epilepsy into dedicated registers, and also better comparison data from pregnant women without epilepsy, from pregnant women with epilepsy that is not treated with antiepileptic drugs, and also from pregnant women taking antiepileptic drugs to treat disorders other than epilepsy. Even if such data could be collected in sufficient quantity, under present conditions its accumulation would probably take a considerable period of time. During this period, the situation in relation to the currently available antiepileptic drugs might become increasingly clear, but by the time these drugs have become better understood, they may also have become increasingly superseded as new antiepileptic drugs come into greater use. Medicine could possibly find itself in the situation of finally having the knowledge that enables it to be better able to employ in pregnant women certain antiepileptic drugs only when these drugs are disappearing from use. It may be necessary to reconcile the desire to amass as much information as possible before studying it, with the consequence of delaying its analysis. Depending on the rate of appearance of new and better antiepileptic drugs, similar considerations are likely to apply in the future for the drugs currently coming into increasing use in pregnant women. It clearly will be important to maintain the existing pregnancy registers as far as is possible and to ensure their continuing financial support. Possibly in some circumstances combining registers might be advantageous, though with the potential disadvantage that this might increasingly distance the data sources from the data collection and analysis personnel.

The role of genetic factors in the responsibility for foetal malformations and neurodevelopmental problems has not been studied to the extent that might have been expected. An increased hazard of a subsequent child being born malformed is known to exist when a mother with epilepsy has had a previous malformed child (Chap. 8), and there is a correlation between the IQs of mother and offspring (Chap. 9). The matter of any possible paternal genetic influence in these situations has gone virtually unexplored. The possible sensitivities in investigating this particular matter, the risk of receiving incorrect or misleading information and the psychological, social and legal difficulties that might arise out of such inquiries have probably deterred the appropriate studies. Nonetheless, a tactful exploration of these matters might be feasible, even if DNA studies were not to prove practicable and ethically acceptable. It would be helpful to know the extent to which inheritable factors contribute to foetal malformation rates and neurodevelopmental issues, while pharmacogenomics studies might reveal correlations with patterns of foetal malformation that could suggest the chemical natures of drug metabolites that could injure the development of the foetus in utero.

The knowledge of associations between intrauterine exposure to antiepileptic drugs and manifestations of impaired neurodevelopment is relatively recent. Although a substantial amount of good-quality work has already been done, the area needs to be explored further, particularly in relation to the newer antiepileptic drugs that are likely to be increasingly used in pregnant women. Despite the logistic difficulties, the childhood populations already studied, or new ones, need to be followed further into adolescence and adult life to gain an appreciation of the possible long-term social and economic consequences of exposure to antiepileptic drugs one or two decades earlier. There is also need for studies specifically planned to determine the stages of pregnancy and postnatal life (the latter in the breastfed infant) when the neurodevelopment begins to go astray, and also the stage when drug exposure no longer does damage. This knowledge will have a bearing on when maternal valproate intake, or intake of any other antiepileptic drug that has been avoided during pregnancy, can be resumed with safety from the offspring's neurodevelopmental standpoint. Is the vulnerable time in relation to neurodevelopment only in early pregnancy and in late pregnancy, or does vulnerability continue into the period of breastfeeding and, if so, for how long?

A further matter that would benefit from immediate attention is the need to make those who are prescribing antiepileptic drugs for pregnant women more widely aware of the currently available information about the appropriate adjustments of drug dosages during and after pregnancy and the hazards these drugs carry, or do not carry, for the foetus. Neurologists and others who treated epilepsy frequently, particularly if they are aware of the existence of the registers and the findings derived from them, should be in a position to handle these drugs optimally by present-day standards. However, the prescription of so-called antiepileptic drugs for indications other than epilepsy in pregnant women, or in women who may become pregnant, appears to be passing increasingly into the hands of those who are, perhaps, not as well aware as they might be of currently available information concerning the drugs and pregnancy.

Another interesting possibility arises from the known dose-related teratogenesis associated with exposure to valproate and the evidence that the heightened teratogenic risk of antiepileptic drug combinations is determined by the presence of valproate in the combinations. The use of valproate sometimes cannot be avoided in women who may become pregnant or are already pregnant. In such cases, could the overall risk of producing foetal malformations be reduced if valproate doses were employed that were low enough to be inadequate to fully control seizures, or if the valproate were employed in conjunction with a second antiepileptic drug that had a low teratogenic potential and was reasonably effective in the type of seizure disorder being treated? Excluding use of topiramate, the combination would be likely to provide a lesser overall teratogenetic hazard than the previous higher valproate dose and still might achieve an acceptable level of seizure control. On the basis of theory, it has often been suggested that, if dosage of a single antiepileptic drug has been taken to its limit of tolerance, combining antiepileptic drugs with different molecular mechanisms of action may produce added antiepileptic effects. However, in the situation envisaged above, when, for instance, a valproate dosage may be well below that drug's limit of tolerance in the woman concerned, the prescription of a second less teratogenic drug, which acted via one or more of the same molecular mechanisms as valproate, might seem not unreasonable and might facilitate reasonable seizure suppression. To investigate such a possibility ethically might require a fairly extensive opportunistic study.

***

At the time of writing, the full story of the employment of antiepileptic drugs in pregnant women has not been told, and probably cannot yet be told, nor its future predicted with any certainty. However, there still may have been some purpose in attempting to assemble the currently available knowledge and to set down an interpretation of the present situation, in that this may serve as a basis for suggesting some of the directions that future progress in the area might take.

Appendix

M.J. Eadie, F.J.E. Vajda, *Antiepileptic Drugs and Pregnancy: A Guide for Prescribers*, DOI 10.1007/978-3-319-21434-4

	Non-pregnant state									Pregnancy		
Drug	F_{PO}	V	% bound	$F_{u(\infty)}$	$T_{1/2}$	Cl	Metabolism	Induces	Inducible	Cl	Mechanism	M-P Ratio
Carbamazepine	High	~1.0	75	0.01	36	0.7–1.8	Oxidation	Y	Y	Slight↑		0.4–0.7
CBZ–epoxide		0.6–1.6	50–60	0.20–0.35	5–11	~7.0	Hydration					
Clonazepam	~1.0	2.0–4.0	85	~0	22–36	6.3	Reduction and oxidation	N	N	↑		0.8
Ethosuximide	~1.0	0.7	0	0.20	54	0.7–1.1	Oxidation	N	Y	No ↕		0.9
Gabapentin	<0.6	0.9	0	0.60	6	~6.0	Nil	N	N			~1.0
Lamotrigine	~1.0	1.25	55	low	25	1.8	Glucuronidation	N	Y	↑↑	Glucuronidation	0.6
Levetiracetam	~1.0	0.6	<10	0.66	6–8	2.5	Hydrolysis	N	N	↑	Renal excretion	1.05
Oxcarbazepine	~1.0	0.7	66	<0.01	2–3	>100	Reduction	Y				
OXC-MHD			40		9.3	~6.4	Hydration and conjugation			↑		0.5
Phenobarbitone	High	0.5	50	0.25	72–96	0.28	Oxidation and N-glucosidation	Y	Y	↑		
Phenytoin	~1.0	0.5–0.8	90	0.05	22	0.02	Oxidation	Y	Y	↑	Oxidation	
Topiramate	~0.9	0.7	9–17	0.6–0.7	20–30	1.3–2.2	Hydroxylation and conjugations	N	Y	↑		0.86–1.0

	Non-pregnant state									Pregnancy		
Drug	F_{PO}	V	% bound	$F_{u(\infty)}$	$T_{1/2}$	Cl	Metabolism	Induces	Inducible	Cl	Mechanism	M-P Ratio
Valproate	~1.0	0.15–0.20	90	0.01	8–15	1.26	Glucuronidation and β-oxidation			Little↕		
Vigabatrin	0.5–0.6	1.2	0	0.5–0.6	5–7	7.5	Nil	N	N			<1.0
Zonisamide	~1.0	1.1–1.8	40–50	0.15–0.30	50–70	0.7	Reduction and acetylation	N	Y	??↑		0.9

Values for pharmacologically active metabolites are shaded

F_{PO} = oral bioavailability fraction, V = apparent volume of distribution (L/kg), $F_{u(\infty)}$ = fraction of oral dose excreted in urine unmetabolised, $T_{1/2}$ = elimination half-life (hours), Cl = clearance/bioavailability (L/h); M-P ratio = milk to maternal plasma ratio; OXC-MHD = oxcarbazepine monohydroxy derivative; ↑= increased; ↕ = no consistent change

Index

M.J. Eadie, F.J.E. Vajda, *Antiepileptic Drugs and Pregnancy: A Guide for Prescribers*, DOI 10.1007/978-3-319-21434-4

MIX
Papier aus verantwortungsvollen Quellen
Paper from responsible sources
FSC® C105338

If you have any concerns about our products,
you can contact us on
ProductSafety@springernature.com

In case Publisher is established outside the EU,
the EU authorized representative is:
Springer Nature Customer Service Center GmbH
Europaplatz 3, 69115 Heidelberg, Germany

Printed by Libri Plureos GmbH
in Hamburg, Germany